Bone Densitometry
in Growing Patients

CURRENT ◊ CLINICAL ◊ PRACTICE

NEIL S. SKOLNIK, MD • SERIES EDITOR

Bone Densitometry in Growing Patients

Guidelines for Clinical Practice

Edited by

Aenor J. Sawyer, MD

Pediatric Bone Health Consortium
and
Children's Hospital & Research Center at Oakland
Oakland, CA

Laura K. Bachrach, MD

Stanford University School of Medicine
Stanford, CA

Ellen B. Fung, PhD, RD

Children's Hospital & Research Center at Oakland
Oakland, CA

With a Foreword by

Sydney Lou Bonnick, MD, FACP

Clinical Research Center of North Texas, Denton, TX

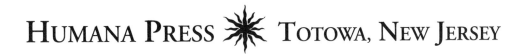

HUMANA PRESS ✳ TOTOWA, NEW JERSEY

© 2007 Humana Press Inc.
999 Riverview Drive, Suite 208
Totowa, New Jersey 07512

www.humanapress.com

Due diligence has been taken by the publishers, editors, and authors of this book to assure the accuracy of the information published and to describe generally accepted practices. The contributors herein have carefully checked to ensure that the drug selections and dosages set forth in this text are accurate and in accord with the standards accepted at the time of publication. Notwithstanding, as new research, changes in government regulations, and knowledge from clinical experience relating to drug therapy and drug reactions constantly occurs, the reader is advised to check the product information provided by the manufacturer of each drug for any change in dosages or for additional warnings and contraindications. This is of utmost importance when the recommended drug herein is a new or infrequently used drug. It is the responsibility of the treating physician to determine dosages and treatment strategies for individual patients. Further it is the responsibility of the health care provider to ascertain the Food and Drug Administration status of each drug or device used in their clinical practice. The publisher, editors, and authors are not responsible for errors or omissions or for any consequences from the application of the information presented in this book and make no warranty, express or implied, with respect to the contents in this publication.

This publication is printed on acid-free paper. ∞
ANSI Z39.48-1984 (American Standards Institute) Permanence of Paper for Printed Library Materials.

Production Editor: Robin B. Weisberg
Cover design: Patricia F. Cleary

Cover illustrations: Photo 1: Pablo Avila, healthy 8-year-old boy with forearm fracture. (Photo taken by Shooting Stars Productions 2005; used with permission from child and parents.) Photo 2: Same child at 9 years old in a Hologic Discovery DXA scanner. (Photo taken by Aenor J. Sawyer 2006; used with permission from child and parents.) Photo 3: Whole body scan of a 12-year-old child with a history of low trauma fractures. (Image acquired on GE Lunar Prodigy by Nicola Crabtree at Birmingham Children's Hospital.)

For additional copies, pricing for bulk purchases, and/or information about other Humana titles, contact Humana at the above address or at any of the following numbers: Tel.: 973-256-1699; Fax: 973-256-8314; E-mail: orders@humanapr.com, or visit our Website: http://www.humanapress.com

Printed in the United States of America. 10 9 8 7 6 5 4 3 2 1
eISBN: 1-59745-211-4

Library of Congress Cataloging-in-Publication Data

Bone densitometry in growing patients : guidelines for clinical practice / edited by Aenor J. Sawyer,
Laura K. Bachrach, Ellen B. Fung.
    p. ; cm. -- (Current clinical practice)
  Includes bibliographical references and index.
  ISBN 1-58829-634-2 (alk. paper)
  1. Bone densitometry. 2. Bones--Growth. 3. Child development. I. Sawyer, Aenor J. II. Bachrach, Laura K.
III. Fung, Ellen B. IV. Series.
  [DNLM: 1. Bone Diseases--radiography. 2. Adolescent. 3. Bone Density. 4. Child. 5. Densitometry--methods.
WS 270 B712 2007]
  RC930.5.B66 2007
  616.7'10757--dc22

                                                                                                2006017180

Series Editor's Introduction

Bone Densitometry in Growing Patients: Guidelines for Clinical Practice, edited by Drs. Sawyer, Bachrach, and Fung, is a milestone book for all health professionals concerned with bone health in growing patients. The book introduces and emphasizes the importance of attending to issues of bone health and development in childhood and adolescence as a way of maintaining such health and decreasing the epidemic of osteoporosis that we are now seeing in older adults. In doing so, the book offers a much-needed first set of standards of bone densitometry in growing patients. Given the numerous reports of serious interpretation errors in densitometry results in children, the development of this body of work is truly important.

It is in this context that *Bone Densitometry in Growing Patients: Guidelines for Clinical Practice* presents the current evidence, including an assessment of the strengths and weaknesses in the data on assessing bone density in childhood and adolescence. In short, the editors and authors have done an outstanding job of organizing not only the key topics in this broad clinical discussion, but also, and most importantly, the evidence within these areas.

Neil S. Skolnik, MD
Associate Director
Family Practice Residency Program
Abington Memorial Hospital
Abington, PA
Professor of Family and Community Medicine
Temple University School of Medicine
Philadelphia, PA

Foreword

In medieval society the idea of childhood did not exist; this is not to suggest that children were neglected, forsaken or despised. The idea of childhood is not to be confused with affection for children; it corresponds to an awareness of the particular nature of childhood, that particular nature which distinguishes the child from the adult, even the young adult...

—Philippe Ariés (Centuries of Childhood, New York: Vintage, 1962)

As a densitometrist for some 20 years, I like to think that I understand bone densitometry and know how to apply it clinically. But to say that children are simply small adults and to proceed accordingly in applying densitometry would be foolhardy. And to assume that expertise in adult densitometry automatically confers expertise in pediatric densitometry would be the height of arrogance. And yet, many of us, well-intended though we may have been, have done just that. But "the particular nature of childhood," in this context, the growing bones of a child that are changing in size, shape, and density, demands approaches to data acquisition, analysis, and interpretation that are unique and distinct from adult densitometry. Current knowledge, although incomplete, makes it clear that this is so. The lower bone densities of a child demand differences in the technical aspects of data acquisition and analysis. Consideration must be given to the effects of the changing size and shape of the bone as the child grows. And the reference databases to which the bone density values are compared and which give those values meaning must be specifically created for the child.

There is much still to be learned in pediatric bone disease and densitometry, just as there is in adult bone disease and densitometry. And we all must continue to learn. To that end, *Bone Densitometry in Growing Patients* is an invaluable source of current information in pediatric densitometry as well as a signpost that pediatric densitometry has come of age. It is time for all of us as densitometrists to leave medieval thinking behind, and recognize that "particular nature of childhood."

Sydney Lou Bonnick, MD, FACP
Clinical Research Center of North Texas
Denton, TX
Author: Bone Densitometry in Clinical Practice:
Application and Interpretation
and co-author: Bone Densitometry for Technologists,
both from Humana Press, Totowa, NJ

Preface

The goal of *Bone Densitometry in Growing Patients: Guidelines for Clinical Practice* is to provide both clinicians and technologists with a practical guide for the use of densitometry in pediatrics. The importance of investigating and improving children's bone health has been established, but the tools to carry out this work are still in development.

At this time, the most available clinical technique is dual-energy x-ray absorptiometry, commonly referred to as DXA. Despite its limitations, DXA is a widely used and well-described method of bone health assessment in adult medicine, and its use is rising rapidly in pediatrics. To date, however, no published texts have adequately addressed the complicated issues encountered when investigating children using DXA. This likely reflects the complexities of performing DXAs in younger patients and the lack of consensus concerning acquisition and interpretation of data in growing children.

Although much information is still needed to optimize the use of DXA in children, we are aware that its use is exponentially increasing and that treatment decisions are often based on the information thus gathered. We therefore felt compelled to merge all available data and expert opinion into a document that will hopefully serve both as a guidebook for centers employing the technique and as a springboard for future developments in this important field.

Work on this book began at the Second International Conference on Children's Bone Health, held in Sheffield, England in 2002. Pediatric bone experts from Europe, Australia, New Zealand, Canada, South Africa, and the United States met to define and address controversies in the acquisition and interpretation of DXA scans in pediatric patients. At subsequent sessions, in conjunction with the American Society for Bone and Mineral Research in 2003 and 2004 and the Third International Pediatric Bone Health meeting in 2005, this working group continued its efforts to discuss best practices in the field of pediatric DXA. As in any field in which research is sparse and opinions are plentiful, there were invigorating debates and fruitful discussions.

Much time was spent outlining numerous uncertainties, including the optimal skeletal sites for scanning, the analysis, the selection of normative data, and the interpretation of the bone mineral data. Each of these variables can affect the results of a study and may lead to misinterpretations of results. When the treatments were limited to optimizing vitamin D and calcium intake and physical activity, the potential for misinterpretation was an important but lesser concern. However, now bisphosphonates and other drugs used to treat osteoporosis in the elderly are being prescribed increasingly in children, despite a lack of data establishing their efficacy and safety in pediatric patients. Many decisions to start these medications are based on the results of DXA scans. When therapeutic decisions rely on erroneous information, such as the diagnosis of "osteoporosis" based upon an adult scanning protocol and normative data (T-scores), there can be serious consequences.

Therefore, although numerous controversies remain, our group of experienced pediatric bone researchers and clinicians agreed on the need to develop guidelines for performing and interpreting DXAs in clinical pediatric practice. Our panel of international of authors has extensive background in pediatric DXA and has published in their areas of expertise. Each chapter has been revised in response to reviews by the editors and an additional panel of four external reviewers to ensure an even broader scope of expertise. We are extremely grateful to all of the valued authors and reviewers cited in the Contributors section.

Bone Densitometry in Growing Patients: Guidelines for Clinical Practice is directed at technologists and clinicians with some prior knowledge of DXA theory and technique. For those less familiar with DXA, we recommend as valuable resources the comprehensive texts written by Dr. Syndey L. Bonnick, *Bone Densitometry in Clinical Practice: Application and Interpretation, Second Edition* and *Bone Densitometry for Technologists, Second Edition* (Humana Press). Although these texts focus on DXA procedures in adults, they provide an essential foundation for work in this field.

This text begins with an introduction of general concepts regarding bone health in children. We have also included a brief overview of all the currently available densitometry techniques used in evaluating children, but we then focus primarily on DXA because it is the most widely used method for bone density assessment in clinical practice. Subsequent chapters discuss the indications for DXA studies in children and the optimal methods for acquiring, analyzing, interpreting, and reporting these scans. Current and future research applications of DXA and other modalities for studying pediatric bone health are also discussed. At the end of each chapter, we have added Key Points to emphasize the themes discussed. Please remember that these are not meant to stand alone—they cannot replace a thorough read of the discussion contained in the text.

Appendices were added to serve as a "resource center," with information including websites, manufacturer details, and pediatric-specific reference data. The Appendices also contain sample requisition forms and information sheets for patients, which have been generously contributed from various existing pediatric DXA centers. We have included some specific information from the three major DXA manufacturers, but we have not tried to recreate operator manuals, which must be followed for optimal DXA performance.

Recommendations throughout the book are evidence-based whenever there are sufficient data to support a conclusion. When conclusive data are lacking, recommendations reflect the consensus opinions of the assembled bone experts who contributed to this book. For some issues, expert consensus has not been achieved. In these instances, two or three common practices are described and supported to allow you to select an appropriate method for your center. When faced with choosing among several recommended techniques, it is important to be consistent once a method is chosen and that it is imperative that the specific method be documented in the patient's report.

Changes in DXA and other densitometry methods are inevitable in coming years, and other noninvasive modalities are likely to emerge to better predict bone strength. However, at this time, DXA remains the gold standard in the clinical setting for assessing bone health in children and adults. Our hope is to optimize the current use of DXA in children as a tool in the clinical management of bone fragility. Ultimately, this may improve the process of identifying and monitoring children at risk for low bone mass, leading to the development of appropriate intervention and treatment programs for this population.

Aenor J. Sawyer, MD
Laura K. Bachrach, MD
Ellen B. Fung, PhD, RD

Acknowledgments

This book reflects the efforts of many dedicated people to whom we owe a great deal of gratitude. First and foremost we would like to thank the chapter authors who represent an international, multidisciplinary panel of pediatric bone density experts. It has been an honor to work with these talented and committed professionals over the past 3 years. Their contributions to this text will certainly make a difference in the lives of many children.

We would like to thank the members of the expert review panel, Maria Luisa Bianchi, Sydney Bonnick, Ailsa Goulding, and Bonnie Specker, for their thoughtful comments and keen criticisms, ensuring the most accurate and timely information available.

In addition, we extend our gratitude to Tom Kelly from Hologic, Ken Faulkner from GE/Lunar, and Tom Sanchez from Cooper Surgical/Norland for providing technical input, instrument specifications, and reference data for each of the widely used densitometers.

We are grateful for the enduring support and valuable input from our mentors Robert Marcus, Mary Bouxsein, James Kasser, Bertrum Lubin, and Elliot Vichinsky and our colleagues John Shepherd, Emily von Scheven, May Wang, Ellen Butensky, Paul Harmatz, Lisa Calvelli, Zahra Pakbaz, and Rita Marie Sten. We are very appreciative of our affiliations with Stanford University, Children's Hospital & Research Center of Oakland, Children's Hospital of Boston, the Foundation for Osteoporosis Research and Education, the Northern California Institute for Bone Health, and the Pediatric Bone Health Consortium.

In the publishing arena, we thank Melinda Griffith. We also thank Cheryl Geels our copyeditor, and the tireless work of Robin Weisberg and Richard Lansing from Humana Press.

Despite all of these resources, talent, and commitment, we would not have been able to make this text a reality without generous sponsorship. We thank Hologic and Merck for educational grants during this process. We are very grateful for the fund-raising efforts of Elliott Schwartz and the generosity of the S.D. Bechtel Jr. Foundation, the major sponsor of this project.

And last, but certainly not least, we are deeply indebted to our families for their unconditional love and support, providing each of us the encouragement, strength, and additional time needed to accomplish this work. We hope that what we have borrowed from them is an investment in the health and happiness of many families.

Aenor J. Sawyer, MD
Laura K. Bachrach, MD
Ellen B. Fung, PhD, RD

Dedication

As an editorial trio, we have worked together seamlessly over the past few years to bring this book to fruition. However, at this time a dedication is in order that requires a bit of a mutiny. Ellen, Aenor, and all involved would like to take this opportunity to dedicate this book to the person we consider our teacher, mentor, role model, and inspiration, Dr. Laura K. Bachrach. She has our utmost professional respect for her pioneering work in the field of pediatric bone density and bone health. Beyond that, Laura is the standard bearer for professional and personal integrity and is tirelessly devoted to helping children in her work and at home. She exemplifies a strong work ethic, attention to detail, commitment to accuracy, and dedication to needed research and compassionate clinical care. Beyond all of these admirable qualities, Laura has redefined modesty and humility, which would have prevented the inclusion of this paragraph had we allowed her to proof this section. On behalf of those who worked on this book, as well as those who are so fortunate to train with you, be treated by you or benefit from your research, we salute you, Laura, and extend our deepest gratitude.

Aenor J. Sawyer, MD
Ellen B. Fung, PhD, RD

Contents

Series Editor's Introduction v

Foreword vii

Preface ix

Acknowledgments xiii

Dedication xiv

Contributors xvii

Acronyms xviii

1. Rationale for Bone Densitometry in Childhood and Adolescence 1
   Aenor J. Sawyer and Laura K. Bachrach

2. Tools for Measuring Bone in Children and Adolescents 15
   Kate A. Ward, Zulf Mughal, and Judith E. Adams

3. Dual-Energy X-Ray Absorptiometry 41
   Nicola J. Crabtree, Mary B. Leonard, and Babette S. Zemel

4. Clinical Indications for the Use of DXA in Pediatrics 59
   *Laura K. Bachrach, Michael A. Levine, Christopher T. Cowell,
   and Nicholas J. Shaw*

5. Acquisition of DXA in Children and Adolescents 73
   Nicola J. Crabtree, Kyla Kent, and Babette S. Zemel

6. Analysis 93
   *Moira Petit, Kyla Kent, Mary B. Leonard, Heather McKay,
   and Babette S. Zemel*

7. Evaluation 115
   Babette S. Zemel and Moira Petit

8 . Reporting DXA Results 127
   *Ellen B. Fung, Laura K. Bachrach, Julie N. Briody,
   and Christopher T. Cowell*

9. Children With Special Considerations 137
   Laurie J. Moyer-Mileur, Zulf Mughal, and Ellen B. Fung

10. Research Considerations 159

    Mary B. Leonard and Moira Petit

11. Looking to the Future of Pediatric Bone Densitometry 173

    Nicholas J. Bishop, Aenor J. Sawyer, and Mary B. Leonard

Appendix A: *Resources* 179

Appendix B: *Equations and Calculations* 197

Appendix C: *Pediatric Normative Data* 199

Appendix D: *Forms and Handouts* 213

Index 223

Contributors

JUDITH E. ADAMS, MBBS, FRCR, FRCP • Clinical Radiology, Imaging Science & Biomedical Engineering, University of Manchester, Manchester, UK

LAURA K. BACHRACH, MD • Division of Endocrinology, Stanford University School of Medicine, Stanford, CA

MARIA LUISA BIANCHI, MD • Bone Metabolism Unit, Istituto Auxologico, Italiano IRCCS, Milano, Italy

NICHOLAS J. BISHOP, MD • Department of Pediatric Bone Health, University of Sheffield, Sheffield, UK

SYDNEY BONNICK, MD, FACP • Clinical Research Center of North Texas and University of North Texas, Denton, TX

JULIE N. BRIODY, MBiomedENG, BSc • Department Nuclear Medicine, The Children's Hospital at Westmead, Westmead, New South Wales, Australia

CHRISTOPHER T. COWELL, MD • Institute of Endocrinology and Diabetes, The Children's Hospital at Westmead, Westmead, New South Wales, Australia

NICOLA CRABTREE, PhD, MSc, BSc(HONS) • Department Nuclear Medicine, Queen Elizabeth Hospital, Edgbaston, Birmingham, UK

ELLEN B. FUNG, PhD, RD • Children's Hospital & Research Center at Oakland, HEDCO Health Science Center, Oakland, CA

AILSSA GOULDING, PhD, FACN • Department of Medical and Surgical Sciences, University of Otago, Dunedin, New Zealand

KYLA KENT, MD • Musculoskeletal Research Laboratory, Palo Alto Veterans Affairs Hospital, Palo Alto, CA

MARY B. LEONARD, MD, MSCE • Department of Pediatrics and Epidemiology, The Children's Hospital of Philadelphia, University of Pennsylvania, School of Medicine, Philadelphia, PA

MICHAEL A. LEVINE, MD • Department of Pediatrics, The Children's Hospital, the Cleveland Clinic, Cleveland Clinic Lerner College of Medicine, Case Western Reserve University, Cleveland, OH

HEATHER MCKAY, PhD • School of Human Kinetics, University of British Columbia Vancouver, British Columbia

LAURIE J. MOYER-MILEUR, PhD, RD • Department of Pediatrics, University of Utah, Salt Lake City, UT

ZULF MUGHAL, MB ChB • Department of Pediatrics, St. Mary's Hospital, Manchester, UK

MOIRA PETIT, PhD • School of Kinesiology, University of Minnesota, Minneapolis, MN

AENOR J. SAWYER, MD • Pediatric Bone Health Consortium and Children's Hospital & Research Center at Oakland, Oakland, CA

NICHOLAS J. SHAW, MB ChB • Department of Endocrinology, Birmingham Children's Hospital, Birmingham, UK

BONNIE L. SPECKER, PhD • Martin Program in Human Nutrition, South Dakota State University, Brookings, SD

KATE A. WARD, PhD • Clinical Radiology, Imaging Science & Biomedical Engineering, University of Manchester, Manchester, UK

BABETTE S. ZEMEL, PhD • Division of Gastroenterology, Hepatology and Nutrition, The Children's Hospital of Philadelphia, Department of Pediatrics, University of Pennsylvania School of Medicine, Philadelphia, PA

aBMD	areal bone mineral density	LDS	low density software
AMI	axial moment of inertia	LS	lumbar spine
AP	anterior-posterior	LSC	least-significant change
BA	bone area	MRI	magnetic resonance imaging
BMAD	bone mineral apparent density	MTI	monitoring time interval
BMC	bone mineral content	NAI	nonaccidental injury
BMD	bone mineral density	NIH	National Institutes of Health
BMDCS	Bone Mineral Density in Childhood Study	OI	osteogenesis imperfecta
		OR	odds ratio
BUA	broadband ultrasonic attenuation	PA	posteroanterior
CSA	cross-sectional area	pDXA	peripheral dual-energy x-ray absorptiometry
CSMI	cross-sectional moments of inertia	pQCT	peripheral quantitative computed tomography
CT	computed tomography		
CV	coefficient of variation	PVC	polyvinyl chloride
2-D	two-dimensional	QCT	quantitative computed tomography
DOS	disk operating system	QUS	quantitative ultrasound
DPA	dual-photon absorptiometry	rad	radiation absorbed dose
DXA	dual-energy x-ray absorptiometry	REM	roentgen-equivalent-man
DXR	digital x-ray radiogrammetry	ROC	receiver operating characteristic
ESD	entrance surface dose	ROI	region of interest
ESP	European Spine Phantom	RUS	radius, ulna, short bone
FDA	Food and Drug Administration	sBMD	standardized BMD
GE	General Electric	SD	standard deviation
Gy	gray	SOS	speed of sound
HSA	Hip Structural Analysis	SPA	single-photon absorptiometry
HR	hazard ratio	SSI	stress-strain index
HU	Hounsfield units	SXA	single x-ray absorptiometry
IJO	idiopathic juvenile osteoporosis	vBMD	volumetric bone mineral density
IRB	Institutional Review Board	VOS	velocity of sound
ISCD	International Society of Clinical Densitometry	WHO	World Health Organization

1

Rationale for Bone Densitometry in Childhood and Adolescence

Aenor J. Sawyer, MD
and Laura K. Bachrach, MD

CONTENTS

INTRODUCTION ADULT BONE HEALTH CRISIS
PEDIATRIC BONE HEALTH CONCERNS
BONE MINERAL ACCRUAL
IMPORTANCE OF PEAK BONE MASS
DETERMINANTS OF BONE ACQUISITION AND PEAK BONE MASS
THE CHALLENGE OF DIAGNOSIS
SUMMARY
REFERENCES

INTRODUCTION

Bone health in children is a rapidly growing area of clinical concern. The recent interest in this field is a response to the rising incidence of childhood fractures as well as the concept that early bone development could be a major determinant of adult osteoporosis and fragility fractures. In the past few years, there has been a marked increase in the use of bone densitometry in children and adolescents, primarily using dual-energy x-ray absorptiometry (DXA). Although a valuable tool, the use of DXA to evaluate children has highlighted its limitations. By recognizing the shortcomings, yet exploiting the strengths of DXA, this noninvasive, low-risk, readily available tool could aid in identifying children at risk for inadequate bone development and monitoring treatment.

To underscore the importance of assessing bone health in children, this chapter reviews the epidemic of adult osteoporosis and the bone health concerns in pediatrics. Current concepts regarding the determinants and importance of optimal bone mineral acquisition are discussed as well. Finally, the challenges of measuring bone health in growing patients are briefly outlined here but are discussed in greater detail in subsequent chapters.

From: *Current Clinical Practice: Bone Densitometry in Growing Patients: Guidelines for Clinical Practice*
Edited by: A. J. Sawyer, L. K. Bachrach, and E. B. Fung © Humana Press Inc., Totowa, NJ

ADULT BONE HEALTH CRISIS

Osteoporosis is a worldwide epidemic, affecting approximately 75 million people in the United States, Europe, and Japan *(1)*. In 2003, Melton et al. estimated the annual European cost of osteoporotic fractures at 25 billion *(2)*. It is expected that approximately 12 million people in the United States over age 50 will be diagnosed with osteoporosis by the year 2010; currently, more than 1.5 million Americans sustain osteoporotic fractures each year *(3,4)*. An estimated 30–50% of women and 15–30% of men have a lifetime risk of sustaining a fracture related to osteoporosis *(5)*. In adults, a history of prior fracture is associated with as much as an 86% increased risk of fracture at any site *(6)*.

In 1990, osteoporosis was defined as "a disease characterized by low bone mass, microarchitectural deterioration of bone tissue, and a consequent increase in fracture risk" *(7)*. Osteoporosis was redefined in 2000 as "a skeletal disorder characterized by compromised bone strength, predisposing to an increased risk of fracture" *(8)*, terminology that emphasizes the importance of factors in addition to bone mass that contribute to bone strength.

PEDIATRIC BONE HEALTH CONCERNS

Fractures in healthy children have often been accepted as common childhood injuries, without concern for underlying health risks, other than child abuse. The incidence and type of pediatric fractures vary by gender, age group, and site. Throughout growth, there is a 2.7:1 ratio of boys to girls who sustain a fracture *(9)*. From infancy to adulthood, there is an increasing rate of fractures, with a peak incidence during the adolescent growth spurt. Although theories regarding increased sports participation or high-risk behavior have been postulated, one possible explanation for this high fracture rate in the peripubertal period is that peak height velocity precedes the peak velocity of bone acquisition by 0.5 to 0.7 yr, as demonstrated by Bailey et al. (Fig. 1 *[10]*).

A growing body of literature on pediatric fractures has raised questions of possible underlying bone health deficiencies in "normal" children. Epidemiological studies from the United States and Finland revealed an increase in fractures of 35% in boys and 60% in girls *(11,12)*, with similar findings seen in Sweden *(13)*, Australia *(14)*, and Japan *(15)*. Goulding et al. *(16)*, in New Zealand, showed a lower bone mass in girls with forearm fractures, indicating that childhood fractures may signal underlying skeletal strength deficits in children who, otherwise, have no known illness. Goulding also observed that girls who had fractured were heavier and had greater total percent body fat as compared with controls *(17)*. These findings are of concern given the growing epidemic of childhood obesity worldwide.

Frequent or low-trauma fractures, long recognized in pediatric patients with osteogenesis imperfecta, have been reported in association with myriad other chronic childhood conditions such as rheumatological disorders, inflammatory bowel disease, and childhood malignancies. Low bone mass and the occurrence of fractures in these patients may be the result of a combination of their underlying systemic illness and adverse effects of drugs or radiation used to treat them.

As the survival rates of even the most catastrophic pediatric illnesses continue to improve, we are faced with the long-term effects of these diseases and their treatments *(18)*. It is critical that the potentially deleterious effects on the skeleton be defined, monitored, and treated when possible. For example, children with acute lymphoblastic

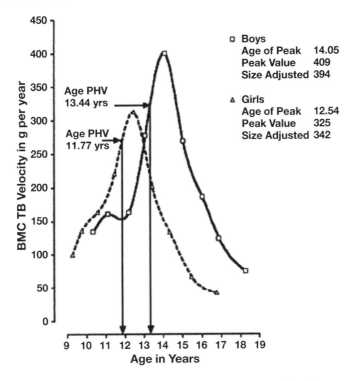

Fig.1. Total body peak BMC velocity curve illustrating velocity at peak and ages at peak BMC and peak height velocities by chronological age for boys and girls. (From ref. *10*.)

leukemia (ALL), the most common pediatric malignancy, have a sixfold greater fracture risk than controls and a marked decrease in total body bone mineral density (BMD) during the course of chemotherapy. Although these negative skeletal effects and increased fracture rates persisted for at least 6 mo after cessation of treatment, a 10-yr follow-up study found improvement of BMD in these patients, with some approximating their healthy peers *(19)*. Interventions of nutrition and exercise programs are now being implemented with ALL patients, but published results are not yet available.

The prevention of childhood fractures in healthy and ill children is obviously of great importance. Additionally, an increased focus on acquisition of optimal bone size, geometry, and mass during childhood and adolescence appears to be critical in establishing a foundation for bone health throughout life.

BONE MINERAL ACCRUAL

Growth curves, which track height and weight, have long been used as an indication of a child's general health. As an analogue to the growth curve, the bone acquisition curve, as shown in Fig. 2 *(20)*, is a helpful framework for understanding changes in bone mass during growth. In addition to the longitudinal and circumferential enlargement of developing bone, changes also occur in composition, which allow the skeleton to withstand mechanical loads experienced from weight bearing and muscular force.

Heaney et al. *(20)*, in a detailed review article, summarized the patterns of gain in bone mineral throughout childhood and adolescence. Nonlinear gains in bone mass throughout

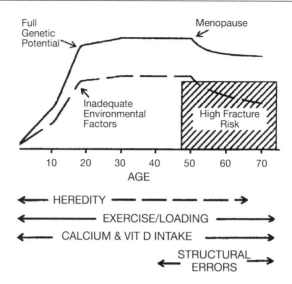

Fig. 2. Diagrammatic representation of the bone mass life-line in individuals who achieve their full genetic potential for skeletal mass and in those who do not. (The magnitude of the difference between the curves is not intended to be to scale.) Along the bottom of the graph are arrayed several of the factors known to be of particular importance. (From ref. *20*; copyright © Robert P. Heaney, 1999.)

the first two decades of life are described, with the most rapid rise seen in the four peripubertal years, specifically between pubertal stages 2 and 4. Before the onset of puberty, boys and girls develop bone mass at similar rates. Beyond that, however, boys tend to acquire greater bone mass than girls. Gains in total body bone mineral during adolescence approximate 30–40% *(10,21)*, twice that which is gained from birth to the onset of puberty and more than the amount lost in later life *(21)*. The rate of bone acquisition slows toward the end of puberty, but consolidation of bone continues until peak bone mass (PBM) is fully achieved, near age 30.

PBM is defined as the total amount of bone tissue amassed by the end of skeletal maturation *(22)*. Although it is estimated that 80–90% of PBM is acquired in the first two decades of life *(21,22)*, studies on the timing of bone accrual reveal a site-specific phenomenon that varies with the unit of measurement. As an example, BMD of the proximal femur peaks by age 20, whereas total-body bone mineral content (BMC) peaks approximately 10 years later *(21)*.

IMPORTANCE OF PEAK BONE MASS

Dent, as early as 1973, described osteoporosis as a disease of adulthood with its roots in childhood *(23)*. According to this model, bone mass achieved by early adulthood is a key determinant of the risk of developing osteoporosis and fragility fractures later in life *(24)*. As illustrated in Fig. 2, a higher PBM is felt to confer greater protection against future fragility fractures *(20)*. Suboptimal PBM is thought to contribute even more than subsequent bone loss to the lifetime risk of osteoporotic fracture *(25)*.

The risk of adult osteoporosis has been linked to exposure to unfavorable environments during critical stages of growth and development. Javaid and Cooper *(26)* have proposed that maternal factors shaping the *in utero* environment for the fetus may have long-lasting or permanent effects on bone mass, bone size, and body composition during childhood or adult life. Similarly, childhood and adolescence are critical periods when diet, activity, and other modifiable variables can influence the growth and strength of bones. Although far from fully defined, a phenomenon has been described in which bone mass acquired early in life may track as a child matures *(21)*; prepubertal children with higher-than-average bone mass typically exhibit higher-than-average bone mass postpuberty *(27,28)*, barring any environmental insult.

As stated by Kreipe *(29)*, "the prevention of osteoporosis, often deemed a geriatric disorder, may now be considered the legitimate domain of pediatricians." The concept that bone mineral accrual in childhood determines PBM, which then may predict adult bone density and strength, remains theoretical due to the lack of requisite but difficult large-cohort, multidecade longitudinal studies. However, this paradigm may offer a valuable construct for early intervention or prevention strategies addressing bone health in children and adults.

DETERMINANTS OF BONE ACQUISITION AND PEAK BONE MASS

Bone mineral accrual and PBM appear to be influenced by many factors, including genetics, nutrition, mechanical loading, puberty, illness, and certain medications. The complex positive and negative effects of these variables individually and in combination are beyond the scope of this chapter but have been reviewed by Heaney et al. *(20)* and Bonjour et al. *(30)*. Some general concepts are discussed in brief here.

Heritability

An estimated 60–80% of the variability in PBM between individuals has been attributed to heritable factors, as demonstrated in adult and adolescent twin studies *(31–35)*. Parent–child studies also reveal a pattern of heritability in bone health. In an observational study of more than 400 family participants, there was a 3.8-fold increase in a son's chance of low bone density if his father presented with low bone density. The daughter's risk was increased 5.1-fold if her mother had low bone density *(36)*.

Although the genes responsible for determining bone size, mineral accrual, and resorption have not been established with certainty, several candidate genes have been implicated including the *vitamin D receptor polymorphisms, estrogen receptor* gene, *Collagen Ia1* gene, *transforming growth factor-β1* gene, and *apolipoprotein E* gene *(37–41)*, to name a few. The specific mechanisms by which each would affect skeletal health are still not well defined. There are numerous studies underway using genome scanning as well as candidate gene techniques to better identify gene loci associated with low bone density or strength, and ultimately, risk of fracture. The genetic potential for peak mass, however, can only be reached when the modifiable factors that contribute to bone acquisition are favorable.

Modifiable Risk

Modifiable or environmental factors, such as diet, activity, body composition, and general health, are thought to explain anywhere from 20 to 40% of the variability seen in PBM. Defining the contribution of each of these factors is a necessary first step in designing strategies to optimize bone health. Modifiable influences can also adversely affect developing bone, as discussed in Chapter 4.

NUTRITION

CALCIUM

Calcium is a key nutrient for skeletal health throughout the life span, allowing for optimal gains in bone mass during the growing years and reducing bone loss in later life *(20)*. For optimal bone health, calcium intake must be sufficient to meet the demands of bone mineral accrual and to compensate for losses in urine, feces, and sweat. Calcium has been described as a threshold nutrient; skeletal mass increases with increasing calcium until intake reaches the level at which gains are constant. Although this concept is widely accepted, the definition of the calcium "threshold" for children of varying ages remains in dispute *(42)*. Estimates of the requirement for calcium come from studies of calcium balance, mineral accrual, and fractures. Some of the most revealing data come from randomized controlled trials of calcium supplementation.

Calcium supplementation in children and adolescents has resulted in short-term gains in bone mineral, but the skeletal effects have varied with the amount and source of calcium supplement, the skeletal region, and the age and maturity of the child *(42–46)*. Gains are greater at sites rich in cortical rather than trabecular bone. Benefits may be greater in pre- or early pubertal children than in later stages of puberty but some studies have shown a benefit in adolescents as well *(42,46,47)*. Physical activity may also modify the skeletal response to calcium supplementation, with synergistic gains at weight-bearing sites *(47,48)*. Another key question is the sustainability of benefit from calcium supplementation. To date, most, but not all studies have found that gains in bone mass are lost by 2 yr following discontinuation of the supplement *(42,49)*. Further research is needed to determine optimal calcium intake throughout the growing years and the best form of supplementation for those children who do not meet these needs through diet alone. Whether calcium influences bone size or mineral accrual must also be determined *(44)*. The ultimate goals are daunting—to test the effects of calcium intake not only on short-term bone mineral changes, but on PBM and lifetime fracture risk.

PHOSPHOROUS

Despite the fact that phosphate makes up at least half of bone mineral mass, it generates much less concern than calcium. This is likely because, as a nutrient, it is generally found in adequate amounts in the diet. Therefore, there are greater concerns for possible overexposure from high intakes of soft drinks. Wyshak et al. *(50)* showed a correlation between the number of carbonated beverages consumed and the incidence of fractures in adolescent girls. The link between soft drinks and poor bone health is likely not the result of adverse effects from soda, but from the displacement of milk from diet *(51)*.

VITAMIN D

It has long been recognized that vitamin D is essential for efficient absorption of calcium *(52)*, yet it is not readily available in the diet. Infants and small children are typically supplemented with this micronutrient, whereas older children and teens are not. Vitamin D deficiency can result from a lack of sun exposure, but also from low intakes of milk, which is typically fortified with vitamin D *(53)*. During adolescence, the period of most rapid bone accrual, calcium absorption needs to be most efficient. Unfortunately, many teenagers, especially females, consume inadequate amounts of milk, resulting in inadequate vitamin D intake, thus decreased calcium absorption and retention in puberty *(54)*. In children on dairy-restricted regiments such as macrobiotic diets, both calcium and vitamin D intakes may be markedly low, leading to reduced bone acquisition (55). Studies of bone acquisition in relation to vitamin D are few, but Jones and Dwyer (56) did note a positive effect of winter solar exposure on the bone density of 8-yr-old Tasmanian children. In adults, it has been shown that low 25(OH)D concentrations increase parathyroid hormone activity, with a subsequent increase in bone resorption (57,58), although this is less well established in children. Combined supplementation of calcium and vitamin D in postmenopausal women has a positive effect on BMD (59) and in elderly women has been shown to decrease hip fracture rates (60).

Severe vitamin D deficiency in children results in nutritional rickets with marked physeal abnormality and osteomalacia. This condition, rarely seen in North America, still remains a major health problem in developing countries in which vitamin D-fortified foods are not available. Milder forms of vitamin D deficiency, which are asymptomatic, may result in children not meeting their full genetic potential with regards to PBM.

PROTEIN

The influence of dietary protein on bone health has been reviewed; both deficiencies and excess may have adverse effects on the skeleton (61). In a cohort of 200 adolescents, a positive association of bone mass gain and protein intake was noted in both genders and was most notable from prepuberty through midpuberty (62). Children with inadequate protein and caloric intake exhibited growth retardation and decreased formation of cortical bone, as reported by Garn (63). As with other nutrients, further research is needed to determine the optimal amounts and form of protein for bone health.

EXERCISE

The mechanical loading of bone is a proven stimulus to increased bone size and density, just as the chronic removal of mechanical stress on bone leads to bone loss (64,65). In developing bones, gains in BMD over time have been shown to be greater in children with increased daily physical activity (66). Bailey et al. (10,67) noted greater bone mass accruals across puberty in an observational study comparing more active and less active youth. Greater bone mineral accrual even during the third decade can has been linked to greater physical activity (68). The benefits of activity have also been demonstrated in side-to-side studies of children and teens engaged in racket sports, with greater bone size and mass in the playing arm.

The skeletal benefits of activity are perhaps most convincingly shown in intervention studies, eliminating any selection bias in subjects (69–74). As mentioned earlier, increasing calcium intake can have synergistic effects with activity on bone health in growing children (75).

Exercise involving relatively intense loading with impact forces has been shown in athlete studies to have the greatest effect on increasing bone mass. For example, the bone mass in gymnasts was much higher than would be expected for age (despite amenorrhea in some) and was greater than that seen in runners, who appear to have greater bone mass than swimmers (76,77).

Although the benefits of regular exercise, which extend beyond the skeletal system, are well known, there is an unfortunate pattern of decreasing activity levels as grade levels advance. The US Surgeon General's report on physical activity revealed a dramatic decrease in activity levels at the beginning of adolescence, with girls at more risk for inactivity during puberty than boys. Approximately half of US youth between the ages of 12 and 21 engage in no vigorous physical activity. These numbers are of great concern in light of the available information regarding the effects of loading or unloading the skeleton during development *(78)*.

Other important environmental influences that can have profoundly negative effects on developing bone, such as chronic illnesses immobility, delayed puberty, malnutrition, and specific medications, are presented in detail in Chapter 4.

This discussion of determinants of bone mass illustrates possible positive and negative influences on children during bone development. With a greater understanding of the impact of environmental risk factors, as well as the expression of polygenetic determinants of bone development, the opportunity to optimize bone health increases greatly. Proper measurement techniques for assessing bone characteristics in children are essential to evaluate the effects of these and other influences.

THE CHALLENGE OF DIAGNOSIS

DXA in Adults

In adults, the advent of noninvasive bone densitometry has offered a means to identify and treat individuals with bone fragility before they fracture and to monitor their response to therapy with parameters other than fracture. Of the available densitometry techniques, DXA is currently the preferred method for detecting adults at risk for osteoporosis. Its widespread use as a clinical tool is in part because of its low radiation exposure, excellent precision, ease of testing, and affordability.

For postmenopausal women, much work has been done to establish disease severity thresholds and even fracture risk based on DXA. In this group, fracture risk has been correlated to low bone density as measured by DXA. The World Health Organization has developed criteria for the diagnosis of "osteoporosis" in postmenopausal Caucasian women based on a BMD that is 2.5 standard deviations or more below the average value for a young adult (i.e., T-score < -2.5).

A significant limitation of DXA is that while it uses density as a surrogate for strength, it does not truly measure all parameters of bone that determine fracture risk. For example, the reduction in fracture rates observed after initiation of bisphosphonate therapy exceeds that predicted by gains in BMD *(79–81)*. This observation illustrates the importance of factors other than bone mineral that contribute to bone strength. The size, shape, geometry, microarchitecture of bone and the rates of bone turnover are important modifiers of bone strength and fracture risk.

In contrast to that of postmenopausal women, the diagnosis of bone fragility in men, younger women, and especially children is more complex and controversial *(82)*. The indications for bone DXA in these patients and the clinical implications of their results are still being debated. Experts in the bone field have proposed guidelines for testing and interpreting DXA results in men, young women, and children, based on opinion where data were lacking *(83)*. Another panel of bone experts have criticized these recommendations, citing the lack of objective data to support the opinions *(84)*. In short, considerable controversy surrounds the optimal approach to identify risk for bone fragility in men and younger individuals.

DXA in Children and Adolescents

Children present the most challenging population for assessing skeletal health, primarily because of the numerous variables of growth. Measurement techniques in the pediatric setting would ideally be safe, painless, of short duration, and would provide valuable information. In comparison with other bone measurement systems, DXA best fits these criteria. However, there are difficulties that are unique to children and adolescents when using this tool. This discussion serves as a very brief introduction to topics that are the focus of this text.

Bones change in size, shape, and mass throughout the first two decades of life, and the tempo of change varies by skeletal site and individual. Measurements of bone mass by DXA are two-dimensional (i.e., areal) and are strongly influenced by bone size, pubertal stage, and bone age *(85,86)*. Children with smaller bones may appear to have low BMD, and, in serial testing, changes resulting from increased bone size can be misconstrued for increased bone density. For this reason, areal BMD can be a source of confusion in the pediatric population, and the concept of volumetric density may be more appropriate.

When using DXA with children, it may be that different units of measurement will be more useful than those for adults. For example, BMC and BMD are often used interchangeably to denote mass, although they are very different parameters. It appears that BMC measured by DXA is more sensitive to change in bone acquisition than is areal BMD, especially in early- and prepubertal children *(86)*.

Another difficulty encountered in the use of DXA is the lack of universal pediatric reference data for determining normal from abnormal bone mass. Until recently, DXA software programs automatically generated a T-score, comparing the data of the subject, regardless of his or her age, with that of healthy young adults. This is an inappropriate comparison for those under age 20 who have not yet achieved PBM.

Even when comparing children to their age- and gender-matched peers, there is difficulty because the tempo of growth, sexual maturation, and bone mineral accrual can vary among individuals and can be altered by chronic illness. These factors must be considered as well in determining if bone mineral is "normal."

The complexity of obtaining and interpreting bone densitometry in children and adolescents has led to confusion and misdiagnoses in children. In one recent study, more than half of the subjects referred for a evaluation of pediatric "osteoporosis" had been misdiagnosed with low bone mass, with the most frequent error resulting from the use of a T-score in pediatric patients *(87)*. As this is a developing field, DXAs are frequently performed and interpreted by specialists with expertise in adult osteoporosis but with limited experience with pediatric densitometry. Misleading information about bone mass can result from the use of inappropriate software or improper positioning during acquisition, as well as from an interpretation of results that does not account for known confounding variables.

The consequences of these errors can be costly. Pediatric patients may be inappropriately labeled as "osteoporotic," producing anxiety in parents and children. Physicians may respond to these reports by restricting physical activity or by prescribing drugs for osteoporosis that are, to date, untested for safety and efficacy in children. In addition, if the results of these studies are confusing or are thought to be unreliable, the clinician is less likely to initiate skeletal health assessment in children using DXA, missing an opportunity to identify and correct deficits in developing bone.

SUMMARY

There is an ever-expanding body of knowledge regarding the positive and negative influences on developing bone. Despite this, we are observing worrisome trends in childhood such as poor nutrition, sedentary lifestyle, and obesity, all of which are associated with low bone mass. Beyond that, increasing rates of childhood fractures have been reported on several continents. In addition, more children are surviving significant illnesses and treatment regiments that can have profound deleterious effects on bone.

Aside from immediate concerns in children, the model of PBM as a determinant of adult osteoporosis and fragility fracture implies that the first two decades of life represent a "window of opportunity" in which to implement upstream prevention and intervention strategies that may impart enduring effects on the bone health of an individual.

It follows that this same period represents a "window of vulnerability" and a time during which increased scrutiny of bone development is essential.

It is therefore critical that we expand our ability to measure bone health parameters in the growing patient, to identify markers of inadequate gain, and to monitor effectiveness of interventions. This requires a noninvasive, safe, and available instrument with good precision, short test time, and useful output. As DXA, even with its limitations, is currently the best fit for bone health assessment in children, it is imperative that the clinical utility of DXA be maximized so that we can recognize indications of bone fragility and identify trajectories of bone acquisition that may predispose a child to a lifetime of poor bone health.

Development of these guidelines for the clinical use of DXA in pediatric patients will hopefully improve the quality of densitometry data and reduce the frequency of misdiagnosis in the clinical setting while research continues to advance the usefulness of this and other tools.

REFERENCES

1. EFFO and NOF 1997. Who are candidates for prevention and treatment for osteoporosis? Osteoporos Int 1997;7(1):1–6.
2. Melton LJ 3rd,Gabriel SE, Crowson CS, Tosteson AN, Johnell O, Kanis JA. Cost-equivalence of different osteoporotic fractures. Osteoporos Int 2003;14(5):383–388.
3. NOF. America's bone health: the state of osteoporosis and low bone mass in our nation., 2002.
4. Riggs BL, Melton LJ 3rd. The worldwide problem of osteoporosis: insights afforded by epidemiology. Bone 1995;17(5 Suppl):505S–511S.
5. Randell A, Sambrook PN, Nguyen TV, et al. Direct clinical and welfare costs of osteoporotic fractures in elderly men and women. Osteoporos Int 1995;5(6):427–432.
6. Kanis JA, Johnell O, De Laet C, et al. A meta-analysis of previous fracture and subsequent fracture risk. Bone 2004;35:375–382.
7. Consensus Development Conference. Prophylaxis and treatment of osteoporosis. Am J Med 1991;90:107–110.
8. NIH Consensus Statement. Osteoporosis Prevention, Diagnosis, and Therapy. Baltimore, MD: NIH, 2000;17:1–36.
9. Cheng JC, Shen WY. Limb fracture pattern in different pediatric age groups: A study of 3350 children. J Orthoped Trauma 1993;7:15–22.
10. Bailey DA, McKay HA, Minwald RL, Crocker PRE, Faulkner RA. A six-year longitudinal study of the relationship of physical activity to bone mineral accrual in growing children: The University of Saskatchewan Bone Mineral Accrual Study. J Bone Miner Res 1999;14:1672–1679.

11. Landin LA. Fracture patterns in children. Acta Orthop Scan 1983;54(suppl 202):1–109.

12. Khosla S, Melton LJ III, Dekutoski MB, Achenbach SJ, Oberg AL, Riggs BL. Incidence of childhood distal forearm fractures over 30 years: A population-based study. JAMA 2003;290:1479–1485.

13. Bengner U, Johnell O. Increasing incidence of forearm fractures. A comparison of epidemiologic patterns 25 years apart. Acta Orthopaedica Scandinavia 1985;56(2):158–160.

14. Sherker S, Ozanne-Smith J. Are current playground safety standards adequate for preventing arm fractures? MJA 2004;180:562–565.

15. Hagino H, Yamamoto K, Ohshiro H, Nose T. Increasing incidence of distal radius fractures in Japanese children and adolescents. J Orthopaedic Science 2000;5(4):356–360.

16. Goulding A, Cannan R, Williams SM, Gold EJ, Taylor RW, Lewis-Barned NJ. Bone mineral density in girls with forearm fractures. J Bone Miner Res 1998;13:143–148.

17. Goulding A, Grant AM, Williams SM. Bone and body composition of children and adolescents with repeated forearm fractures. J Bone Miner Res 2005;20(12):2090–2096.

18. Strauss AJ, Su JT, Dalton VM, Gelber RD, Sallan SE, Silveran LB. Bony morbidity in children treated for acute lymphoblastic leukemia. J Clin Oncol 2001;19,3066–3072.

19. van der Sluis I, van den Heuvel-Eibrink M, Hahlen K, Krenning E, de Muinck Keizer-Schrama S. Bone mineral density, body composition, and height in long-term survivors of acute lymphoblastic leukemia in childhood. Med Pediatr Oncol 2000;35:415–420.

20. Heaney RP, Abrams S, Dawson-Hughes B, et al. Peak bone mass. Osteoporosis Int 2000;11:985–1009.

21. Matkovic V, Jelic T, Wardlaw GM, et al. Timing of peak bone mass in Caucasian females and its implication for the prevention of osteoporosis. Inference from a cross-sectional model. J Clin Invest 1994;93:799–808.

22. Bonjour JP, Theintz G, Buchs B, Slossman D, Rizzoli R. Critical years and stages of puberty for spine and femoral bone mass accumulation during adolescence. J Clin Endocrinol Metab 1991;73:555–563.

23. Dent CE. Keynote address: Problems in metabolic bone disease. In: Frame B, Parfitt M, Duncan H, eds. Clinical aspects of metabolic bone disease. Amsterdam: Exerpta medica, 1973; 1–7.

24. Hansen MA, Overgaard K, Riis BJ, Christiansen C. Role of bone mass and bone loss in postmenopausal osteoporosis: 12 year study. BMJ 1991;303:961–964

25. Hui SL, Slemenda CW, Johnston CC. The contribution of bone loss to post menopausal osteoporosis. Osteoporosis Int 1990;1:30–34.

26. Javaid MK, Cooper C. Prenatal and childhood influences on osteoporosis. Best Pract Res Clin Endocrinol Metab 2002;16;349–367.

27. Ferrari S, Rizzoli R, Slosman D, Bonjour J-P. Familial resemblance for bone mineral mass is expressed before puberty. J Clin Endocrinol Metab 1998;83:358–361.

28. Dertina D, Loro ML, Sayre J, Kaufman F, Gilsanz V. Child bone measurements predict values at young adulthood. Bone 1998;23:S288.

29. Kreipe RE. Bones of today, bones of tomorrow. Am J Dis Child 1992;146:22–25.

30. Bonjour JP, Chevalley, T, Ferrari S, Rizzoli R. Peak Bone Mass and Its Regulation. In: Glorieux F, Pettifor J, Juppner H, eds. Pediatric Bone: Biology and Disease. San Diego, CA: Academic Press, 2003, pp.235–248.

31. Eisman JA. Genetics of osteoporosis. Endocrine Rev 1999;20: 788-804.

32. Pocock NA, Eisman JA, Hopper JL, Yeates MG, Sambrook PN, Eberl S. Genetic determinants of bone mass in adults: A twin study. J Clin Invest 1987;80:706–710.

33. Albagha OME, Ralston SH. Genetic determinants of susceptibility to osteoporosis. Endocrinol Metab Clin N Am 2003;32:65-81.

34. Dequeker J, Nijs J, Verstaeten A, Geudens P, Gevers G. Genetic determinants of bone mineral content at the spine and the radius: A twin study. Bone 1987;8:207–209.

35. Young D. Hopper, JL, Nowson CA, et al. Determinants of bone mass in 10- to 26-year-old females: A twin study. J Bone Min Res 1995;10:558–567.

36. Jouanny P ,m Guillemin F, Kuntz C, Jeandel C, Pureel J. Environmental and genetic factors affecting bone mass: Similarity of bone density among members of healthy families. Arthritis Rheum 1995;38:61–67.

37. Spector TD, Keen RW, Arden NK, et al. Influence of vitamin D receptor genotype on bone mineral density in postmenopausal women: A twin study in Britain. BMJ 1995;310:1357–1360.

38. Sano M, Inoue S, Hosoi T, , et al. Association of estrogen receptor dinucleotide repeat polymorphism with osteoporosis. Biochem Biophys Res Commun 1995;217:378–383.

39. Grant SFA, Reid DM, Blake G, Herd R, Fogelman I, Ralston SH. Reduced bone density and osteoporosis associated with a polymorphic Sp2 binding site in the collagen type Ia1 gene. Nature Genet 1996;14:203–205.

40. Bertoldo F, D'Agruma L, Furlan F, et al. Transforming growth factor-beta1 gene polymorphism, bone turnover, and bone mass in Italian postmenopausal women. J Bone Miner Res 2000;15:634–649.

41. Shiraki M, Shiraki Y, Aoki C, et al. Association of bone mineral density with apolipoprotein E phenotype (abstract). J Bone Miner Res 1996;10:S436.

42. Wosje KS, Specker BL. Role of calcium in bone health during childhood. Nutrition Rev 2000;58:253–268.

43. Johnston CC, Miller JZ, Slemenda CW, et al. Calcium supplementation and increased in bone mineral density in children. N Engl J Med 1992;327:119–120.

44. Bonjour JP, Carrie AL, Ferrari S, et al. Calcium-enriched foods and bone mass growth in prepubertal girls: A randomized , double-blind, placebo-controlled trial. J Clin Invest 1997;99:1287–1294.

45. Cadogan J, Eastell R, Jones N, Barker ME. Milk intake and bone mineral acquisition in adolescent girls: Randomised, controlled intervention trial. BMJ 1997;315:1255–1260.

46. Bonjour J-P. Is peripuberty the most opportune time to increase calcium intake in health girls? BoneKEy-Osteovision 1005;2:6–11.

47 Johannsen N, Binkley T, Englert V, Neiderauer G, Specker B. Bone response to jumping is site-specific in children: a randomized trial. Bone 2003;33:533–539

48. Iuliano-Burns S, Saxon L, Naughton G, Gibbons K, Bass SL. Regional specificity of exercise and calcium during skeletal growth in girls: a randomized controlled trial. J Bone Miner Res 2003; 18:156–162.

49. Lee WT, Leung SS, Leung DM, Cheng JC. A follow-up study on the effects of calcium-supplement withdrawal and puberty on bone acquisition of children Am J Clin Nutr 1996;64:71–77.

50. Wyshak G, Frisch RE. Carbonated beverages, dietary calcium, the dietary calcium/phosphorous ratio, and bone fractures in girls and boys. J Adolesc Health 1994;15:210–215.

51. Fitzpatrick L, Heaney RP. Got soda? J Bone Miner Res 2003; 18:1570–1572.

52. Wosje KS, Specker BL. Role of calcium in bone health during childhood. Nutrition Rev 2000;58:253–268.

53. Holick MF. Sunlight and vitamin D for bone health and prevention of autoimmune diseases, cancers and cardiovascular disease. Am J Clin Nutr 2004;80(suppl):1678S–1688S.

54. Abrams SA, Stuff JE. Calcium metabolism in girls: Current dietary intakes lead to low rates of calcium absorption and retention during puberty. Am J Clin Nutr 1994;60:739–743.

55. Dagnelie PC, Vergote F, Staveren WA, van den Berg H, Dingian P, Hautvast J. High prevalence of rickets in infants on macrobiotic diets. Am J Clin Nutr 1990;51:202–208.

56. Jones G, Dwyer T. Bone mass in prepubertal children: Gender differences and the role of physical activity and sunlight exposure. J Clin Endocrinol Metab 1998;83:4274–4279.

57. Chapuy M-C, Preziosi P, Maamer M, et al. Prevalence of vitamin D insufficiency in an adult normal population. Osteoporos Int 1997;7:439–443.

58. Thomas MK, Lloyd-Jones DM, Thadhani RI, et al. Hypovitaminosis D in medical inpatients. N Engl J Med 1998;338:777–783.

59. Shea B, Wells G, Cranney A, et al; Osteoporosis Methodology Group and The Osteoporosis Research Advisory Group. Meta-analyses of therapies for postmenopausal osteoporosis. VII. Meta-analysis of calcium supplementation for the prevention of post menopausal osteoporosis. Endocr Rev 2002;23:552–529.

60. Chapuy MC, Arlot ME, Cuboeuf F, et al. Vitamin D3 and calcium to prevent hip fractures in the elderly women. N Engl J Med 1992;327:1637–1642.

61. Rizzoli R, Bonjour J-P. Dietary protein and bone health. J Bone Miner Res 2004;19:527–531.

62. Bonjour J-P, Rizzoli R. Bone Acquisition in adolescence. In: Marcus R, Feldman D, Kelsey J, eds. Osteoporosis. San Diego, CA: Academic Press, 1996,465–476.

63. Garn SM. The Earlier Gain and the Later Loss of Cortical Bone. Springfield, IL: C.C. Thomas, 1970.

64. Rubin CT, Lanyon LE. Regulation of bone formation by applied dynamic loads. J Bone Joint Surg 1984;66:397–402.

65. Rubin CT, Lanyon LE. Regulation of bone mass by mechanical strain magnitude. Calcif Tissue Int 1985;37:41–47.

66. Slemenda CW, Miller JZ, Hui SL, Reister TK, Johnston CC Jr. Role of physical activity in the development of skeletal mass in children. J Bone Miner Res 1991;6:1227–1233.

67. Bailey DA, Mirwald RL, Crocker PE, Faulkner RA. Physical activity and bone mineral acquisition during the adolescent growth spurt. Bone 1998;23:S171.

68. Recker RR, Davies KM, Hinders SM, Heaney RP, Stegman MR, Kimmel DB. Bone gain in young adult women. JAMA 1992;268:2403–2408.
69. Bass S, Pearce G, Bradney M, Hendrich E, Delmas PD, Harding A, Seeman E. Exercise before puberty may confer residual benefits in bone density in adulthood studies in active prepubertal and retired female gymnasts. J Bone Miner Res 1998;13:500–507.
70. Bass SL, Saxon L, Daly RM, et al. The effect of mechanical loading on the size and shape of bone in pre-, peri-, and post pubertal girls: A study in tennis players. J Bone Miner Res 2002;17:2274–2280.
71. Kannus P, Haapasalo H, Sankelo M, et al. Effect of starting age of physical activity on bone mass in the dominant arm of tennis and squash players. Ann Intern Med 1995;123:27–31.
72. Khan K, McKay HA, Haapasalo H, et al. Does childhood and adolescence provide a unique opportunity for exercise to strengthen the skeleton? J Sci Med Sport 2000;3:150–164.
73. MacKelvie KJ, Khan KM, McKay HA. Is there a critical period for bone response to weight-bearing exercise in children and adolescents? A systematic review. Br J Sports Med 2002;36:250–257.
74. Janz KF, Burns TL, Levy SM, et al. Everyday activity and bone geometry in children: The Iowa bone development study. Med Sci Sports Exerc 2004;36:1124–1131.
75. Specker B, Binkley T. Randomized trial of physical activity and calcium supplementation on bone mineral content in 3 to 5 year old children. J Bone Miner Res 2003;18:885–892.
76. Robinson, TL, Snow-Harter C, Jaffe DR, Gillis D, Shaw J, Marcus R. Gymnasts exhibit higher bone mass than runners despite similar prevalence of amenorrhea. J Bone Miner Res 1995:10:26–35.
77. Jaffe DR, Snow-Harter C, Conolly DA, Robinson TL, Marcus R. Differential effects of swimming versus weight-bearing activity on bone mineral status of eumenorrheic athletes. J Bone Miner Res 1995;10:586–593.
78. US Department of Health and Human Services. Physical Activity and Health: A Report of the Surgeon General. Atlanta, GA: DHHS, Centers for Disease Control NS Prevention, National Center for Chronic Disease Prevention and Health Promotion, 1996.
79. Cummings SR, Karpf DB, Harris F, et al. Improvement in spine bone density and reduction in risk of vertebral fractures during treatment with antiresorptive drugs. Am J Med 2002;112:281–289.
80. Wasnich RD, Miller PD. Anti-fracture efficacy of antiresorptive agents are related to changes in bone density. J Clin Endocrinol Metab 2000;85 231–236.
81. Watts NB, Cooper C, Lindsay R, et al. Relationship between changes in bone mineral density and vertebral fracture risk associated with risedronate: Greater increases in bone mineral density do not relate to greater decreases in fracture risk. J Clin Densitom 2004;7:255–261.
82. Leweicki EM, Miller PD, Leib ES, Bilezikian JP. Response to "the perspective of the international osteoporosis foundation on the official positions of the international society for clinical densitometry," by John A. Kanis et al. J Clin Densitom 2005;8(2):143–144.
83. Lieb E, Lewiecki EM, Binkley N, Hamdy RC. Official position of the International Society for Clinical Densitometry. J Clin Densitom 2004;7:1–5.
84. Kanis JA, Seeman E, Johnell O, Rizzoli R, Delmas P. The perspective of the International Osteoporosis Foundation on the Official Positions of the International Society for Clinical Densitometry. J Clin Densitom 2005;8:145–147.
85. Lloyd T, Rollings N, Andon MB, et al. Determinants of bone density in young women. I. Relationships among pubertal development, total body bone mass, and total body bone density in premenarchal females. J Clin Endocrinol Metab 1992;75:383–387.
86. Wren, TA, Liu X, Pitukcheewanont P, Gilsanz V. Bone acquisition in healthy children and adolescents: Comparisons of dual-energy x-ray absorptiometry and computed tomography measures. J Clin Endo Metab 2005;90(4):925–928.
87. Gafni RI, Baron J. Overdiagnosis of osteoporosis in children due to misinterpretation of dual-energy x-ray absorptiometry (DEXA). J Pediatr 2004;144(2):253–257.

2

Tools for Measuring Bone in Children and Adolescents

Kate A. Ward, PhD,
Zulf Mughal, MBChB, FRCP, FRCPCM, DCM
and Judith E. Adams, MBBS, FRCR, FRCP

CONTENTS

INTRODUCTION
WHAT ARE WE MEASURING WITH BONE DENSITOMETRY?
DUAL-ENERGY X-RAY ABSORPTIOMETRY
QUANTITATIVE COMPUTED TOMOGRAPHY
QUANTITATIVE ULTRASOUND
MAGNETIC RESONANCE IMAGING
RADIOGRAMMETRY
COMPARISON BETWEEN CENTRAL AND PERIPHERAL TECHNIQUES
SUMMARY
SUMMARY POINTS
REFERENCES

INTRODUCTION

This chapter provides an overview of the current densitometry techniques that are used in children. The strengths and limitations of each of the techniques are discussed. Dual-energy x-ray absorptiometry (DXA) is discussed only briefly, as the remainder of this book concentrates on this technique in detail. Table 1 provides a technical overview of costs, uses, precision, and radiation exposure associated with densitometry methods. Radiation doses associated with other imaging modalities and with natural background sources are provided for comparison in Table 2.

WHAT ARE WE MEASURING WITH BONE DENSITOMETRY?

Bone densitometry offers a tool with which pediatric bone status can be assessed. As the child grows, the skeleton will increase in size and mineral content and will change in shape. When interpreting measurements from bone densitometry scanners, it is imperative that these changes in bone size, shape, and mass are taken into account *(20,21)*. For

From: *Current Clinical Practice: Bone Densitometry in Growing Patients: Guidelines for Clinical Practice*
Edited by: A. J. Sawyer, L. K. Bachrach, and E. B. Fung © Humana Press Inc., Totowa, NJ

Table 1
A Technical Overview of Currently Available Bone Densitometry Techniques

Technique	Costs[a]	Sites	Clinical/research	Radiation dose (μSv)	Precision (CV %)
DXA	$72–180K	Lumbar spine	Both	0.4–4	<1
	£39–99K	Total body	Both	0.02–5	1–2
	€59–147K	Proximal femur	Both	0.15–5.4 (not inc. Lunar Expert)	0.15–5.4
AXIAL QCT	Scanner (Software)	Spine	Both	3-D 55	0.8–1.5[1]
	$630–900K ($18–22K)	Femur	Research	2-D 50–60	
	£345–493K (£10–12K)			3-D 10–20	<1[3]
	€516–736 (€15–18K)				
Peripheral QCT	$45–252K	Radius	Research	<1.5–4 per scan	0.8–1.5
	£25–138K	Tibia	Research	<1.5–4 per scan	3.6–7.8 for ages 3–5[4]
	€37–206K				1.3–1.8 for 12-year-olds[5]
					1.2–4[6]
QUS	$27–36K	Femur	Research	None	BUA 1.6–5[7,8]
	£15–20K	Calcaneus			
	€22–29K	Phalanges			SOS 0.5–1.2[9–12]
		Radius			
		Tibia			
MRI	Scanner (Software)	Tibia	Research	None	0.12–1.02[13]
	$1.8–2.7 million ($18–22K)	Humerus			0.55–3.63
	£1–1.5 million (£10–12K)	Femur			
	€1.5–2.2 million (€15–18K)				
Radiogrammetry	Software	Metacarpal	Research	0.17	<1[14]
	$18–22K				
	£10–12K				
	€15–18K				

[a]Calculated from US dollar ($) at conversion rate $1 USD = £0.55 GBP, ¤ 0.82 Euros. These figures are subject to currency fluctuations, and prices are approximations.

BUA, broadband ultrasonic attenuation; DXA, dual-energy x-ray absorptiometry; MRI, magnetic resonance imaging; QCT, quantitative computed tomography; QUS, quantitative ultrasound; SOS, speed of sound.

16

Table 2
An Overview of Radiation Exposures for Comparison With Bone Densitometry
Techniques

	Effective dose (μSv)
Return transatlantic flight[15]	80
Annual naturally occurring background radiation[16]	
North America	3000
United Kingdom	2000
Australia	1500
Hand radiograph[17]	0.17
Chest radiograph[18]	12–20
Planar lumbar spine radiograph[18]	700
Radioisotope bone scan[19]	4000

example, changes in bone density over time could reflect changes in bone size, mineral content, or a combination of these. The quantitative measures that can be obtained from most densitometry techniques include bone area (BA; cm^2), bone mineral content (BMC; g), and bone mineral density (BMD; g/cm^2).

A model based on the biological organization of bone was proposed by Rauch and Schonau *(22)* to help in understanding and interpreting the measurements obtained from bone densitometry and to relate these changes to the physiological changes that occur during bone development (*see* Fig. 1). The model describes separate definitions for the material, compartment, and total densities of bone, and each of these will be discussed briefly:

1. *Material mineral density.* This reflects the degree of mineralization of the organic bone matrix. Material density can be determined only within a very small volume occupied only by bone matrix, exclusive of marrow spaces, osteonal canals, lacunae, and canaliculi. The resolution required to measure $BMD_{material}$ is not possible with current noninvasive densitometric techniques; $BMD_{material}$ can be determined from specimens taken at bone biopsy, an invasive procedure. These specimens can be analyzed by mineral/ash weight, contact radiography, backscatter electron microscopy, or laser-ablated mass spectrometry. Measurement of $BMD_{material}$ is not routinely assessed in clinical practice.

2. *Compartment mineral density.* The $BMD_{compartment}$ is the amount of mineral contained within the trabecular or cortical compartments (i.e., the mass of mineral per unit volume of trabecular or cortical bone). Quantitative computed tomography (QCT) measures cortical and trabecular bone separately, and can therefore measure $BMD_{compartment}$ in both types of bone. DXA measurements are a composite of trabecular and cortical bone, and so the technique is not able to separate the two components at most sites. $BMD_{compartment}$ can be determined by DXA in skeletal sites such as the diaphyses of the femur and the radius, both of which are comprised of cortical bone. Radiogrammetry measures the cortical $BMD_{compartment}$ of the metacarpals.

3. *Total mineral density.* BMD_{total} is the mineral density of all of the material contained within the periosteal envelope and articular surfaces. QCT and DXA measure BMD_{total}. Calculations are required to estimate bone volume from DXA scans because this technique measures areal density only. Bone mineral apparent density (BMAD) is an example

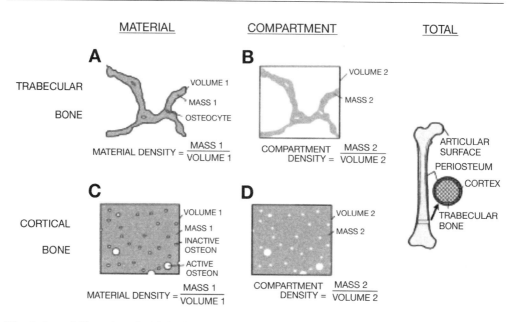

Fig. 1. A model based on the biological organization of bone proposed by Rauch and Schonau*(22)* to help in understanding and interpreting the measurements obtained from bone densitometry and to relate these changes to the physiological changes that occur during bone development. The model describes separate definitions for the material, compartment, and total densities of bone.

of a volumetric density calculated using BMD_{total}. This density is sometimes inappropriately referred to in the literature as "true bone density."

Table 3 summarizes which of the aforementioned BMD measurements can be determined using the densitometry techniques discussed in this chapter; quantitative ultrasound (QUS) and magnetic resonance imaging (MRI) do not measure BMD.

DUAL-ENERGY X-RAY ABSORPTIOMETRY

DXA has been available since the late 1980s and now is used extensively for diagnosis and monitoring of osteoporosis *(23–25)*. The fundamental principle of DXA is the measurement of the transmission of x-rays through the body at high and low energies. The use of two energies allows discrimination between soft tissue and bone; low-energy photons are attenuated by soft tissue, and the high-energy photons by bone and soft tissue.

By subtracting the soft tissue from soft tissue and bone, it is possible to quantify the amount of bone within the x-ray scan path. Pixel-by-pixel attenuation values are converted to areal BMD (aBMD; g/cm^2) by comparison with a bone mineral phantom. In most clinical and research reports, aBMD is designated simply as BMD. Bone area is calculated by summing the pixels within the bone edges, as defined by software algorithms. BMC is calculated by multiplying mean aBMD by BA. DXA may be applied to the whole body or to the skeletal regions of interest, for example, the spine, the proximal femur, and the radius.

DXA is the most widely available bone densitometry technique for measurement of bone status in children *(26)*. The advantages and limitations of the technique are discussed more extensively in subsequent chapters. Briefly, the advantages of DXA include

Table 3
A Summary of What Each Technique[a] Measures in Relation to the Bones' Biological
Organization (22)

| Method | BMD$_{material}$ | BMD$_{compartment}$ | | BMD$_{total}$ |
		Cortical	Trabecular	
DXA	No	Yes	No	Yes
QCT	No	Yes	Yes	Yes
Radiogrammetry	No	Yes	No	No

[a]Magnetic resonance imaging and quantitative ultrasound do not measure bone mineral density; they provide measurement of parameters related to the structure of the bone but not bone mineral density by definition.

DXA, dual-energy x-ray absorptiometry; QCT, quantitative computed tomography.

rapid scan times, a low ionizing radiation dose, and the availability of pediatric reference data. Also, the cost of running a DXA service is relatively inexpensive. DXA can be used to assess body composition and is currently the only technique that can be applied to the hip region in children.

Although DXA has many advantages, the limitations of the method must be considered. BMD measurements provided by DXA are size-dependent because they are based on two-dimensional (2D) projections of three-dimensional (3D) structures that do not adjust for the depth of the bone. As a consequence, even if volumetric bone density is identical in two children, aBMD will be less in the smaller child and greater in the larger one. Growth between scans should be taken into account when interpreting longitudinal data. There are several methods to correct DXA data for size dependence (27–34) , as discussed further in Chapter 3. DXA measurements are also influenced by changes in body composition, and due consideration must be given to such changes when interpreting data. Overall, DXA remains the primary bone densitometry tool for clinical pediatric bone assessments and an important research tool.

QUANTITATIVE COMPUTED TOMOGRAPHY

Axial Quantitative Computed Tomography

Axial QCT of the spine was first described in the late 1970s (35) and became more widely used during the 1980s (36). With the introduction of DXA in 1988, the use of QCT declined. However, there has been renewed interest in QCT as investigators recognize the importance of bone size and geometry in assessing pediatric bone status. QCT is particularly useful in children because it measures volumetric density (g/cm^3), which is not size-dependent. Recent technical developments (such as spiral and spiral multislice computed tomography [CT]) add to the potential information available from QCT. Use of QCT for clinical and research purposes will probably increase in the future (37,38).

QCT of the spine requires that the patient lie supine on the scanner table with legs flexed and supported on a pad to flatten out the natural lumbar lordosis (Fig. 2A). The height of the scanner table should be kept constant. A bone mineral-equivalent phantom is placed under the patient in the site to be scanned. A water or soft-tissue-equivalent pad should be placed between the patient and the phantom if there is a significant air gap (Fig. 2B).

The original phantoms were filled with variable-concentration fluid dipotassium hydrogen phosphate (K_2HPO_4), which enabled the bone region of interest, measured in Hounsfield units (HU), to be transformed into bone mineral equivalents in mg/cm^3. The reliability of fluid phantoms declined with time as a result of transpiration of fluid through the Plexiglas material, allowing development of air bubbles in the phantom and causing alterations in K_2HPO_4 concentration. Therefore, solid hydroxyapatite phantoms are now favored.

Some CT manufacturers provide their own software and phantoms (e.g., Siemens AG, Munich, Germany); alternatively, software and phantoms can be purchased separately (e.g., from Mindways Software Inc., Austin, TX). For comparable results in longitudinal studies, the same phantom (and scanner) should be used. Similarly to DXA instrumentation *(39,40)*, if scanners or phantoms must be changed during longitudinal studies, then cross-calibration with patients and a phantom, such as the European Spine Phantom (ESP) *(41)*, must be performed to make results comparable.

For 2D spine measurements, an initial lateral scan projection radiograph is obtained (Fig. 2C). A 10-mm section is then performed through the midplane of the vertebrae to be measured and parallel to the vertebral endplates. The section is confirmed to be in the correct plane when the area of the basivertebral vein is identified. For 2D QCT in adults, generally, four vertebrae are scanned (T12–L3 or L1–L4) to ensure that at least two to three vertebrae are available for analysis at follow-up scans, should it be necessary to exclude vertebrae that have fractured between measurements. Because vertebral fractures occur less commonly in children, and because the ionizing radiation dose should be minimized, generally, only two adjacent vertebrae (between L1 and L3) are scanned. Vertebrae should be matched to those scanned in the reference database used because BMD differs among vertebrae. If longitudinal studies are performed, it is essential to scan the identical vertebrae examined at baseline.

QCT results are expressed as a mean volumetric BMD (vBMD; mg/cm^3). The trabecular vBMD, measured by QCT, is a composite of the amount of bone and marrow per voxel. The measurement is composite because of the relatively small size of trabeculae compared to the voxel, resulting in marrow being included in the measurement. Because marrow fat is limited in children, age-related marrow changes in fat composition should not confound spinal vBMD measurements in children as significantly as they do in adults *(42)*.

The original body CT scanners used rotate-translate technology and permitted only 2D slices to be obtained; the procedure took about 15 min. Over the past decade, there have been steady technical developments in CT with the introduction of continuous spiral rotation of the x-ray tube and multiple rows of detectors *(43)*. Such developments have permitted very rapid (i.e., less than a minute) 3D volume scanning. With this type of scanning, L1–L3 are scanned, and the 2D section used for analysis can be selected from this 3D volume of tissue. These developments improve precision (with coefficients of variation of less than 1%) and have advantages in children in that they reduce movement

---

Fig. 2. *(opposite page)* **(A)** Standard position for quantitative computed tomography of the spine; **(B)** The Mindways Spine Phantom positioned under a patient with a gel bag to eliminate air gaps between patient and phantom; **(C)** A lateral scan projection radiograph to locate the centers of the vertebral bodies, where volumetric trabecular density will be measured.

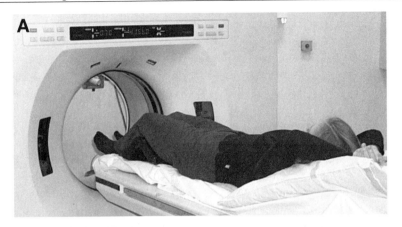

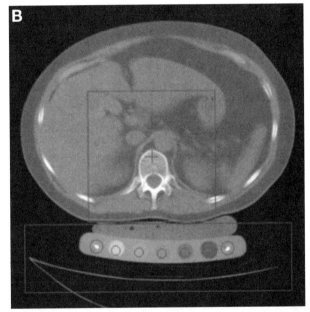

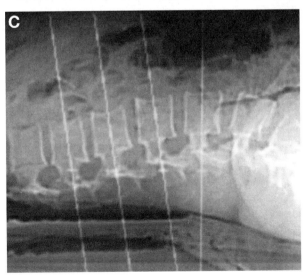

artifacts. As quantitative skeletal assessment does not require the optimization of image quality needed for conventional CT, a low-dose technique can be employed to minimize the radiation dose *(44,45)* (Table 1). The results are expressed as standard deviations (SDs) from the mean for appropriate age-, race-, and sex-matched reference data (i.e., a Z-score). The most frequently used normative data for spinal QCT are those reported by Gilsanz and colleagues *(1,46,47)* (Table 4).

QCT offers several advantages as a densitometric technique. Whereas DXA measures integral (i.e., cortical and trabecular) bone density, QCT provides separate measures of cortical and trabecular BMD. As trabecular bone is generally more metabolically active than cortical bone, trabecular vBMD as measured by QCT is more sensitive to change in BMD *(65)*. The BMD provided is volumetric and not influenced by bone size, in contrast to DXA, which provides an areal density. QCT also provides true morphometric dimensions of bones and, in the shafts, can measure cross-sectional area of bone, cortical thickness and density, and periosteal and endosteal circumference. These parameters can be used to calculate estimates of biomechanical bone strength including the stress-strain index (SSI) and the moment of inertia. QCT also has the potential to be applied to peripheral skeletal sites, such as the radius, the tibia, and the mid-femur, with lower associated radiation exposure than spinal QCT *(66)*.

The limitations of QCT include an approximately 10- to12-fold greater dose of ionizing radiation than DXA for spine scans. Access to QCT may be problematic because many radiology departments lack the appropriate phantoms and software to perform bone studies. Furthermore, CT equipment is often in great demand for other diagnostic purposes. Currently, there are very few commercial analysis packages for QCT that require little setup (Mindways Software Inc. produces one such package). Therefore, some centers have resorted to developing their own analysis software *(67)*. As with other bone densitometry techniques, QCT requires skilled and dedicated technical staff to perform the scans to optimize precision. Finally, there are fewer published pediatric reference data for QCT than for DXA; the most widely used norms were derived from a cohort of only 101 children *(46)*.

Peripheral Quantitative Computed Tomography

Peripheral QCT (pQCT) first became commercially available in the early 1990s *(68–70)*. The most commonly used pQCT scanner (the XCT 2000, Stratec, Pforzheim, Germany) utilizes the original rotate-translate technology, which generates only single 2D slices (1–2 mm thick) and requires about 1 min to obtain a single slice. The first high-resolution spiral pQCT machine has recently been released (by SCANCO Medical AG, Basserdorf, Switzerland) and can measure a block of tissue of 10 mm in depth. However, its application in pediatric clinical and research studies has not yet been determined.

The sites of measurement are the radius, the tibia, and the femur. For clinical assessment of a child's bone, the most commonly used site is the distal 4% of the forearm or tibia length proximal to the distal growth plate. In children, it is important to avoid the section including the growth plate, which produces falsely high measures as a result of the zone of provisional calcification.

To locate the appropriate scan slice, a scanogram is performed. For the forearm, the reference line is placed bisecting the medial border of the radius (Fig 3Ai); the scanner automatically moves 4% of the forearm length from this reference location and performs the scan in the prescribed site. For the tibia, the reference line location varies but is usually

Table 4
An Overview of Reference Data Currently Available With Machines

Technique	Reference data	Source	n	Age range (years)
DXA	Spine	• Hologic[48,49a,50 b]	218c, 666, 1444	1–19, 8–17, 3–20
		GE Lunar[30,51–55] and unpublished manufacturer data	>1100	3 mo to 19
	Proximal femur	• Norland[56,57]	778	2–20
		Hologic[49a,50b]	892, 1047	8–17, 5–20
		GE Lunar[30,51–57] and unpublished manufacturer data	>1100	4–27
	Total body	• Norland[56,57]	778	2–20
		Hologic[49,50]	977, 1948	8–17, 3–20
		GE Lunar[30,51–55] and unpublished manufacturer data	>1100	4–27
		• Norland Argentina[56,57]	778	2–20
QCT	Spine	• GE CT 9800[46]	101	2–19
	Radius	• Stratec XCT-2000[58]	371	5–18
	Tibia	• Stratec NIH, to be published	N/A	N/A
QUS	Calcaneus	• McCue CUBA	367	6–17
		• GE Lunar Achilles[9,56,60]	311	6–20
		• UBIS	491	6–21
	Phalanges	• IGEA[61,62]	1328, 1083	3–17,3–21
	Radius, tibia	• Sunlight[63]	1095	0–18
Radiogrammetry	Metacarpals	• Sectra-Pronosco X-Posure—Not currently available	N/A	N/A

Note: Databases listed above are those currently provided by the manufacturer; there are many other databases derived from research groups for their own ethnic- and population-specific purposes. In certain cases, use of these may be appropriate, but caution should be taken regarding the machine type and origin of data; in longitudinal studies, the same database should always be used.

[a]Provided only with approval by Institutional Review Boards in the United States.

[b]Version 12.1 onwards.

[c]These data are not gender specific.

[d]Cross calibration performed (64), reference data provided with Mindways; software for Philips SR4000 and newer generation CT scanners.

DXA, dual-energy x-ray absorptiometry; QCT, quantitative computed tomography; QUS, quantitative ultrasound.

A

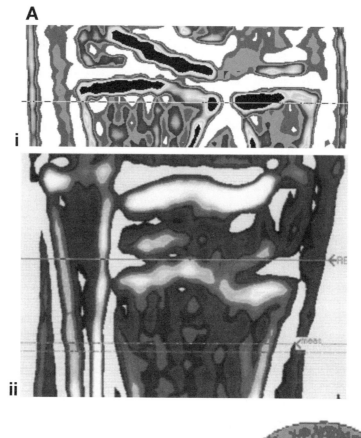

i

ii

B

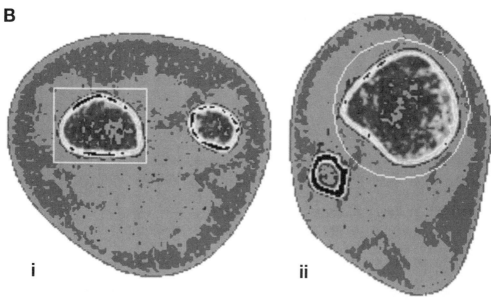

i   ii

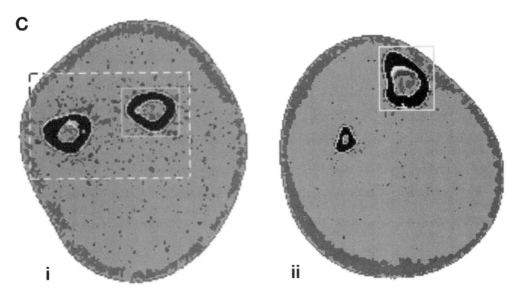

Fig. 3. Peripheral quantitative computed tomography. The scan site is located by a scanogram of **(Ai)** the distal radius and ulna and **(Aii)** the distal tibia and fibula. Total, cortical and subcortical, and trabecular volumetric bone mineral densities and areas are measured at the distal site; examples of scans of **(Bi)** the distal radius and ulna and **(Bii)** the distal tibia and fibula are given. Bone geometry, density, strength, and muscle area are measured at diaphyseal sites using peripheral quantitative computed tomography. Examples of scans at **(Ci)** 50% radius and **(Cii)** 65% tibia are shown. Cortical bone is in black, the pale gray is muscle, and the dark gray is intramuscular and subcutaneous fat.

placed on the metaphysis; again, the scanner moves to the measurement site from this point (Fig. 3Aii). Upon closure of the growth plate at skeletal maturity, the distal surface of the epiphysis is used for placement of the reference line. Radial abnormalities such as Madelung's deformity (i.e., dorsolateral distortion of the lower end of the radius) may cause difficulties in positioning the reference line. In children treated with bisphosphonates, the reference line must be positioned to ensure that the growth arrest lines (residual of the provisional zone of calcification) are avoided in the measurement.

The low radiation dose of pQCT allows multiple site measurements to be made. Often, research protocols include sections taken at 4, 14, 20, 38, and 66% of the leg length and, in the forearm sections, at 4, 50, and 65% of the forearm length. Multiple site measurements allow site-specific changes in bone and soft tissue to be studied. The scan time can take between 2 and 3 min per slice; typically, a single slice is obtained at each site. Therefore, the technique is more successful in older children who are able to remain still during the relatively long scan procedure.

pQCT offers the benefits of axial QCT. vBMD is measured, and, because it is not size-dependent, it will not be influenced by the growth of a child. pQCT is able to separate trabecular from cortical bone. Both trabecular and cortical vBMD remain consistent with age when measured by pQCT *(58,71)*. As the technique is only applicable to the peripheral skeleton, these measurements are obtained at much lower cost and radiation exposure (Table 1) than axial QCT. pQCT also allows assessments of bone geometry, parameters related to bone strength, and muscle cross-sectional areas (a surrogate for muscle strength).

In order to measure these parameters, the sites of measurement by pQCT are optimized. The 4% site at the distal end of the radius (Fig. 3Bi) or tibia (Fig 3Bii) assesses total and trabecular vBMD. In the mid-diaphyseal portion of the bone, measurements are made of cortical vBMD, BA, cortical thickness, periosteal circumference, endosteal circumference, and muscle cross-sectional area (Fig. 3Ci,ii). Parameters related to bone strength are also measured at the mid-diaphyseal site; these include the axial moment of inertia (AMI) and the SSI. The AMI is the distribution of bone material around the center of the bone, and the SSI is a combination of the AMI and the vBMD of the cortex; both parameters relate well to the fracture load *(72,73)*. The study of the adaptation of bone to loading from muscle is possible using pQCT. By calculating the ratio of bone to muscle, it is possible to investigate whether the bones have adequately adapted to the mechanical stresses to which they are exposed *(74)*. Inadequate development of bone strength can contribute to bone fragility.

Clinical Research Applications of pQCT

pQCT has been used in pediatric research to assess bone development in healthy children *(4,22,58,75–77)* and those at risk for poor bone health *(78–84)* The technique has also been used to study the effects of exercise and calcium on bone mass and geometry *(85–87)* At present, pQCT is used primarily for research, rather than for clinical studies, for several reasons. There have been challenges in achieving adequate precision, controversies related to the optimum site of scanning of bone for pediatric studies, and a paucity of pediatric reference data. However, a model for the use of pQCT in the assessment of clinical conditions has been proposed *(74)* and could also be applicable to DXA measurements of lean mass and BA or BMC.

QUANTITATIVE ULTRASOUND

The first QUS scanner was developed in 1984 *(88)* for the assessment of calcaneal bone status in adults. The measurements obtained from QUS are based on the attenuation of the ultrasound beam as it passes through the specified region of interest. Most commonly, the broadband ultrasound attenuation (BUA; dB/MHz), the speed of sound (SOS; m/s), or the velocity of sound (VOS; m/s) are measured. These measurements are related to both BMD and parameters of bone quality and strength.

The majority of ultrasound scanners developed to date have been designed to transmit the ultrasound wave through the bone, with a receiver measuring the attenuated wave at the other side (Fig. 4Ai,ii). However, more recently, a technique called ultrasound critical-angle reflectometry, which uses only a single probe, has been developed (Fig. 4B). The ultrasonic wave travels along the cortical bone, and the reflected wave is measured to give a value for SOS.

Ultrasound may be applied to measure only the peripheral skeleton at sites such as the calcaneus, the radius, the phalanges, the patella, and the tibia. Axial sites cannot be measured by QUS because of the large amount of soft tissue and muscle that surround

---

Fig. 4. *(opposite page)* Examples of quantitative ultrasound scanners: **Ai, Aii,** fixed calcaneal ultrasound scanners; **B**, critical angle reflectometry method being used with a neonate; **Ci,** imaging calcaneal ultrasound device; and **Cii**, image.

A

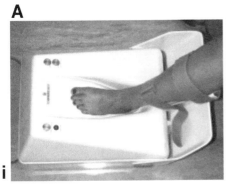

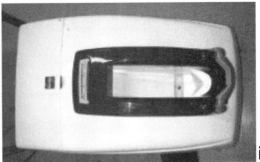

i ii

B

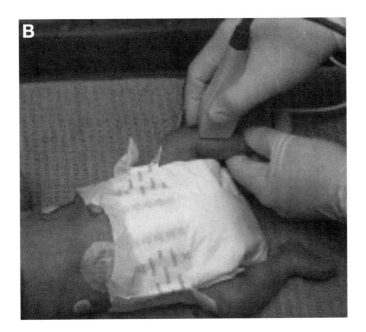

C

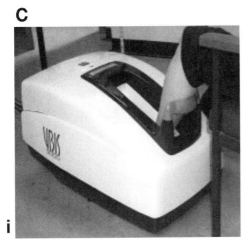

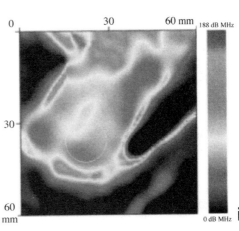

i ii

these sites and impede the ultrasound wave signal. The most commonly measured site is the calcaneus because it is rich in metabolically active trabecular bone, has little surrounding soft tissue, and reflects the effects of weight bearing on the skeleton (9,59,60,89). Ultrasound has been applied in children and neonates, measuring the properties of the cortical bone in the tibia, the radius, and the phalanges (63,90–92).

QUS does not involve ionizing radiation, an obvious advantage in the assessment of bone status in children. The equipment is relatively small and portable and less costly to operate than other bone densitometry methods. Like DXA, QUS has proven useful in predicting osteoporotic fracture in adults. Several studies have shown that QUS parameters predict fractures of the hip, wrist, or other sites in women (93–96) and men (93). Its ability to predict fracture in children has yet to be established (97).

The application of calcaneal ultrasound in children has been problematic for several reasons. Many of the calcaneal ultrasound scanners have fixed transducers and molded foot wells that are designed to fit an adult foot. When used to scan the smaller feet of children, these devices may not allow proper alignment of transducers for capturing the appropriate region of the heel.

Newer machines have addressed this problem by providing shims to reposition small feet in the heel well or portable transducers that can be applied directly to the heel. Other ultrasound devices overcome the problem of selecting the appropriate region of interest by allowing imaging, alteration, and movement of the size of the region of interest (Fig. 3Ci,ii). The newer devices are more suitable for measurement in pediatrics and measure the phalanges, the radius, and the tibia.

To date, the clinical utility of ultrasound in children has not been adequately assessed. However, it has been used in varying clinical research populations to detect differences between bone status in children with disease and that in normal children (7,90,91). At present, QUS should be used as a tool to complement other bone densitometry techniques.

MAGNETIC RESONANCE IMAGING

MRI is the most recently developed technique for skeletal assessment in children. Quantification of an MRI scan is based on the resonance and relaxation of protons in lipids and water; different tissues will have varying quantities of water and lipids, thus allowing imaging and differentiation of various anatomical structures. In bone, the marrow provides the signal with little contribution from bone; therefore, the image formed shows marrow as white and bone as black (Fig. 5A,B). In MRI, varying sequences can be used, but in all (T1- or T2-weighted) scans, bone has a low or absent signal and muscle has an intermediate one. In validation studies, bone quantification using MRI has been shown to correlate well to ash weight and 3D QCT scans (98).

Fig. 5. *(opposite page)* **(A)** A sagittal magnetic resonance image (195×195×500 μm) for assessment of calcaneal trabecular bone structure in a 7-yr-old boy; **(B)** trabecular structure of the distal radius acquired on a 3T scanner using the Mayo wrist coil; Multiplanar capabilities of MRI shown by **(Ci)** coronal and **(Cii)** axial images of the shoulder. Images can also be taken in the sagittal plane. Bone has no signal (black), muscle has an intermediate signal (dark gray), and fat, a high signal (white). Images are normally taken in the midshaft of the long bones for bone geometry analysis. A&B Image courtesy of Sharmila Majumdar, PhD and Thomas Link, MD, University of California San Francisco, San Francisco, CA.

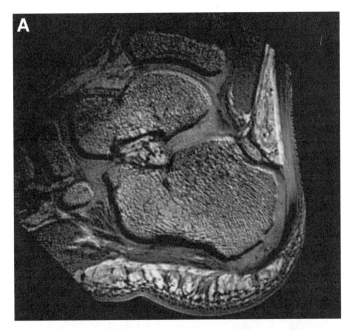

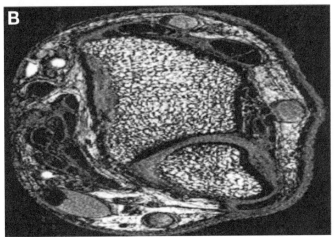

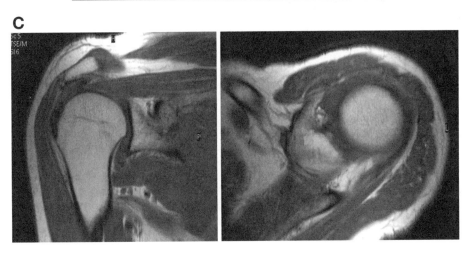

MRI offers several potential advantages. The technique provides a volumetric measure of bone without using ionizing radiation. Imaging in multiple anatomical planes is possible without having to reposition the subject (Fig. 5Ci,ii). Simultaneous scanning of several limbs is also feasible. Similarly to QCT, MRI distinguishes trabecular from cortical bone compartments and provides measures of bone morphometry, from which parameters of bone strength can be calculated. By scanning whole bones, MRI offers the possibility to study comprehensively the differential growth patterns of the bones *(99,100)*. The technique is applicable to both the axial *(101)* and appendicular skeleton *(13,99–103)*. There are a few limitations of MRI. The equipment is noisy for the subject, and scanning can take as long as 20–30 min with positioning and a scout scan, depending on the imaging sequence used. Lying in the long, horizontal gantry of the scanner can be distressing to claustrophobic individuals (1–2% of subjects). Keeping children still without sedation may be a problem. However, in several published research studies, sedation was not used and the children tolerated the scan process well (100,103,104). The environment of the scanner room is not as child-friendly as that for other densitometry techniques, and parents cannot remain with the child during scanning. Accurate in vivo measurement of trabecular bone structure (trabecular thickness is 0.05–0.2 mm) is technically challenging and is still being developed *(105–112)*. The optimization of sequence, field strength, and receiver coils is imperative for the quality of imaging required. To date, MRI has been used only in research protocols; its applicability in clinical practice has yet to be assessed.

RADIOGRAMMETRY

Radiogrammetry has been used for more than 40 yr to assess skeletal status from hand radiographs using various measures of the metacarpal cortex *(113–115)*. The method is commonly applied to the midpoint of the second metacarpal or to the middle three metacarpals of the nondominant hand. Measurements of the total width of a bone and its medullary width can be used to calculate various indices of bone status such as metacarpal cortical thickness and index. Measurements by radiogrammetry are most sensitive to cortical bone changes (i.e., periosteal apposition and endosteal resorption) and provide information on changes in bone during growth and aging *(116,117)*.

Despite the wide availability and relatively low costs of radiogrammetry, the poor precision of this method has limited its use as a clinical or research tool *(118)*. Measurements of cortical thickness gave intra- and interobserver errors of up to 8–10% and 8–11%, respectively *(118)*. Precision improved during the 1970s with the use of more accurate measurement tools *(119,120)*. Some investigators have found hand radiogrammetry to be problematic in younger children in whom epiphyseal fusion is less advanced, whereas others have successfully applied the technique in those over age 5.

The potential value of radiogrammetry for assessing bone status is being considered with the progression of computer-aided analysis in diagnostic medical imaging, for example, using active shape or appearance modeling *(121,122)*. Radiogrammetry may also be valuable in facilities in which axial DXA may be limited.

Digital (or computed) x-ray radiogrammetry (DXR) uses computer image processing to reduce the errors that previously limited radiogrammetry by automating the location and placement of regions of interest for analysis of metacarpals on hand radiographs (Fig. 6). Inter- and intra-operator errors were considerably reduced to approximately 1%

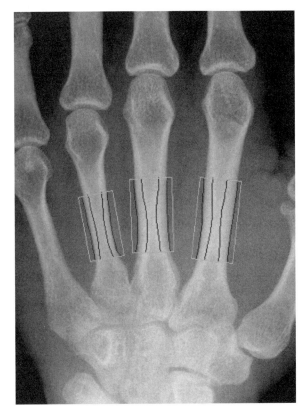

Fig. 6. Digital x-ray radiogrammetry of the hand. The figure shows a hand radiograph with regions of interest positioned, from which metacarpal index, bone width, bone mineral density, and cortical thickness can be calculated.

when compared to with manual analysis *(123)*. Using a digitizer further improved the method's sensitivity *(124)*. The active shape models used for the SECTRA X-posure system were based on adult hand radiographs and therefore may present problems when used with younger children. However, DXR has been used to investigate differences among patient groups and healthy children and also to study bone development in healthy children *(125–127)*. The applicability of DXR is currently as a research tool.

COMPARISON BETWEEN CENTRAL AND PERIPHERAL TECHNIQUES

In adults, measurements of bone mass at both axial and peripheral sites have proven to predict future osteoporotic fracture *(128)*. In older adults, osteoporosis is defined in terms of bone densitometry as a T-score (i.e., the SD from the mean of ethnic- and sex-matched peak BMD) of –2.5 or below using axial DXA in the lumbar spine and proximal femur. The agreement in classification by the various densitometric techniques has been studied in adults *(129–131)*, and each performs well in differentiating osteoporosis or osteopenia from normal bone status. However, each technique identifies different people as osteoporotic or osteopenic; hence, the diagnostic agreement among the methods is poor (i.e., a κ* score of 0.4). As an exception to the rule, several studies have shown that the agreement between trabecular vBMD (measured by QCT) and lateral DXA BMD has a κ score of 0.75 *(131)*. The reasons for poor agreement among different bone density methods and at different sites are likely to include differences in the ability of the technique to measure integral or separate cortical and trabecular bone *(132,133)*, differing patterns of regional bone loss (e.g., in the spine versus the radius), and differential disease-specific effects on bone. Differences in scanner technology will also be relevant in contributing to the poor agreement among methods. Whether BMD is measured in adults or in children, the agreement among different techniques is likely to be of similar magnitude (*r* between 0.4 and 0.9).

Because there may be regional differences in bone mass and strength, selection of skeletal site to scan is important. For example, in children with juvenile idiopathic arthritis, who are most likely to suffer a vertebral crush fracture *(134,135)*, measurement of spinal trabecular bone should be a priority. Any measurement that does not include the spine is less likely to be sensitive to the bone changes that occur. Diagnostic agreement between axial and peripheral skeletal sites may also differ depending on the child's phase of skeletal development. A large change in DXA spinal BMD with no change in radius trabecular BMD may be caused by the increase in bone size due to the pubertal growth spurt rather than being due to the change in volumetric bone mineral density. The relationship between the peripheral and axial bone densitometry techniques and fractures has not been studied in children.

Several studies have been performed that investigate the ability of peripheral measurement to predict osteoporotic fracture in adults *(128,136,137)*. Site-specific measurements have proven to be the best predictors of fractures at that site; for example, hip BMD will predict hip fracture better than radial or spinal BMD measurements. However, BMD measurements by peripheral techniques do predict spine and hip fracture in adults, thus providing useful information if an axial BMD measurement is not available.

The forearm is the most common site of fracture in children. Goulding et al. *(138)* have shown that children who have had fractures generally have lower BMD in the whole skeleton. Some studies have confirmed an association between low BMD and all upper limb fractures *(139)*, whereas others have observed reductions in hip and spine but not whole-body bone measurements in children who have fractured *(140,141)*. In the only prospective study of childhood fracture to date, low BMD, as measured by axial DXA, was predictive of the likelihood of a child to refracture within 4 yr of the initial fracture date *(142)*. The correlation between BMD and childhood fractures has been reviewed *(143)*. In young people, lower bone density at the spine or whole body has been linked to fractures only at the forearm but not at other skeletal sites. These findings suggest that low BMD may be a contributing factor to childhood fracture, just as it is in adults. However, there are insufficient data to establish a "fracture threshold" in children and young adults. Furthermore, comparisons among different scanning techniques for childhood fractures have not yet been made.

---

* A κ score is a measurement of agreement between two methods when the measurements are measured on the same categorical (i.e., 0 or 1) scale. For example, category 1 is Z-score < −2 (osteopenia) and category 0 is Z-score > −2 (normal). Degree of agreement ranges from 0 to 1, with 1 being excellent, 0.8 good, and so forth.

Table 5
A Summary of the Main Advantages and Limitations of Each of the Bone Measurement Techniques in Children, as Discussed in This Chapter

Technique	Advantages	Limitations
DXA	1. Rapid scan times 2. Relatively low cost 3. High precision 4. Availability of pediatric reference data 5. Low ionizing radiation dose 6. Clinical applications have been established 7. Can assess body composition 8. Can be used to assess hip region	1. Size-dependent measurements 2. Sensitive to body composition changes 3. Software and reference data changes 4. Integral measurement of trabecular and cortical bone
Axial QCT	1. Size-independent 2. Separate measure of cortical and trabecular bone 3. Measures bone geometry 4. Imaging of trabecular bone structure feasible 5. Measures muscle and fat 6. Applicable to central and peripheral sites	1. Relatively high-ionizing radiation dose 2. Relatively high cost 3. Access to equipment can be problematic 4. Operation requires skilled staff 5. Specialist acquisition and analysis software limited 6. Limited pediatric reference data
Peripheral QCT	1. Same advantages as 1–5 for axial QCT 2. Low radiation dose 3. Lower cost than axial QCT	1. Long scan time 2. Only applicable to peripheral sites
QUS	1. Nonionizing, noninvasive 2. Portable equipment for community use 3. Applicable in neonates 4. Low costs	1. Relatively low precision 2. Scanners are not designed for children 3. Only applicable to peripheral sites 4. Sensitive to scan environment
MRI	1. Nonionizing, noninvasive 2. Size-independent 3. Can image in multiple planes without moving the patient 4. Applicable to axial and peripheral sites 5. Measures muscle and fat	1. Noisy 2. Long scan time 3. Claustrophobia in some individuals 4. Parents cannot be in room with children
Digital radiogrammetry	1. Retrospective analysis 2. Low radiation dose 3. Speed 4. Centralized analysis 5. Low costs 6. Widely available	1. Applicable to hand radiographs only 2. Cortical measurements only

DXA, dual-energy x-ray absorptiometry; QCT, quantitative computed tomography; QUS, quantitative ultrasound; MRI, magnetic resonance imaging.

33

SUMMARY

DXA is currently the most widely available and acceptable clinical tool for the assessment of bone status in children. With appropriate use and consideration of its limitations, DXA provides valuable information of the bone status of an individual. The following chapters provide details regarding the acquisition, interpretation, and reporting of DXA in children to provide the best possible clinical service. The other densitometry techniques discussed in this chapter remain predominantly research tools. However, their use in clinical practice is likely to increase in the future as a means of assessing bone geometry and the site-specific effects of diseases. It should be remembered that all bone densitometry techniques were designed for use in adults; the application and interpretation of all of the methods described in this chapter are much more difficult in children and adolescents.

SUMMARY POINTS

- X-rays have been used in many different imaging modalities, from simple radiographic images to highly sophisticated spiral computer tomography, which can provide 2D cross-sectional and 3D volume images of the body and its organs.
- The absorption of x-irradiation by tissues is determined by the energy (or wavelength) of the radiation and the composition (i.e., electron density and atomic number) of the tissue through which it passes.
- Table 5 summarizes the advantages and limitations of the techniques discussed in this chapter.
- DXA is currently the most accepted bone densitometry technique for clinical application in children. Other densitometry techniques discussed in this chapter remain predominantly research tools.

REFERENCES

1. Gilsanz V, Boechat MI, Roe TF, Loro ML, Sayre JW, Goodman WG. Gender differences in vertebral body sizes in children and adolescents. Radiology 1994;190:673–677.
2. Hangartner T, Gilsanz V. Evaluation of cortical bone by computed tomography. J Bone Miner Res 1996;11:1518–1525.
3. Kovanlikaya A, Loro ML, Hangartner TN, Reynolds RA, Roe TF, Gilsanz V. Osteopenia in children: CT assessment. Radiology 1996;198:781–784.
4. Binkley T, Specker B. pQCT measurement of bone parameters in young children—Validation of technique. J Clin Densitom 2000;3:9–14.
5. Moyer-Mileur L, Xie B, Pratt T. Peripheral quantitative computed tomography (pQCT) assessment of tibial bone mass change in preadolescent girls. Federation of American Societies for Experimental Biology 2000: 14 (4):A265. Abstract No. 183.4..
6. Sievanen H, Koskue V, Rauhio A, Kannus P, Heinonen A, Vuori I. Peripheral quantitative computed tomography in human long bones: evaluation of in vitro and in vivo precision. J Bone Miner Res 1998;13:871–882.
7. Mughal M, Langton C, Utretch G, Morrison J, Specker B. Comparison between broad-band ultrasound attenuation of the calcaneum and total body bone mineral density in children. Acta Paediatrica 1996;85:1–3.
8. Wilmshurst S, Ward K, Adams J, Langton C, Mughal M. Mobility status and bone density in cerebral palsy. Arch Dis Child 1996;75:164–165.
9. Schonau E. The determination of ultrasound velocity in the os calcis, thumb and patella during childhood. Eur J Pediatr 1994;153:252–256.
10. Lappe JM, Recker RR, Malleck MK, Stegman MR, Packard PP, Heaney RP. Patellar ultrasound transmission velocity in healthy children and adolescents. Bone 1995;16:251S–256S.
11. Jaworski M, Lebiedowski M, Lorenc RS, Trempe J. Ultrasound bone measurement in pediatric subjects. Calcif Tissue Int 1995;56:368–371.

12. Halaba Z, Pluskiewicz W. The assessment of development of bone mass in children by quantitative ultrasound through the proximal phalanxes of the hand. Ultrasound Med Biol 1997;23:1331–1335.

13. Bass SL, Saxon L, Daly RM, Turner CH, Robling AG, Seeman E, Stuckey S. The effect of mechanical loading on the size and shape of bone in pre-, peri-, and postpubertal girls: a study in tennis players. J Bone Miner Res 2002;17:2274–2280.

14. Ward KA, Cotton J, Adams JE. A technical and clinical evaluation of digital x-ray radiogrammetry. Osteoporos Int 2003;14:389–395.

15. NRPB. (National Oncologic Protection Board, Oxon).

16. World Nuclear Association. Radiation and the nuclear fuel cycle. http://world-nuclear.org/info/inf05.htm, accessed March 2006.

17. Huda W, Gkanatsios N. Radiation dosimetry for extremity radiographs. Health Phys 1998;75:492–99.

18. Hart D, Wall B. 31 (National Radiological Protection Board, Oxon, 2002). www.phls.co.uk/radiation/publications/w_series_reports/2002/nrpb_w4.pdf

19. Ebdon-Jackson S, Hamlet R, Wall B. Diagnostic radiology: a necessary evil? The Magazine of the Health Protection Agency, 2005.

20. Parfitt AM. A structural approach to renal bone disease. J Bone Miner Res 1998;13:1213–1220.

21. Nelson D, Koo W. Interpretation of absorptiometric bone mass measurements in the growing skeleton: issues and limitations. Calcif Tissue Int 1999;65:1–3.

22. Rauch F, Schonau E. Changes in bone density during childhood and adolescence: an approach based on bone's biological organization. J Bone Miner Res 2001;16:597–604.

23. Mazess RB, Barden HS. Bone densitometry for diagnosis and monitoring osteoporosis. Proc Soc Exp Biol Med 1989;191:261–271.

24. Compston JE, Cooper C, Kanis JA. Fortnightly review: bone densitometry in clinical practice. BMJ 1995;310:1507–1510.

25. Genant HK, Engelke K, Fuerst T, et al. Noninvasive assessment of bone mineral and structure: state of the art. J Bone Miner Res 1996;11:707–730.

26. Adams JE, Shaw N, eds. A practical guide to bone densitometry in children. Bath: National Osteoporosis Society, 2004 (position statement).

27. Carter D, Bouxsein M, Marcus R. New approaches for interpreting projected bone densitometry data. J Bone Miner Res 1992;7:137–145.

28. Crabtree NJ, Kibirige MS, Fordham JN, et al. The relationship between lean body mass and bone mineral content in paediatric health and disease. Bone 2004;35:965–972.

29. Hogler W, Briody J, Woodhead HJ, Chan A, Cowell CT. Importance of lean mass in the interpretation of total body densitometry in children and adolescents. J Pediatr 2003;143:81–88.

30. Kroger H, Kontaniemi A, Vainio P, Alhava E. Bone densitometry of the spine and femur in children by dual-energy x-ray absorptiometry. Bone Miner 1992;17:75–85.

31. Molgaard C, Thomsen B, Prentice A, Cole T, Michealsen K. Whole body bone mineral content in healthy children and adolescents. Arch Dis Child 1997;76:9–15.

32. Prentice A, Parsons T, Cole T. Uncritical use of bone mineral density in absorptiometry may lead to size-related artifacts in the identification of bone mineral determinants. Am J Clin Nutr 1994;60:837–842.

33. Warner JT, Cowan FJ, Dunstan FD, Evans WD, Webb DK, Gregory JW. Measured and predicted bone mineral content in healthy boys and girls aged 6–18 years: adjustment for body size and puberty. Acta Paediatrica 1998;87:244–249.

34. Nevill AM, Holder RL, Maffulli N, Cheng JC, Leung SS, Lee WT, Lau JT. Adjusting bone mass for differences in projected bone area and other confounding variables: an allometric perspective. J Bone Miner Res 2002;17:703–708.

35. Isherwood I, Rutherford R, Pullan B, Adams P. Bone mineral estimation by computed assisted transverse axial tomography. Lancet 1976;2:712–715.

36. Guglielmi, G., Lang, T.F., Cammisa, M., et al. Quantitative computed tomography at the axial skeleton, in Genant HK, Guglielmi G, and Jergas M, eds. Bone Densitometry and Osteoporosis. Berlin: Springer, 1998; pp. 335–343.

37. van Rijn RR, van der Sluis IM, Link TM, et al. Bone densitometry in children: a critical appraisal. Eur Radiol 2003;13:700–710.

38. Mughal M, Ward K, Adams J. Assessment of bone status in children by densitometric and quantitative ultrasound techniques, in Carty H, Brunelle F, Stringer DA, Kao SCS, eds. Imaging Children, Second Edition. Edinburgh: Churchill Livingstone, 2004, pp. 477–486.

39. Faulkner K, McClung M. Quality control of DXA instruments in multicentre trials. Osteoporos Int 1995;5:218–227.

40. Genant HK, Grampp S, Gluer CC, et al. Universal standardization for dual energy -ray absorptiometry: patient and phantom cross-calibration results. J Bone Miner Res 1994;9:1503–1514.

41. Kalender WA, Felsenberg D, Genant HK, Fischer M, Dequeker J, Reeve J. European Spine Phantom—a tool for standardization and quality control in spinal bone mineral measurements by DXA and QCT. Eur J Radiol 1995;20:83–92.

42. Gilsanz V. Bone density in children: a review of the available techniques and indications. Eur J Radiol 1998;26:177–182.

43. Kalender W. Computed Tomography. Munich: Publicis MCD Verlag, 2000.

44. Cann C. Low dose CT scanning for quantitative spinal bone mineral analysis. Radiology 1981;140:813–815.

45. Kalender W. Effective dose values in bone mineral measurements by photon absorptiometry and computed tomography. Osteoporos Int 1992;2:82–87.

46. Gilsanz V, Gibbens DT, Roe TF, et al. Vertebral bone density in children: effect of puberty. Radiology 1988;166:847–850.

47. Mora S, Gilsanz V, eds. Bone Densitometry in Children. Berlin: Springer-Verlag, 1998.

48. Southard RN, Morris JD, Mahan JD, et al. Bone mass in healthy children: measurement with quantitative DXA. Radiology 1991;179:735–738.

49. Faulkner RA, Bailey DA, Drinkwater DT, McKay HA, Arnold C, Wilkinson AA. Bone densitometry in Canadian children 8–17 years of age. Calcif Tissue Int 1996;59:344–51.

50. Zemel, B. et al. Reference data for the whole body, lumbar spine and proximal femur for American children relative to age, gender and body size. J Bone Miner Res 2004;19(S1):S231.

51. Kroger H, Kotaniemi A, Kroger L, Alhava E. Development of bone mass and bone density of the spine and femoral neck—a prospective study of 65 children and adolescents. Bone Miner 1993;23:171–182.

52. Lu PW, Briody JN, Ogle GD, et al. Bone mineral density of total body, spine, and femoral neck in children and young adults: a cross-sectional and longitudinal study. J Bone Miner Res 1994;9:1451–1458.

53. Matkovic V, Jelic T, Wardlaw GM,. Timing of peak bone mass in Caucasian females and its implication for the prevention of osteoporosis. Inference from a cross-sectional model. J Clin Invest 1994;93:799–808.

54. Boot AM, de Ridder MAJ, Pols HAP, Krenning EP, de Muinck Keizer-Schrama SM.. Bone mineral density in children and adolescents: relation to puberty, calcium intake, and physical activity. J Clin Endocrinol Metab 1997;82:57–62.

55. Maynard LM, Guo SS, Chumlea WC,et al. Total-body and regional bone mineral content and areal bone mineral density in children aged 8–18 y: The Fels Longitudinal Study. Am J Clin Nutr 1998;68:1111–1117.

56. Zanchetta JR, Plotkin H, Filgueira MLA. Bone mass in children: normative values for the 2–20-year-old population. Bone 1995;16:393S–399S.

57. Plotkin H, Nunez M, Alvarez Filgueira ML, Zanchetta JR. Lumbar spine bone density in Argentine children. Calcif Tissue Int 1996;58:144–149.

58. Neu C, Manz F, Rauch F, Merkel A, Schonau E. Bone densities and bone size at the distal radius in healthy children and adolescents: a study using peripheral quantitative computed tomography. Bone 2001;28:227–232.

59. Mughal MZ, Ward KA, Qayum N, Langton C. Assessment of bone status using the contact ultrasound bone analyser. Arch Dis Child 1997;76:535–536.

60. Sawyer A, Moore S, Fielding KT, Nix DA, Kiratli J, Bachrach LK. Calcaneus ultrasound measurements in a convenience sample of healthy youth. J Clin Densitom 2001;4:111–120.

61. Barkmann R, Rohrschneider W, Vierling M, et al. German pediatric reference data for quantitative transverse transmission ultrasound of finger phalanges. Osteoporos Int 2002;13:55–61.

62. Baroncelli GI, Federico G, Bertelloni S, de Terlizzi F, Cadossi R, Saggese G. Bone quality assessment by quantitative ultrasound of proximal phalanxes of the hand in healthy subjects aged 3–21 years. Pediatr Res 2001;49:713–718.

63. Zadik Z, Price D, Diamond G. Pediatric reference curves for multi-site quantitative ultrasound and its modulators. Osteoporos Int 2003;14:857–862.

64. Cann C. Quantitative CT applications: comparison of current scanners. Radiology 1987;162:257–261.

65. Genant H, Cann C, Ettinger B, Gordan G. Quantitative computed tomography of vertebral spongiosa: a sensitive method for detecting early bone loss after oophorectomy. Ann Intern Med 1982;97:699–705.

66. Ward K, Alsop C, Caulton J, Rubin C, Adams J, Mughal Z. Low magnitude mechanical loading is osteogenic in children with disabling conditions. J Bone Miner Res 2004;19:360–369.

67. Lang T, LeBlanc A, Evans H, Lu Y, Genant H, Yu A. Cortical and trabecular bone mineral loss from the spine and hip in long-standing spaceflight. J Bone Miner Res 2004;19:1006–1012.

68. Schneider P, Borner W. Peripheral quantitative computed tomography for bone mineral measurement using a new special QCT-scanner. Methodology, normal values, comparison with manifest osteoporosis. Rofo Fortschr Geb Rontgenstr Neuen Bildgeb Verfahr 1991;154:292–299.

69. Ruegsegger P, Durand E, Dambacher MA. Localization of regional forearm bone loss from high resolution computed tomographic images. Osteoporos Int 1991;1:76–80.

70. Ruegsegger P, Durand EP, Dambacher MA. Differential effects of aging and disease on trabecular and compact bone density of the radius. Bone 1991;12:99–105.

71. Fujita T, Fujii Y, Goto B. Measurement of forearm bone in children by peripheral computed tomography. Calcif Tissue Int 1999;64:34–39.

72. Schiessl H, Ferretti J, Tysarczyk-Niemeyer G, Willnecker J. Noninvasive bone strength index as analysed by peripheral quantitative computed tomography, in: Schoenau E, ed. *Paediatric Osteology: New Developments in Diagnostics and Therapy.* Amsterdam: Elsevier, 1996;141–146.

73. Augat P, Iida H, Jiang Y, Diao E, Genant HK. Distal radius fractures: mechanisms of injury and strength prediction by bone mineral assessment. J Orthop Res 1998;16:629–635.

74. Schonau E, Neu C, Beck B, Manz F, Rauch F. Bone mineral content per muscle cross-sectional area as an index of the functional muscle-bone unit. J Bone Miner Res 2002;17:1095–1101.

75. Schonau E. The development of the skeletal system in children and the influence of muscular strength. Horm Res 1998;47:27–31.

76. Schonau E, Neu C, Rauch F, Manz F. Gender-specific pubertal changes in volumetric cortical bone mineral density at the proximal radius. Bone 2002;31:110–113.

77. Leonard MB, Shults J, Elliott DM, Stallings VA, Zemel BS. Interpretation of whole body dual energy x-ray absorptiometry measures in children: comparison with peripheral quantitative computed tomography. Bone 2004;34:1044–1052.

78. Schonau E, Matkovic V. The funcitonal muscle-bone-unit in health and disease. In Schonau E, Matkovic V, eds. *Paediatric Osteology. Prevention of Osteoporosis—A Paediatric Task.* Singapore: Elsevier, 1998;191–202.

79. Schweizer R, Martin DD, Schwarze CP, et al. Cortical bone density is normal in prepubertal children with growth hormone (GH) deficiency, but initially decreases during GH replacement due to early bone remodelling. J Clin Endocrinol Metab 2003;88:5266–5272.

80. Lima EM, Goodman WG, Kuizon BD, et al. Bone density measurements in pediatric patients with renal osteodystrophy. Pediatr Nephrol 2003;18:554–559.

81. Moyer-Mileur LJ, Dixon SB, Quick JL, Askew EW, Murray MA. Bone mineral acquisition in adolescents with type 1 diabetes. J Pediatr 2004;145:662–669.

82. Brennan BM, Mughal Z, Roberts SA, et al. Bone mineral density in childhood survivors of acute lymphoblastic leukemia treated without cranial irradiation. J Clin Endocrinol Metab 2005;90:689–694.

83. Roth J, Palm C, Scheunemann I, Ranke MB, Schweizer R, Dannecker GE. Musculoskeletal abnormalities of the forearm in patients with juvenile idiopathic arthritis relate mainly to bone geometry. Arthritis Rheum 2004;50:1277–1285.

84. Bechtold S, Ripperger P, Bonfig W, Pozza RD, Haefner R, Schwarz HP. Growth hormone changes bone geometry and body composition in patients with juvenile idiopathic arthritis requiring glucocorticoid treatment: a controlled study using peripheral quantitative computed tomography. J Clin Endocrinol Metab 2005;90:3168–3173.

85. Heinonen A, Sievanen H, Kannus P, et al. High-impact exercise and bones of growing girls: a 9-month controlled trial. Osteoporosis International 2000;11:1010–1017.

86. Specker BL, Binkley TL. Randomized trial of physical activity and calcium supplementation on bone mineral content in 3- to 5-year-old children. J Bone Miner Res 2003;18:885–892.

87. Ward KA, Roberts SA, Adams JE, Mughal MZ. Bone geometry and density in the skeleton of prepubertal gymnasts and school children. Bone 2005;36:1012–1018.

88. Langton CM, Palmer SB, Porter RW. The measurement of broadband ultrasonic attenuation in cancellous bone. Eng Med 1984;13:89–91.

89. Wunsche K, Wunsche B, Fahnrich H, et al. Ultrasound bone densitometry of the os calcis in children and adolescents. Calcif Tissue Int 2000;67:349–355.

90. Damilakis J, Galanakis E, Mamoulakis D, Sbyrakis S, Gourtsoyiannis N. Quantitative ultrasound measurements in children and adolescents with type 1 diabetes. Calcif Tissue Int 2004;75:424–428.

91. Hartman C, Brik R, Tamir A, Merrick J, Shamir R. Bone quantitative ultrasound and nutritional status in severely handicapped institutionalized children and adolescents. Clin Nutr 2004;23:89–98.

92. Eliakim A, Nemet D, Wolach B. Quantitative ultrasound measurements of bone strength in obese children and adolescents. J Pediatr Endocrinol Metab 2001;14:159–164.

93. Khaw KT, Reeve J, Luben R, et al. Prediction of total and hip fracture risk in men and women by quantitative ultrasound of the calcaneus: EPIC-Norfolk prospective population study. Lancet 2004;363:197–202.

94. Bauer DC, Gluer CC, Cauley JA, et al. Broadband ultrasound attenuation predicts fractures strongly and independently of densitometry in older women. A prospective study. Study of Osteoporotic Fractures Research Group. Arch Intern Med 1997;157:629–634.

95. Pluijm SM, Graafmans WC, Bouter LM, Lips P. Ultrasound measurements for the prediction of osteoporotic fractures in elderly people. Osteoporos Int 1999;9:550–556.

96. Stewart A, Torgerson DJ, Reid DM. Prediction of fractures in perimenopausal women: a comparison of dual energy x-ray absorptiometry and broadband ultrasound attenuation. Ann Rheum Dis 1996;55:140–142.

97. Fielding KT, Nix DA, Bachrach LK. Comparison of calcaneus ultrasound and dual x-ray absorptiometry in children at risk of osteopenia. J Clin Densitom 2003;6:7–15.

98. Hong J, Hipp JA, Mulkern RV, Jaramillo D, Snyder BD. Magnetic resonance imaging measurements of bone density and cross-sectional geometry. Calcif Tissue Int 2000;66:74–8.

99. Hogler W, Blimkie CJ, Cowell CT, et al. A comparison of bone geometry and cortical density at the mid-femur between prepuberty and young adulthood using magnetic resonance imaging. Bone 2003;33:771–778.

100. Macdonald HM, Heinonen H, Khan KM, et al. Geometric characteristics of the developing tibia in early pubertal girls; a qualitative MRI study. J Bone Miner Res 2003: 18(suppl 1): S66, Abstract #F091.

101. Kroger H, Vainio P, Nieminen J, Kotaniemi A. Comparison of different models for interpreting bone mineral density measurements using DXA and MRI technology. Bone 1995;17:157–159.

102. Heinonen A, McKay H, Whithall K, Forster B, Khan K. Muscle cross-sectional area is associated with specific site of bone in prepubertal girls: a quantitative magnetic resonance imaging study. Bone 2001;29:388–392.

103. Daly RM, Saxon L, Turner CH, Robling AG, Bass SL. The relationship between muscle size and bone geometry during growth and in response to exercise. Bone 2004;34:281–287.

104. McKay HA, Sievanen H, Petit MA, et al. Application of magnetic resonance imaging to evaluation of femoral neck structure in growing girls. J Clin Densitom 2004;7:161–168.

105. Herlidou S, Grebe R, Grados F, Leuyer N, Fardellone P, Meyer ME. Influence of age and osteoporosis on calcaneus trabecular bone structure: a preliminary in vivo MRI study by quantitative texture analysis. Magn Reson Imaging 2004;22:237–243.

106. Boutry N, Cortet B, Dubois P, Marchandise X, Cotten A. Trabecular bone structure of the calcaneus: preliminary in vivo MR imaging assessment in men with osteoporosis. Radiology 2003;227:708–717.

107. Link TM, Vieth V, Stehling C, et al. High-resolution MRI vs multislice spiral CT: which technique depicts the trabecular bone structure best? Eur Radiol 2003;13:663–671.

108. Newitt DC, van Rietbergen B, Majumdar S. Processing and analysis of in vivo high-resolution MR images of trabecular bone for longitudinal studies: reproducibility of structural measures and microfinite element analysis derived mechanical properties. Osteoporos Int 2002;13:278–287.

109. Laib A, Newitt DC, Lu Y, Majumdar S. New model-independent measures of trabecular bone structure applied to in vivo high-resolution MR images. Osteoporos Int 2002;13:130–136.

110. Wehrli FW, Hilaire L, Fernandez-Seara M, et al. Quantitative magnetic resonance imaging in the calcaneus and femur of women with varying degrees of osteopenia and vertebral deformity status. J Bone Miner Res 2002;17:2265–2273.

111. Wehrli FW, Saha PK, Gomberg BR, et al. Role of magnetic resonance for assessing structure and function of trabecular bone. Top Magn Reson Imaging 2002;13:335–355.

112. Wehrli FW, Leonard MB, Saha PK, Gomberg BR. Quantitative high-resolution magnetic resonance imaging reveals structural implications of renal osteodystrophy on trabecular and cortical bone. J Magn Reson Imaging 2004;20:83–89.

113. Barnett E, Nordin B. The radiological diagnosis of osteoporosis. Clin Radiol 1960;11:166–174.

114. Meema H. The occurrence of cortical bone atrophy in old age and osteoporosis. J Can Assoc Radiol. 1962;13:27–32.

115. Meema H, Meema S. Measurable roentgenologic changes in some peripheral bones in senile osteoporosis. J Am Geriatr Soc 1963;11:1170–1182.

116. Garn S, Poznanski A, Nagy J. Bone measurement in the differential diagnosis of osteopenia and osteoporosis. Radiology 1971;100:509–518.

117. Ashby R, Ward K, Mughal M, Adams J. Age related changes in metacarpal morphometry and areal bone mineral density in children assessed by digital x-ray radiogrammetry (DXR). J Bone Miner Res 2002;17:S297.

118. Adams P, Davies G, Sweetnam P. Observer error and measurements of the metacarpal. Br J Radiol 1969;42:192–197.

119. Dequeker J. Quantitative radiology: radiogrammetry of cortical bone. Br J Radiol 1976;49:912–920.

120. Saville PD, Heaney RP, Recker RR. Radiogrammetry at four bone sites in normal middle-aged women. Their relation to each other, to calcium metabolism and to other biological variables. Clin Orthop Relat Res 1976;307–315.

121. Cootes T, Hill A, Taylor C, Haslam J. The use of active shape models for locating structures in medical images. Image Vision Comput 1994;6:276–285.

122. Cootes T, Taylor C, Cooper D, Graham J. Active shape models: their training and application. Comput Vision Image Understanding 1995;1:38–59.

123. Derisquebourg T, Dubois P, Devogelaer JP, et al. Automated computerized radiogrammetry of the second metacarpal and its correlation with absorptiometry of the forearm and spine. Calcif Tiss Int 1994;54:461–465.

124. Kalla A, Meyers O, Parkyn N, Kotze T. Osteoporosis screening—radiogrammetry revisited. Br J Rheumatol 1989;28:511–517.

125. Mentzel HJ, John U, Boettcher J, et al. Evaluation of bone-mineral density by digital x-ray radiogrammetry (DXR) in pediatric renal transplant recipients. Pediatr Radiol 2004;35:489–494.

126. van Rijn RR, Grootfaam DS, Lequin MH, et al. Digital radiogrammetry of the hand in a pediatric and adolescent Dutch Caucasian population: normative data and measurements in children with inflammatory bowel disease and juvenile chronic arthritis. Calcif Tissue Int 2004;74:342–350.

127. Malich A, Freesmeyer MG, Mentzel HJ, et al. Normative values of bone parameters of children and adolescents using digital computer-assisted radiogrammetry (DXR). J Clin Densitom 2003;6:103–111.

128. Marshall D, Johnell O, Wedel H. Meta-analysis of how well measures of bone mineral density predict occurrence of osteoporotic fractures. BMJ 1996;312:1254–1259.

129. Martin JC, Campbell MK, Reid DM. A comparison of radial peripheral quantitative computed tomography, calcaneal ultrasound, and axial dual energy x-ray absorptiometry measurements in women aged 45–55 yr. J Clin Densitom 1999;2:265–273.

130. Kroger H, Lunt M, Reeve J, et al. Bone density reduction in various measurement sites in men and women with osteoporotic fractures of spine and hip: The European quantitation of osteoporosis study. Calcif Tissue Int 1999;64:191–199.

131. Grampp S, Genant HK, Mathur A, et al. Comparisons of noninvasive bone mineral measurements in assessing age-related loss, fracture discrimination, and diagnostic classification. J Bone Miner Res 1997;12:697–711.

132. Eastell R, Wahner HW, O'Fallon WM, Amadio PC, Melton LJ 3rd, Riggs BL. Unequal decrease in bone density of lumbar spine and ultradistal radius in Colles' and vertebral fracture syndromes. J Clin Invest 1989;83:168–174.

133. Faulkner KG, Gluer CC, Majumdar S, Lang P, Engelke K, Genant HK. Noninvasive measurements of bone mass, structure, and strength: current methods and experimental techniques. AJR 1991;157:1229–1237.

134. Elsasser U, Wilkins B, Hesp R, Thurnham DI, Reeve J, Ansell BM. Bone rarefaction and crush fractures in juvenile chronic arthritis. Arch Dis Child 1982;57:377–380.

135. Varonos S, Ansell B, Reeve J. Vertebral collapse in juvenile chronic arthritis: its relationship with glucocorticoid therapy. Calcif Tiss Int 1987;41:75–78.

136. Black DM, Cummings SR, Genant HK, Nevitt MC, Palermo L, Browner W. Axial and appendicular bone density predict fractures in older women. J Bone Miner Res 1992;7:633–638.

137. Gardsell P, Johnell O, Nilsson BE, Gullberg B. Predicting fractures in women by using forearm bone densitometry. Calcif Tiss Int 1989;44:235–242.

138. Goulding A, Cannan R, Williams SM, Gold EJ, Taylor RW, Lewis-Barned NJ. Bone mineral density in girls with forearm fractures. J Bone Miner Res 1998;13:143–148.

139. Ma D, Jones G. The association between bone mineral density, metacarpal morphometry, and upper limb fractures in children: a population-based case-control study. J Clin Endocrinol Metab 2003;88:1486–1491.

140. Kalkwarf H, Laor T, Bean J. Bone mass, density, and dimensions and forearm fracture risk among injured children. Bone 2005;36:S40.

141. Mobley S, et al. Children and bone fragility fractures have reduced bone mineral areal density at the forearm and hip and higher percent body fat. J Bone Miner Res 2005;20.

142. Goulding A, Jones IE, Taylor RW, Manning PJ, Williams SM. More broken bones; A 4-year double cohort study of young girls with and without distal forearm fractures. J Bone Miner Res 2000; 15: 2011–2018.

143. The Writing Group for the ISCD Position Development Conference. Diagnosis of osteoporosis in men, premenopausal women, and children. J Clin Densitometry 2004; 7: 17–26.

3

Dual-Energy X-Ray Absorptiometry

Nicola J. Crabtree, PhD, MSc, BSc(Hons)
Mary B. Leonard, MD, MSCE, Babette S. Zemel, PhD

CONTENTS

    HISTORY
    PRINCIPLES OF DXA
    DEVELOPMENT
    PRECISION
    STRENGTHS OF DXA
    LIMITATIONS OF DXA
    SUMMARY POINTS
    REFERENCES

HISTORY

Early attempts at bone densitometry used conventional x-rays with a step wedge made from an aluminum or ivory phantom included in the field of view as a means of calibration. The bone density was calculated by a visual comparison of the density of the bone and the known densities of the each of the steps on the phantom.

The next advancement in the field of bone density was the invention of single-photon absorptiometry (SPA) by Cameron and Sorenson in 1963 *(1)*. This technique used a radioactive source of either iodine (I-125) or americium (Am-241), with energies of 27 keV and 60 keV, respectively. The subject placed his or her arm in a water bath to provide a uniform path length through which the gamma rays would pass. This process allowed the calculation of the amount of bone tissue in the region scanned by means of subtraction of the photons attenuated by the soft tissue from the photons attenuated by bone and soft tissue. This technique proved to be very useful in terms of bone quantification, but it was limited to a peripheral site.

To measure bone density at axial sites (i.e., the spine or hip), in which the soft tissue is of variable thickness, gamma rays of two different energies are required to distinguish soft tissue from bone. Dual-photon absorptiometry (DPA) allowed this, providing the simultaneous transmission of gamma rays with photon energies of 44 keV and 100 keV from gadolinium-153 *(2)*. Estimates of bone and soft tissue were then derived using algebraic equations.

From: *Current Clinical Practice: Bone Densitometry in Growing Patients: Guidelines for Clinical Practice*
Edited by: A. J. Sawyer, L. K. Bachrach, and E. B. Fung © Humana Press Inc., Totowa, NJ

Since the late 1980s, the expensive and potentially hazardous radioactive sources used in both SPA and DPA have been superseded by single x-ray absorptiometry (SXA) *(3)* and dual-energy x-ray absorptiometry (DXA). Similarly to DPA, the fundamental principle of DXA is the measurement of the transmission of x-rays, produced from a stable x-ray source, at high and low energies. The advantages of using x-rays instead of SPA or DPA include a shorter acquisition time and improved accuracy and precision as a result of the increased photon flux. Improvements in precision and resolution have been coupled with a decrease in radiation exposure *(4)*. With the increased availability of DXA, there has been a dramatic rise in its use in pediatric research and clinical practice (Fig. 1).

PRINCIPLES OF DXA

The x-rays used in diagnostic imaging and densitometry must have sufficient energy to pass through the body and still be detectable by sensors after passage. X-ray beam energy is attenuated or reduced with the passage through tissue. The extent of attenuation varies with the energy of the photons and the density and thickness of the material through which they pass.

Attenuation will follow an exponential pattern often observed in other biological situations. For monoenergetic radiation (i.e., from photons with the same energy) this pattern of attenuation can be described using the following formula:

$$I = I_0 e^{-\mu M}$$

where I = measured intensity of the x-ray; I_0 = initial intensity of the x-ray beam; μ = mass attenuation coefficient $(cm^2 g^{-1})$; and M = area density (g/cm^2)

In other words, for a given beam intensity level, each tissue will have a unique attenuation property such that the attenuation is a function of a constant (i.e., the mass attenuation coefficient) specific to that tissue and the mass of the tissue. Because bone is surrounded by soft tissue, a more complex model is required to be able to distinguish the density of the bone from the surrounding tissue.

The fundamental principle of DXA is the measurement of transmission of x-rays with high- and low-energy photons through the body. The mathematics used to calculate bone density values can be explained using an exponential equation that assumes the body to be a two-compartment model consisting of bone mineral and soft tissue. Bone mineral is a physically dense material mainly made up of phosphorus and calcium molecules that have relatively high atomic numbers. Soft tissue is a mixture of muscle, fat, skin, and water. It has a lower physical density and a lower effective atomic number because its main chemical constituents are hydrogen, carbon, and oxygen. At the same photon energy, soft tissue and bone will have different mass attenuation coefficients, so the exponential equation becomes:

$$I = I_0 \exp{-(\mu_B M_B + \mu_S M_S)}$$

Where B = bone and S = soft tissue.

For the different x-ray energies, the mass attenuation coefficient will be different, leading to two equations, one for low-energy photons and one for high-energy photons:

$$I^L = I^L_0 \exp(-\mu_B{}^L M_B - \mu_S{}^L M_S)$$

$$I^H = I^H_0 \exp(-\mu_B{}^H M_B - \mu_S{}^H M_S)$$

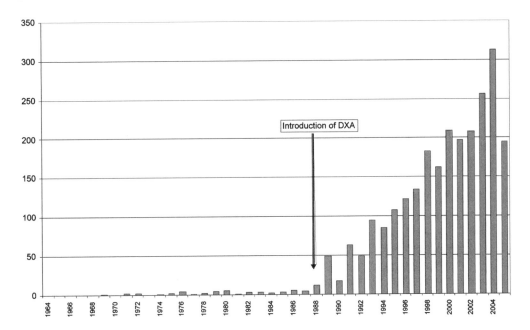

Fig. 1. Number of publications on pediatrics and bone mineral density from 1965 to 2005 (using citations in PubMed).

where L = low-energy photons and H = high-energy photons.

These equations are solved for M_B (i.e., the area density of bone)

$$M_B = \frac{Ln\ (I^L_0 / I^L) - k\ Ln\ (I^H_0 / I^H)}{\mu^L_B - k\mu^H_B}$$

where $k = \mu^L_S / \mu^H_S$.

The ratio k can be derived from the patient measurement by measuring the transmitted intensity of the beam at points at which there is no bone (i.e., at which $M_B = 0$). Once the ratio k is determined, the equation can be solved to calculate the area bone density, M_B.

The bone density is determined for each point, or each pixel, of the area being scanned. As the source and detector move linearly across the scanned area, a bone profile is generated on a pixel-by-pixel basis. The bone density image is then made up of many linear passes.

After acquisition, the machine's software employs an edge-detection algorithm to evaluate the bone profile and to identify the pixels that represent where the bone edge begins and ends within the area scanned. The bone density is then calculated as the average M_B across the bone profile (Fig. 2). From the pixel-by-pixel density image, the software sums the number of pixels containing bone to calculate the bone area (BA) that was scanned. Using the mean bone mineral density (BMD) value and the BA, it is possible to calculate the actual amount of bone mineral content (BMC) within the image:

$$BMC\ (g) = BMD\ (g/cm^2) \times BA\ (cm^2)$$

DXA is a projectional technique in which three-dimensional objects are analyzed as two-dimensional. DXA provides an estimate of areal BMD in g/cm^2. This BMD is not a measure of volumetric density (in g/cm^3) because it provides no information about the

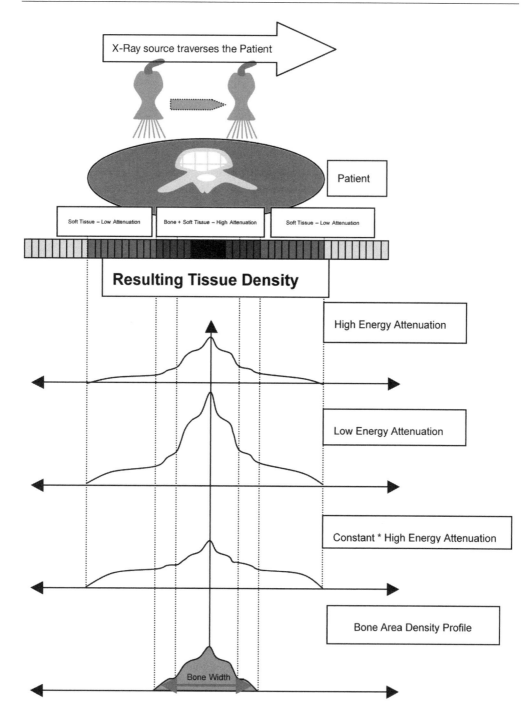

Fig. 2. Bone profile, observed as the x-ray moves linearly across the patient, and the corresponding tissue density profiles.

depth of bone. Given two bones of identical volumetric BMD, the smaller bone will have a lower areal BMD than the larger one because the influence of bone thickness is not factored. This would mean that areal BMD in a small child would be lower than areal BMD in a taller child even if they had identical volumetric bone densities. Numerous strategies have been proposed to estimate volumetric BMD from areal BMD results *(5,6)*; these are described in detail in Chapter 10.

DXA measurements represents the sum of cortical and trabecular bone within the projected BA, concealing the distinct structural characteristics. Therefore, the influence of disease processes or medications that differentially affect cortical vs trabecular bone may be obscured or difficult to detect by DXA.

Other potential problems arise when the DXA software is unable to detect the difference between bone and soft tissue. This typically occurs in patients with undermineralized bones, as may occur in younger or sicker children. Bone densitometry manufacturers have tried to tackle this issue with the introduction of low-density software for better edge detection of the bone *(7)*. As detailed under "Limitations of DXA: Bone Detection Algorithms," it is important to recognize the limitations of this software and the potential for further underestimation of BMD.

DEVELOPMENT

Since the introduction of clinical DXA, there have been changes in the technique for acquiring the information required to calculate bone density. New technology has allowed more stable x-ray units to be made and more-sensitive detectors to be utilized. However, the most significant change has been the introduction of the fan beam and narrow fan beam systems.

Pencil Beam vs Fan Beam Scanners

Originally, the scanners used a highly collimated beam of x-rays in conjunction with sequential detectors or a single detector that moved in a raster pattern (i.e., in a series of thin parallel lines) across the patient. This pencil beam system produces the most geometrically correct information, with little or no magnification of the area being scanned.

The newer fan beam systems use a slit collimator to generate a beam that diverges in two directions in conjunction with a linear array of solid-state detectors, so bone measurements can be made with a single sweep of the x-ray arm. The fan beam systems use higher energy photon intensities and a greater photon flux, thus producing a better-resolution image considerably faster than the older pencil beam machines. The lumbar spine can be scanned in 30 seconds with the fan beam, as compared with the 3–10 min required for the pencil beam system.

The trade-off for improved image resolution with the fan beam is a higher radiation exposure. Additionally, the geometry associated with this technique leads to magnification of the image in one direction *(8,9)*. The degree of magnification will depend on the distance of the bone or tissue away from the source: the closer the body part is to the source, the greater the magnification.

The most recent advance has been the introduction of the narrow fan beam bone densitometer. This machine uses a narrow fan beam x-ray source in conjunction with semiconductor detectors. It scans in a rectilinear raster fashion, much like the original pencil beam machines. However, because the beam is wider than the original pencil beam machine, it can cover the body in a much faster time, typically 30 s. Recent cross-

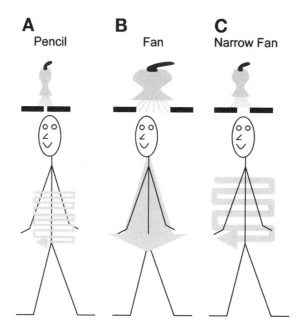

Fig. 3. Scanning by (A) pencil beam, (B) fan beam, and (C) narrow fan beam. The path of the x-ray beams is represented with the arrow.

calibration studies demonstrated no detectable magnification effect between the old-generation pencil beam scanner and the new narrow fan beam machine *(10)* (Fig. 3).

Radiation

The amount of radiation exposure in DXA is extremely low compared to many other x-ray imaging techniques. It has been difficult to directly estimate the degree of risk associated with these very low levels of radiation except by extrapolation from studies that involved distinctly higher levels of radiation exposure. Presently, studies have not been able to establish a link between health risk and the low levels of radiation exposure that are typical of DXA. According to the Health Physics Society, the risks of health effects for exposures less than 5–10 rem (Roentgen Equivalent Man) "are either too small to be observed or are nonexistent" *(11)*.

Health effects of radiation have been demonstrated at doses above 5–10 rem (greater than 50,000–100,000 μSv) *(11)*. The principal risk due to radiation is random x-ray interactions with the body, which can result in carcinogenic or genetic effects. Typically, carcinogenic effects will not manifest in an individual for several decades following an exposure *(12)*. This is an important consideration when scanning children because they have a longer amount of time for expression of an effect than adults *(12)*. Because the majority of the children scanned will still be fertile, the potential genetic effects of radiation exposure are a theoretical consideration *(13)*. However, as shown in Table 1, radiation exposures from DXA are approximately 10,000 times less than the radiation doses at which health effects occur.

Estimates of risk from radiation exposure are expressed in terms of effective dose, in units of sieverts or rems, where 1 mrem equals 10 μSv. The effective dose is calculated from the magnitude of exposure, the type of radiation causing the exposure, the organs

Table 1

Effective Dose and Entrance Surface Doses for the Commonly Available Bone Densitometers

		Scan Type			
		Spine		Whole Body	
Manufacturer and Instrument	Beam type	Effective Dose (μSv)	Entrance Surface Dose (μGy)	Effective Dose (μSv)	Entrance Surface Dose (μGy)
Hologic QDR 1000 and QDR 2000	Pencil	0.5[14]	60[14]	4.6[14]	18[14]
Lunar DPX series	Pencil	0.2[15]	10.3[15]		0.2
Norland XR-46	Pencil		4.7[17]		0.2[17]
Norland XR-26	Pencil		44[17]		0.5[17]
Hologic QDR 2000	Fan	0.4–2.9[14]	57–432[14]	3.6[14]	11[14]
Hologic QDR4500 series	Fan	8.0[16]	200[16]		10[a]
Lunar Expert	Fan	31[15]	895[15]		50[a]
Lunar Prodigy	Narrow Fan	0.7[a]	37[a]	<1.0[a]	0.4[a]

Note: effective dose estimations are for adults with functioning reproductive organs.
1 mrem = 10 μSv; 1 mrad = 10 μGy.
[a]Manufacturer's reported values.

47

exposed, and their relative radiosensitivities. The resulting value can be compared to other scanning techniques (Chapter 2, Table 1), to naturally occurring background radiation (8.6 μSv/day), or to a round trip transatlantic flight (80 μSv).

The more commonly cited unit of radiation exposure is the entrance surface dose (ESD) in units of gray (Gy); 10 μGy = 1 mrad (i.e., 1 Gy = 100 rad). ESD is a measure of the radiation on the surface of the patient, before it passes through and is absorbed by the body. It is an easier measure to obtain as it requires only a simple measure of the x-ray output detected at the skin surface. It will be approximately the same for any patient scanned at any one exposure level, irrespective of the region scanned. The ESD will be higher than the effective dose. Although ESD gives the operator an indication of the exposure levels, it does not take into account the organs being exposed and the relative radiosensitivities of the irradiated organs.

Table 1 lists both the effective and entrance surface doses of ionizing radiation doses associated with the more commonly used densitometers. As a result of limited published pediatric data, the doses in the table refer to estimates for adults.

In summary, the radiation exposure associated with DXA is acceptable for pediatric use. However, efforts should always be made to minimize lifetime radiation exposure through the judicious selection of patients and skeletal sites for DXA scanning (Chapter 4) and through optimal densitometry technique (Chapter 5).

PRECISION

The precision of a diagnostic test such as DXA is an indication of the reproducibility of replicate measurements. Precision determines the certainty about the initial quantitative measurements as well as the ability to detect small changes with future measurements. The precision of DXA measurements is determined by factors related to the machine, the software, and the operator. Precision can determined for short-term and long-term replicate measurements. It is expressed as the percent coefficient of variation (%CV) and is the percentage of variation of the measurement compared to the mean value for replicate measurements.

$$\%CV = \frac{(\text{Standard Deviation [SD] of the Measurement}) \times 100}{\text{Mean Value of the Measurements}}$$

Short-Term Machine Precision

Machine precision is calculated from repeat scanning of a single phantom, without moving the phantom between scans. Usual protocol for the measurement of machine precision requires scanning a phantom 10 times on the same day. For newer DXA models, the CV for this procedure is typically less than 1%.

Long-Term or Temporal Machine Precision

Long-term precision is measured by repeatedly scanning a phantom daily or weekly over months to years to monitor any temporal changes in the machine. These measurements can be used to assess the long-term stability of a scanner; because the measurements from a phantom should theoretically be the same each day, any drift or change would therefore be due to the machine.

$$CV\% = \frac{(\text{Standard Error in the Estimate [SEE]}) \times 100}{\text{Mean Change}}$$

In Vivo Short-Term Precision

In vivo short-term precision is calculated by repeated scanning of subjects a minimum of two times on the same day or within a short time interval. To achieve statistical power, BMD testing must be done three times in each of 15 individuals or twice in each of 30 subjects. The standard deviation for each patient is calculated, and then the root mean square standard deviation for the group is calculated. A good explanation for these calculations can be found on the website of the International Society for Clinical Densitometry (http://www.iscd.org). Because this procedure requires two scans and twice the radiation exposure, in vivo precision testing is considered by some to be clinical research. Regardless of interpretation, all participants should provide written informed consent.

The precision estimates reflect both machine precision and operator precision. For this reason, in vivo testing results in a greater CV (i.e., lower precision) than machine precision using a phantom, but it is more representative of the real scanning situation. The best precision will be achieved if the patients are scanned and analyzed by a single fully trained operator.

Precision studies are most commonly performed in healthy adults. However, precision measured in mature individuals may differ from that measured in children because of the latter's smaller size and variable ability to cooperate. The ability of the software to detect the edges of smaller bones may also affect precision in children. Ideally, pediatric data should be gathered when possible. One multicenter study of DXA precision in 155 children, ages 6–15 yr, demonstrated coefficient of variation values of 0.64–1.03 for spine and 0.66–1.20 for whole-body BMD, depending on the age range *(18)*.

Long-Term In Vivo Precision

This measure is obtained by repeat scanning of a group of patients over a period of time. It is harder to evaluate because, unlike a phantom, which maintains stable bone density over time, the patient's bone density may increase or decrease. For children, this is particularly difficult to estimate due to the expected changes in bone measures in growing children.

Least Significant Change

The least significant change (LSC) is the smallest percent difference that can be detected by the technique from repeat measurement of a patient. This value is usually expressed as $2.8 \times \%CV$.

STRENGTHS OF DXA

Accessibility

Although availability of DXA may vary from country to country, this technique is now widely available in both general hospitals and academic medical centers. In some areas, mobile units are also available, reducing the need for the patient to travel long distances to the nearest machine.

Radiation Dose

Although any radiation exposure results in a degree of risk to the patient, DXA has one of the lowest effective doses of all the ionizing radiation imaging techniques, being equivalent to approximately less than 1 d naturally occurring radiation in most cases.

Precision

Much work has been done by the manufacturers of DXA machines to produce a stable x-ray source and an efficient detector system, thereby making DXA a precise technique for measuring bone. The average coefficient of variation for a spine DXA scan is 1.5% or less, compared to as much as 5% for an average calcaneus ultrasound scan *(19)*. Additionally, sophisticated analysis software packages are used, which, for a large proportion of DXA scans, require little or no operator intervention, thus further improving precision.

Short Scan Time

Recent advances in DXA hardware have drastically shortened scan times. Whole-body DXA scans can be completed in 3 min or less, and spine scans in less than 1 min, which minimizes the possibility of movement artifacts in young children.

Normative Data

As a result of the wide availability and relatively low radiation dose, DXA data have been collected on samples of healthy infants, children, and adolescents in several countries (Chapter 2, Table 4; *see* Appendix C at end of volume). These data have been used clinically as reference values to identify children with "normal" vs "abnormal" bone density. However, caution should be used in applying these reference data for several reasons: (1) the manufacturer, model, and software version will affect DXA results, so data on healthy children used for comparison should all be acquired and analyzed in a similar fashion; (2) these data are derived from convenience samples that may not provide adequate representation of all age and gender groups; (3) reference data that do not provide gender-specific norms are likely to overestimate bone deficits in boys compared to girls *(20)*; and (4) most reference data provide means and standard deviations relative to age, and there are no guidelines on how to account for children with delayed skeletal age or altered body size. These issues are discussed in further detail in Chapter 7.

Interpretation of DXA Results

DXA is widely accepted as a quantitative measurement technique for assessing skeletal status. In elderly adults, DXA BMD is also a sufficiently robust predictor of osteoporotic fractures, that it can be used to define the disease. The World Health Organization criteria for the diagnosis of osteoporosis in adults is based on a T-score, the comparison of a measured BMD result with the average BMD of young adults at the time of peak bone mass *(21)*. A T-score of –2.5 standard deviations (SD) or less below the mean peak bone mass is used for the diagnosis of osteoporosis, and a T-score of –2.5 SD or less with a history of a low-impact fracture is classified as severe osteoporosis.

In adults, each SD decrease in the T-score is associated with an average increase of fracture risk by 1.5- to 3-fold *(22)*. Measurements of BMD in anatomic regions that are likely to fracture—such as the spine, hip, or forearm—provide the best prediction of risk of fracture at that site. For example, the Study of Osteoporotic Fractures showed that at the femoral neck, each SD decrease in bone density increased the age-adjusted risk of hip fracture 2.6 times (95% confidence interval [CI] 1.9, 3.6). Low hip bone density was a stronger predictor of hip fracture than bone density measurements of the spine, radius, or calcaneus *(23)*.

Ongoing epidemiological studies in adults have demonstrated that the relationship between T-score and fracture risk is age-dependent; for a given T-score, the risk of fracture increases with age (24). In addition, other risk factors, such as previous fracture, maternal history of hip fracture, greater height, impaired cognition, slower walking speed, nulliparity, type 2 diabetes mellitus, Parkinson's disease, and poor depth perception also contribute independently to the risk of hip fracture in older women (25). These observations reflect the fact that bone mass is only one factor contributing to the risk of fracture in adults. Bone quality and geometry and the risk of falling also contribute to the likelihood of bone fracture. In children, less is known about the risk factors for fractures and whether they are age-dependent.

Because of the predictive value of the T-score in adults, it is a standard component of DXA BMD reporting software. However, it is clearly inappropriate to compare the bone mineral status of a child with adults who have reached peak bone mass. Instead, the bone density of children should be expressed as a Z-score, the number of standard deviations from the mean for age and gender. Additional adjustments for body size or body composition are recommended by some, as discussed in Chapter 7. Despite the growing body of published normative data utilizing DXA in children, there are no evidence-based guidelines for the definition of osteoporosis, osteopenia, or fracture risk based upon BMD in children. Further discussion of this important consideration and the relationship between DXA BMD and fracture risk can be found in Chapters 7 and 10.

LIMITATIONS OF DXA

Confounding by Bone Size

DXA provides only two-dimensional measurements of BMC and BA for the three-dimensional bone. Thus, BMD is not a measure of volumetric density (g/cm^3) because it provides no information about bone depth. Bones of larger width and height are also thicker. As shown in Fig. 4, the BMD of bones with identical volumetric BMD but varying size will differ substantially in areal BMD. Smaller bones will have a lower areal BMD than larger bones because bone thickness is not factored into DXA results. The lower areal BMD of children when compared with adults is due, in part, to their smaller bone size. In addition, children who are small for their age will have a lower areal BMD than their same-age peers, even if their volumetric BMD is identical.

Because of the confounding by bone size, several investigators have suggested that the use of BMC adjusted for body size is preferable to conventional units of areal BMD, especially in children (26–29). Others have suggested that volumetric BMD can be estimated from the BMC and BA values obtained from DXA by calculating bone mineral apparent density (5,30,31). For whole-body DXA scans, BA relative to height may provide additional information about bone dimensions and strength (27,29). The clinical utility of these approaches remains to be determined. Further details are given in Chapter 10, describing how these techniques are being evaluated in research.

Projection Artifacts

An additional limitation of DXA is that it may introduce artifacts into the measurement of bone size (i.e., the projected area) and density in children with abnormal body composition (9,32). Hologic scanners are configured such that the fan beam is projected from

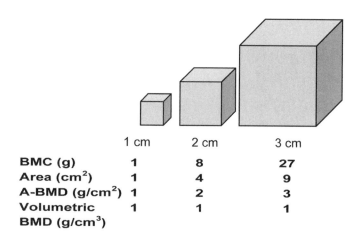

	1 cm	2 cm	3 cm
BMC (g)	1	8	27
Area (cm²)	1	4	9
A-BMD (g/cm²)	1	2	3
Volumetric BMD (g/cm³)	1	1	1

Fig. 4. The difference between volumetric and areal bone mineral density in differently sized bones, as assessed by dual-energy x-ray absorptiometry.

below the patient, with a linear array of detectors above the patient. The portion of the body that is closest to the source of the beam is magnified more than if the same region were closer to the detector. Subsequently, thinner individuals will appear to have a disproportionately greater BA and BMC. This has important implications for longitudinal studies because children will increase in length and thickness as they grow. Moreover, increases in soft-tissue thickness associated with glucocorticoid therapy may result in the erroneous impression of decreased BMC and BA as the bone is lifted further from the x-ray source.

Changes in the surrounding soft tissues may also impact bone detection algorithms. Given that many children for whom poor bone mineral accrual is a concern also have altered body size and composition, these effects are likely to be important but have not been quantified. For adults, the effects of weight and body composition changes on the estimation of total-body BMC, BA, and BMD have been evaluated using in vivo and in vitro models. The direction and magnitude of the effects depend on the manufacturer and software version *(33,34)*. For example, with a 16% weight loss in obese adult women, the Lunar DPX system operating in the standard software mode showed losses of 5.3, 3.2, and 2.3% for BMC, BA, and BMD estimations, respectively. For the Hologic 1000 W, a 12% weight loss in obese adult women resulted in losses of 8.3, 6.8, and 1.6% for BMC, BA, and BMD estimations *(33)*. Measurements of whole-body phantoms wrapped in lard confirmed that these observed changes with weight loss in adults were attributable, at least in part, to changes in surrounding soft tissue and distance from the x-ray source and not to actual changes in bone size and density. Across all scanners evaluated, the effects of weight and body composition changes are more pronounced for total-body BMC and BA than they are for BMD. Similar results have been noted for estimation of BMC, BA, and BMD of the spine as well *(33,35)*.

For children with weight and body composition in the normal range, it is fair to assume that the effects of normal growth-related changes in weight and body composition on BMC, BA, and BMD will be comparable to those occurring in the reference population. Thus, the interpretation of reference-based Z-scores should not be affected by these normal, growth-related changes. For children experiencing rapid shifts in weight and body composition, for example, with intentional weight loss regimens or with weight gain through glucocorticoid therapy, the measurement artifacts described previously should be taken into consideration in the interpretation of DXA results.

Bone Detection Algorithms

Pediatric DXA images often could not be analyzed with early-generation software as a result of the failure of the bone edge detection algorithm to identify and measure completely all bones. In one series, the DXA lumbar spine scan could not be analyzed using standard software (QDR 2000, Hologic, Waltham, MA, USA) in 40% of chronically ill children less than 12 yr of age and in younger healthy children, particularly those less than 6 yr of age (7). Although it is possible to use visual inspection to fill in the regions missed by standard software, this reduces precision by introducing greater operator-related variability. It resulted in loss of the systems algorithm threshold definition of bone edge and led to inaccuracies in measurements of bone mineralization.

In an effort to address this limitation, software modifications were developed to improve detection of low-density bone in children and severely osteopenic adults (Hologic, GE Lunar). Although the new software performed well, these modifications increased the detection of low-density bone. Because the bone map included areas of less dense bone (not detectable by standard software), low-density software resulted in a systematic decrease in the BMD measurement compared with the standard analysis (7). Comparable effects were seen with whole body pediatric software analyses (36). Because results acquired using standard and low density software analyses differed by as much as 9–11%, these two software options could not be used interchangeably in studies of BMD in children, For the same reason, reference data must be acquired in the same analysis mode as that used to examine the patient.

More recent software modifications include methods to adjust bone-detection thresholds based on the subject's weight (37). and techniques for improved bone detection in the lumbar spine based on anatomical assumptions. Future studies are needed to evaluate the utility of these new approaches in longitudinal studies and in children with altered body composition. Although these techniques illustrate the advancements that are being made in bone mineral analysis, it must also be remembered that proper comparison to a reference population requires that the same methods be used in subjects and controls.

Lack of Standardized Reference Data

The ability to interpret DXA measurements has also been influenced by the lack of standardized reference data. As noted previously, DXA results vary by manufacturer, model number, and software version. In particular, manufacturers and software versions vary in how the lower BMD of children is detected. Cross-calibration of DXA machines from different manufacturers has been done to establish a set of equations to convert BMD on each machine to a "standardized BMD" (sBMD) (38). These formulae are presented in Appendix B. However, these equations were established for adults, and further research is needed to determine if they are applicable to children. Consequently, careful selection of pediatric reference data that matches the manufacturer, model, and software version is essential.

In addition, utilizing reference data that are based on adequate numbers of children within each age and gender group is crucial for characterizing bone mineral status. Currently, the US National Institutes of Health is conducting a large, mixed longitudinal multiethnic multicenter study to establish national norms for bone mineral density. Until these data are published, other pediatric reference data must be employed (provided in Appendix C).

Pediatric studies of healthy children have identified numerous factors influencing BMD. BMC and BMD are largely influenced by body size (height, weight and body mass index [BMI, weight/height^2]) *(27,31,39–44)*. Gender, sexual maturation *(31,39–46)*, ethnicity *(30,31,44,47,48)*, body composition *(39,40,49)*, nutrient intake *(50,51)*, physical activity *(52,53)*, skeletal age *(40,54)*, and genetics *(48,55,56)* are also important factors. Age, body size and composition, and sexual maturation explain up to 88% of the variability in DXA measures of BMD, especially when study samples consist of children of widely varying ages *(40,42,43,57)*.

Although it is recognized that these are important covariates of bone density, it is unclear how they should be used clinically. For adults, the International Society of Clinical Densitometry recommends the use of a uniform Caucasian reference database for evaluating bone density for all ethnic groups *(58)*. The reasons are that (1) it is not always possible to identify patient ethnicity, and reference data are not available for all ethnic groups; (2) there is insufficient evidence linking BMD to fracture risk in other ethnic groups; and (3) use of Caucasian reference data in African Americans results in a lower prevalence of osteoporosis, which is in accordance with the lower rates of fracture among African Americans. A useful discussion of this topic can be found at the website of the International Society for Clinical Densitometry (http://www.iscd.org/Visitors/positions/official.cfm). Among children, it is unclear if reference norms should follow similar guidelines because even less is know about BMD and fracture risk across different ethnic groups. Similarly, evidence-based pediatric recommendations for adjusting for body size, body composition, and skeletal and sexual maturation are lacking.

SUMMARY POINTS

- The fundamental principle of DXA is the measurement of transmission of x-rays, produced from a stable x-ray source, at high and low energies.
- Since the introduction of DXA, there has been an exponential increase in pediatric research and clinical practice of bone densitometry in pediatrics.
- DXA is a projectional technique in which three-dimensional objects are analyzed as two-dimensional. Problems may arise when the dimensions of the area scanned change with time, as is the case in a growing child.
- DXA technology has numerous strengths as a clinical tool in the field of pediatric densitometry, including its availability, short scan times, minimal radiation exposure, and excellent precision.
- There remain a number of factors that must be considered carefully when interpreting DXA results in pediatrics, including size and projection artifacts, bone detection limitations, and the lack of standardized normative data for children and adolescents.

REFERENCES

1. Cameron JR, Sorenson J. Measurement of bone mineral in vivo: an improved method. Science 1963;11:230–232.
2. Madsen M, Peppler W, Mazess RB. Vertebral and total body bone mineral content by dual photon absorptiometry. Calcif Tissue Res 1976;21 Suppl:361–364.
3. Kelly TL, Crane G, Baran D. Single x-ray absorptiometry of the forearm: precision, correlation, and reference data. Calcif Tissue Int 1994;53:212–218.

4. Kelly TL, Slovik D, Schoenfeld DA, Neer RM. Quantitative digital radiography versus dual photon absorptiometry of the lumbar spine. J Clin Endocrinol Metab 1988;67:839–844.

5. Carter DR, Bouxsein ML, Marcus R. New approaches for interpreting projected bone densitometry data. J Bone Miner Res 1992;7:137–145.

6. Kroger H, Vainio P, Nieminen J, Kotaniemi A. Comparison of different models for interpreting bone mineral density measurements using DXA and MRI technology. Bone 1995;17:157–159.

7. Leonard MB, Feldman HI, Zemel BS, Berlin JA, Barden EM, Stallings VA. Evaluation of low density spine software for the assessment of bone mineral density in children. J Bone Miner Res 1998;13:1687–1690.

8. Cole JH, Scerpella TA, van der Meulen MC. Fan-beam densitometry of the growing skeleton: are we measuring what we think we are? J Clin Densitom 2005;8:57–64.

9. Pocock NA, Noakes KA, Majerovic Y, Griffiths MR. Magnification error of femoral geometry using fan beam densitometers. Calcif Tissue Int 1997;60:8–10.

10. Oldroyd B, Smith AH, Truscott JG. Cross-calibration of GE/Lunar pencil and fan-beam dual energy densitometers—bone mineral density and body composition studies. Eur J Clin Nutr 2003;57:977–987.

11. Radiation Risk in Perspective. Health Physics Society. Accessed May 24, 2006. http://hps.org/documents/radiationrisk.pdf

12. Board statement on diagnostic medical exposures to ionizing radiation during pregnancy and estimates of late radiation effects to the U.K. population. Documents of NRPB4, No 4, 1993.

13. Annals of the ICRP. 1990 Recommendations of the International Commission on Radiological Protection. ICRP Publication 60. 1991; Volume 21: No. 1–3.

14. Lewis MK, Blake GM, Fogelman I. Patient dose in dual x-ray absorptiometry. Osteoporos Int 1994;4:11–15.

15. Njeh CF, Apple K, Temperton DH, Boivin CM. Radiological assessment of a new bone densitometer—the Lunar EXPERT. Br J Radiol 1996;69:335–340.

16. Starritt H C, Elvins D M, Ring F. Radiation dose and the Hologic Acclaim x-ray densitometer, in *Current Research in Osteoporosis and Bone Mineral Measurement*, 4th ed. London: British Institute of Radiology, 1996; pp. 99–100.

17. Zanchetta JR, Plotkin H, Alvarez Filgueira ML. Bone mass in children: normative values for the 2–20-year-old population. Bone 1995;16:393S–399S

18. Shepherd J, Fan B, Sherman M, et al. Pediatric DXA precision varies with age. J Bone Miner Res 2004;19(Suppl 1):234, abstract # SU124.

19. Nejh CF, Hans D, Li J, et al. Comparison of six calcaneal quantitative ultrasound devices: precision and hip fracture discrimination. Osteoporos Int 2000;11(12):1051–1062.

20. Leonard MB, Propert KJ, Zemel BS, Stallings VA, Feldman HI. Discrepancies in pediatric bone mineral density reference data: potential for misdiagnosis of osteopenia. J Pediatr 1999;135:182–188.

21. WHO. The WHO Study Group: assessment of fracture risk and its application to screening for postmenopausal osteoporosis. Geneva, Switzerland, 1994.

22. Marshall D, Johnell O, Wedel H. Meta-analysis of how well measures of bone mineral density predict occurrence of osteoporotic fractures. BMJ 1996;312:1254–1259.

23. Cummings SR, Black DM, Nevitt MC, et al. Bone density at various sites for prediction of hip fractures. The Study of Osteoporotic Fractures Research Group. Lancet 1993;341:72–75.

24. Kanis JA, Johnell O, Oden A, Dawson A, De Laet C, Jonsson B. Ten year probabilities of osteoporotic fractures according to BMD and diagnostic thresholds. Osteoporos Int 2001;12:989–995.

25. Taylor BC, Schreiner PJ, Stone KL, et al. Long-term prediction of incident hip fracture risk in elderly white women: Study of osteoporotic fractures. J Am Geriatr Soc 2004;52:1479–1486.

26. Prentice A, Parsons TJ, Cole TJ. Uncritical use of bone mineral density in absorptiometry may lead to size-related artifacts in the identification of bone mineral determinants. Am J Clin Nutr 1994;60:837–842.

27. Molgaard C, Thomsen BL, Prentice A, Cole TJ, Michaelsen KF. Whole body bone mineral content in healthy children and adolescents. Arch Dis Child 1997;76:9–15.

28. Heaney RP. Bone mineral content, not bone mineral density, is the correct bone measure for growth studies. Am J Clin Nutr 2003;78:350–352.

29. Leonard MB, Shults J, Elliott DM, Stallings VA, Zemel BS. Interpretation of whole body dual energy x-ray absorptiometry measures in children: Comparison with peripheral quantitative computed tomography. Bone 2004;34:1044–1052.

30. Bachrach LK, Hastie T, Wang MC, Narasimhan B, Marcus R. Bone mineral acquisition in healthy Asian, Hispanic, black, and Caucasian youth: A longitudinal study. J Clin Endocrinol Metab 1999;84:4702–4712.

31. Wang MC, Aguirre M, Bhudhikanok GS, et al. Bone mass and hip axis length in healthy Asian, black, Hispanic, and white American youths. J Bone Miner Res 1997;12:1922–1935.

32. Blake GM, Parker JC, Buxton FM, Fogelman I. Dual x-ray absorptiometry: A comparison between fan beam and pencil beam scans. Br J Radiol 1993;66:902–906.

33. Tothill P, Laskey MA, Orphanidou CI, Van Wijk M. Anomalies in dual energy x-ray absorptiometry measurements of total-body bone mineral during weight change using Lunar, Hologic and Norland instruments. Br J Radiol 1999;72:661-669.

34. Tothill P. Dual-energy x-ray absorptiometry measurements of total-body bone mineral during weight change. J Clin Densitometry 2005;8(1):31-38.

35. Tothill P, Avenill A. Anomalies in the measurement of changes in bone mineral density of the spine by dual-energy x-ray absorptiometry. Calc Tissue Int 1998; 63:126-133.

36. Zemel BS, Leonard MB, Stallings VA. Evaluation of the Hologic experimental pediatric whole body analysis software in healthy children and children with chronic disease (Abstract). J Bone Miner Res 2000;15(Supp l1):S400.

37. Kelly TL. Pediatric whole body measurements J Bone Miner Res 2002;17(Suppl 1): Abstract#S296.

38. Hui SL, Gao S, Zhou XH, Johnston CC Jr, Lu Y, Gluer CC, Grampp S, Genant H. Universal standardization of bone density measurements: a method with optimal properties for calibration among several instruments. J Bone Miner Res 1997;12:1463–1470.

39. del Rio L, Carrascosa A, Pons F, Gusinye M, Yeste D, Domenech FM. Bone mineral density of the lumbar spine in white Mediterranean Spanish children and adolescents: Changes related to age, sex, and puberty. Pediatr Res 1994;35:362–366.

40. Glastre C, Braillon P, David L, Cochat P, Meunier PJ, Delmas PD. Measurement of bone mineral content of the lumbar spine by dual energy x-ray absorptiometry in normal children: correlations with growth parameters. J Clin Endocrinol Metab 1990;70:1330–1333.

41. Katzman DK, Bachrach LK, Carter DR, Marcus R. Clinical and anthropometric correlates of bone mineral acquisition in healthy adolescent girls. J Clin Endocrinol Metab 1991;73:1332–1339.

42. Lu PW, Briody JN, Ogle GD, et al. Bone mineral density of total body, spine, and femoral neck in children and young adults: a cross-sectional and longitudinal study. J Bone Miner Res 1994;9:1451–1458.

43. Southard RN, Morris JD, Mahan JD, et al. Bone mass in healthy children: Measurement with quantitative DXA. Radiology 1991;179:735–738.

44. Horlick M, Wang J, Pierson RN Jr, Thornton JC. Prediction models for evaluation of total-body bone mass with dual-energy x-ray absorptiometry among children and adolescents. Pediatrics 2004;114:337–345.

45. Plotkin H, Nunez M, Alvarez Filgueira ML, Zanchetta JR. Lumbar spine bone density in Argentine children. Calcif Tissue Int 1996;58:144–149.

46. Theintz G, Buchs B, Rizzoli R, Slosman D, Clavien H, Sizonenko PC, Bonjour JP. Longitudinal monitoring of bone mass accumulation in healthy adolescents: evidence for a marked reduction after 16 years of age at the levels of lumbar spine and femoral neck in female subjects. J Clin Endocrinol Metab 1992;75:1060–1065.

47. Nelson DA, Simpson PM, Johnson CC, Barondess DA, Kleerekoper M. The accumulation of whole body skeletal mass in third- and fourth-grade children: effects of age, gender, ethnicity, and body composition. Bone 1997;20:73–78.

48. Parfitt AM. Genetic effects on bone mass and turnover-relevance to black/white differences. J Am Coll Nutr 1997;16:325–333.

49. Pietrobelli A, Faith MS, Wang J, Brambilla P, Chiumello G, Heymsfield SB. Association of lean tissue and fat mass with bone mineral content in children and adolescents. Obes Res 2002;10:56–60.

50. Chan GM, Hoffman K, McMurry M. Effects of dairy products on bone and body composition in pubertal girls. J Pediatr 1995;126:551–556.

51. Sentipal JM, Wardlaw GM, Mahan J, Matkovic V. Influence of calcium intake and growth indexes on vertebral bone mineral density in young females. Am J Clin Nutr 1991;54:425–428.

52. Slemenda CW, Christian JC, Williams CJ, Norton JA, Johnston CC. Genetic determinants of bone mass in adult women: a reevaluation of the twin model and the potential importance of gene interaction in heritability estimates. J Bone Miner Res 1991;6:561–567.

53. Bailey DA, McKay HA, Mirwald RL, Crocker PR, Faulkner RA. A six-year longitudinal study of the relationship of physical activity to bone mineral accrual in growing children: The University of Saskatchewan bone mineral accrual study. J Bone Miner Res 1999;14:1672–1679.

54. Magarey AM, Boulton TJ, Chatterton BE, Schultz C, Nordin BE, Cockington RA. Bone growth from 11 to 17 years: relationship to growth, gender and changes with pubertal status including timing of menarche. Acta Paediatrica 1999;88:139–146.
55. Seeman E. From density to structure: growing up and growing old on the surfaces of bone. J Bone Miner Res 1997;12:509–521.
56. Seeman E, Hopper JL, Young NR, Formica C, Goss P, Tsalamandris C. Do genetic factors explain associations between muscle strength, lean mass, and bone density? A twin study. American Journal of Physiology 1996;270:E320–327.
57. Bachrach LK. Acquisition of optimal bone mass in childhood and adolescence. Trends Endocrinol Metab 2001;12:22–28.
58. Leib ES, Lewiecki EM, Binkley N, Hamdy RC. Official positions of the International Society for Clinical Densitometry. J Clin Densitom 2004;7:1–6.

4

Clinical Indications for the Use of DXA in Pediatrics

Laura K. Bachrach, MD,
Michael A. Levine, MD,
Christopher T. Cowell, MD,
and Nicholas J. Shaw, MB, ChB

CONTENTS

INTRODUCTION
RATIONALE FOR DXA STUDIES IN PEDIATRICS
POTENTIAL CANDIDATES FOR DXA
TIMING OF INITIAL DXA STUDIES
OPTIMAL TIMING FOR FOLLOW-UP STUDIES
REFINING INDICATIONS FOR PEDIATRIC DXAS
SUMMARY POINTS
REFERENCES

INTRODUCTION

The demand for bone mineral assessments in pediatrics has grown in the past decade. This trend likely reflects greater awareness of the importance of early bone health for osteoporosis prevention *(1,2)*. An estimated 60% of the variable risk of osteoporosis has been attributed to the magnitude of peak bone mass reached by early adulthood; the remaining 40% is explained by subsequent bone loss. Genetic factors, undernutrition, hormone disorders, medications, immobilization, and chronic illness during childhood and adolescence may compromise the rate at which bone size, mineral content, and quality are accrued *(1–3)*. If not reversed, this results in reduced peak bone, increasing the lifetime risk of osteoporotic fracture. In severely affected children, low-impact or fragility fractures can begin in childhood.

From: *Current Clinical Practice: Bone Densitometry in Growing Patients: Guidelines for Clinical Practice*
Edited by: A. J. Sawyer, L. K. Bachrach, and E. B. Fung © Humana Press Inc., Totowa, NJ

The demand for bone densitometry is not limited to children with chronic illness. At times, bone scans are ordered to evaluate osteopenia noted on conventional radiographs. Densitometry may also be ordered to assess bone mass in otherwise healthy children who sustain recurrent or low-impact fractures. The incidence of childhood fractures has risen by 35% in boys and 60% in girls during the past three decades *(4,5)*. This trend has raised concerns that pediatric bone health may be declining. Recent studies have observed that children who have sustained a forearm fracture have lower bone mass and a greater risk of future fracture than controls *(6–9)*.

The widespread availability, speed, and safety of dual-energy x-ray absorptiometry (DXA) have contributed to its greater use in pediatrics. However, despite the proliferation of pediatric bone studies, the specific indications for bone densitometry in clinical pediatric practice remain controversial. This chapter will review current evidence and expert opinion regarding which children warrant DXA examinations, how often these studies should be repeated, and how the results should be used to guide clinical management.

RATIONALE FOR DXA STUDIES IN PEDIATRICS

Bone densitometry is performed in adults to assess bone mass, a surrogate measure of bone strength and resistance to fracture. DXA results are used to determine if deficits in bone mineral are present, to predict the risk of osteoporotic fracture, to help identify which patients warrant therapy, and to monitor response to treatment. Although the rationale for performing DXAs in pediatrics is similar, the interpretation and clinical significance of bone densitometry in children and adolescents are more challenging than in older adults. As discussed in Chapter 7, the distinction between a normal or abnormal DXA result is dependent not only on the reference data used but also on the application of adjustments, if any, for bone size, weight, pubertal status, or other clinical variables. Furthermore, the clinical implications of low bone density in childhood are less certain than in adults.

The association between low bone mineral density (BMD) and fractures in older adults is sufficiently robust that the World Health Organization (WHO) has developed criteria for "osteopenia" and "osteoporosis" based on BMD T-scores alone (i.e., standard deviations above or below the mean for healthy young adults). The WHO criteria are not appropriate for use in children and young adults who have not yet achieved peak bone mass, as they will normally have negative T-scores *(10)*. There are insufficient data to determine a specific risk of fragility fracture based solely on bone mass in children and young adults. Furthermore, BMD alone does not explain fracture risk. Even in adults, bone quality, rates of bone turnover, and the nature of trauma also contribute to the risk of fracture. It is likely that these other factors are operational in children as well.

As discussed in detail in Chapters 3 and 5, several characteristics of DXA affect the reliability of this technique to assess bone density in growing children. Controversies surround the optimal way to correct for variables of bone size, maturity, and body composition. It would be ideal to select the methods that best predict fractures in childhood. This will be a difficult goal to achieve because the incidence of fractures is low; a very large study cohort would be needed to define the relationship between bone mass and fracture risk in children.

Table 1
Potential Clinical Indications for Dual-Energy X-Ray Absorptiometry
(DXA) Studies in Pediatrics

- Recurrent or low-trauma fracture
- Osteopenia diagnosed on conventional radiograph
- Chronic disease[a]
  - o Chronic inflammatory disease
  - o Hypogonadism
  - o Idiopathic juvenile osteoporosis
  - o Immobilization
  - o Long-term systemic glucocorticoid therapy
  - o Osteogenesis imperfecta
- Need for monitoring treatment effect

[a]Decision to perform DXA in an individual patient with these disorders should be influenced by disease severity and other clinical risk factors for poor bone health.

These complexities make it more challenging to use DXA to identify which children warrant therapy for bone fragility. Once these children are identified, there are challenging decisions regarding therapy because there are no approved pharmacological agents for the treatment of osteoporosis in pediatric patients. None of the drugs used to treat postmenopausal or steroid-induced osteoporosis in older patients have been adequately tested for safety and efficacy in children.

POTENTIAL CANDIDATES FOR DXA

Potential candidates for DXA include children with genetic disorders or chronic diseases associated with low bone mass, children with recurrent low-impact fractures, and those identified as having osteopenia on a standard radiograph (Table 1). This list should not be interpreted as a mandate for screening all young patients with these diagnoses; clinical judgment is needed to determine when DXA studies will influence clinical care for an individual child. Systematic screening for research purposes should be designated as an investigational study with appropriate informed consent.

Genetic Disorders and Chronic Diseases

Table 2 lists several of the genetic and acquired disorders that have been reported as associated with low bone mass and fragility fractures in children and adolescents. Most of the conditions listed in this table have been examined only in small convenience samples, many of which failed to consider delayed growth or maturity in interpreting results. Because of these limitations, it is not possible to predict with certainty the risk of low bone mass or fractures in each condition. It is beyond the scope of this chapter to provide a detailed discussion of these disorders, but reviews are available in the literature *(1,2,11)*, and specific disorder-related references are cited in the table.

Bone fragility in most of the heritable disorders results from defects in the bone matrix that affect the entire skeleton *(12–14)*. Osteogenesis imperfecta (OI) is the best example of these disorders, and given the variable expressivity of these genetic defects, there is a wide range of skeletal effects. Some patients show only asymptomatic low bone mass,

Table 2
Disorders Associated with Low Bone Mass and/or Fragility Fractures in Children and Adolescents

Genetic disorders *(12–14)*

- Ehlers-Danlos syndrome
- Fibrous dysplasia
- Gaucher's disease
- Galactosemia
- Glycogen storage diseases
- Homocystinuria
- Hypophosphatasia
- Marfan's syndrome
- Menke's kinky hair syndrome
- Osteogenesis imperfecta

Chronic disease

- Anorexia nervosa *(1,15–18)*
- Asthma *(19,20)*
- Celiac disease *(21,22)*
- Cystic fibrosis *(23)*
- Hematological diseases (i.e., talasemia and sickle cell anemia *[24]*)
- Inflammatory bowel disease *(25)*
- Malignancy (leukemia *[26–28]*)
- Posttransplantation *(29)*
- Renal failure *(30)*
- Rheumatological disorders *(31,32)*

Endocrine disorders

- Glucocorticoid excess (endogenous or iatrogenic) *(35,36)*
- Growth hormone deficiency *(37)*
- Hyperthyroidism *(38)*
- Hyperparathyroidism *(39)*
- Sex steroid deficiency or resistance *(1,40,41)*
- Type 1 diabetes *(42,43)*

Immobilization

- Cerebral palsy *(45)*
- Muscular dystrophy *(46)*
- Paraplegia *(47)*

Idiopathic juvenile osteoporosis *(48,49)*
Idiopathic adolescent scoliosis *(50)*
Disorders causing osteomalacia *(51)*

- Hypophosphatemic rickets *(52)*
- Vitamin D deficiency *(51)*
- Vitamin D resistance *(51,53)*

whereas others progress to chronic bone pain, recurrent fractures, and progressive skeletal deformity. In patients with fibrous dysplasia, total bone mass is not diminished, but fragility fractures occur at the site of lytic or cystic lesions.

Myriad acquired diseases have also been associated with low bone mass (15–32). Nearly all of these diverse disorders are associated with multiple threats to skeletal health. Malnutrition, vitamin D insufficiency, inadequate calcium intake or retention, immobility, deficiency of or resistance to sex steroids or growth hormone, and increased cytokines complicate many of these conditions (1,11). Glucocorticoids, chemotherapeutic agents, calcineurin inhibitors, and radiation therapy used to treat these disorders have also been implicated in causing poor bone health.

As with the genetic disorders, the severity of deficits in bone quantity and quality in chronic disease varies by diagnosis and within each diagnostic category. For example, children and adults with cystic fibrosis (CF) may have markedly reduced bone mass and low trauma fractures. Mean areal BMD Z-scores in some cohorts of patients with CF range from –1.2 to –1.9 for whole-body and femoral neck regions, with significant reductions in volumetric BMD (i.e., bone mineral apparent density [BMAD]) as well (23). The factors associated with low bone mass included disease severity, glucocorticoid use, hypogonadism, and undernutrition (23). By contrast, well nourished children with CF have normal BMD for age (33), and those with mild to moderate disease are no more prone to fracture than age-matched controls (34). Therefore, the decision to order a DXA scan must be based on clinical judgment of risk factors.

Endocrine Disorders (35–43)

Deficiency or excess of several hormones can limit bone mineral accrual and can contribute to bone loss. Skeletal findings range from mild decreases in bone density among children with type I diabetes (42,43) to clinically apparent fragility fractures among children with endogenous or exogenous glucocorticoid excess (35,36). The most common clinical concern is the skeletal effects of long-term systemic glucocorticoids prescribed for chronic disease, malignancy, or posttransplantation. The dose, route of administration, specific agent, and duration of glucocorticoid therapy influence the severity of the bone deficit. However, factors such as nutrition, activity, inflammation, and genetic variables appear to modify the skeletal response to chronic glucocorticoid excess as well. A recent study demonstrated that children with steroid-responsive nephrotic syndrome treated long-term with high-dose prednisone had similar bone mass to age-matched controls (44). These findings challenge the assumption that glucocorticoid excess inevitably leads to reduced bone mass.

Appropriate treatment to correct endocrine deficits (such as sex steroid therapy for ovarian failure) may be sufficient to prevent or restore deficits in bone mineral. In other cases, the potential for reversing the effects of an endocrine deficit or excess remains questionable.

Immobilization (45–47)

Mechanical loading of bone is a key determinant of bone strength. For children who are immobilized as a result of cerebral palsy, neuromuscular disorders, or congenital or posttraumatic spinal injury, inadequate accrual and increased loss of bone are inevitable. In many of these conditions, the adverse effects of immobilization may be compounded by co-existing deficiencies of calories, protein, calcium, or vitamin D intake and by the use of anticonvulsant therapy. Low bone mass and fragility fractures, particularly of the hip and lower extremities, are common in these disorders.

Idiopathic Juvenile Osteoporosis (48,49)

This rare disorder presents in prepubertal children as bone pain and fragility fractures of spine and long bones; low bone mass has been found when densitometry is performed. The diagnosis of idiopathic juvenile osteoporosis (IJO) is often made when other potential causes for bone fragility have been excluded. Because the etiology of IJO remains elusive, more than one defect may account for the disorder. Standard radiographs may be more helpful than DXA in differentiating IJO from mild OI. Absence of callus at fracture sites and radiolucent bands in metaphyseal regions (i.e., neo-osseus osteoporosis) are characteristic of IJO, whereas callus formation is normal at fracture sites in OI.

Scoliosis (50)

Low bone mass has been associated with spinal deformities in adolescents with idiopathic scoliosis (50). Both areal BMD of the spine and femur (as measured by DXA) and volumetric bone density of the radius and tibia (measured using quantitative computed tomography [QCT]) were reduced in girls with adolescent idiopathic scoliosis with values below −1 standard deviation (SD) in 36–38%. This observation has led to speculation that reduced bone mass may contribute to the development of spinal deformity.

Rickets and Osteomalacia (51–53)

Rickets in children with open epiphyses (or osteomalacia in adults with closed epiphyses) is characterized by delayed or deficient mineralization of newly formed bone matrix. Thus, rickets differs from the conditions listed previously, in which the matrix is mineralized but bone mass is reduced. Worldwide, the most common causes of rickets is vitamin D deficiency. Genetic or acquired causes of phosphorous or calcium deficiency, as well as defects in vitamin D metabolism or action, can also cause rickets.

Rickets cannot be distinguished from osteoporosis by DXA because bone mineral may be reduced for age in both circumstances. Overt skeletal manifestations, including bowing of the legs in younger children, craniotabes, rib cage deformity, and painful swelling of the metaphyses of the most rapidly growing bones (e.g., the distal wrist), may be helpful in identifying rickets. Biochemical markers such as elevated serum alkaline phosphatase or reduced phosphorus, calcium, or 25-hydroxyvitamin D help in the diagnosis. In the absence of these clinical and biochemical findings, it may be necessary to perform a bone biopsy to differentiate between rickets and osteoporosis.

Childhood Fractures

Fractures can occur in otherwise normal children; the distal forearm is the most common site (6–9). The incidence of fractures peaks between 9 and 12 yr of age in females and between 12 and 14 yr in males, coinciding with the pubertal growth spurt (54). Because peak bone growth precedes peak bone mineral accrual by 6–12 mo, the skeleton in early adolescence may be relatively undermineralized and more susceptible to fracture with trauma. Several studies have compared the BMD of "normal" children and adolescents with fractures to that of age-matched controls without fractures. Most (6–9), but not all (55,56), studies have found mean BMD to be significantly lower in children with forearm fractures than in controls. Differences between cases and controls averaged 3–6% at the spine, trochanter, and total body, and a higher percent of those with fractures had BMD Z-scores below –1. Skaggs et al. *(57)* found that bone cross-sectional area (measured by QCT) was also smaller in girls with a history of low-impact forearm fracture than in controls.

Children who sustain one forearm fracture appear to be at increased risk to sustain subsequent fractures. In longitudinal study, Goulding et al. *(7)* found that 29% of the subjects with a fracture at study entry had at least one subsequent fracture during the next 4 yr as compared with only 8% of the control subjects. The risk of future fracture was estimated to increase 1.5- to 2-fold for each SD that total body, spine, or hip BMD fell below the mean *(7,9)*. Other risk factors for future fractures included high body weight and low spine BMAD, an estimate of volumetric BMD *(7)*. Low BMD has been linked to fractures at the forearm but not at the hand, upper arm, or other skeletal sites *(9)*.

Recurrent fractures and fractures that occur with minimal trauma may warrant investigation with DXA. A low-impact fracture is defined as one occurring from standing height or less *(4)*. A detailed history of the nature of the injury is important, however, to assess the direction and magnitude of the force associated with the fracture *(4)*. For example, some fractures from standing height, such as those occurring during soccer or other vigorous sports, involve significant impact or torsion and may not qualify as low-impact.

Vertebral compression fractures are far less common than extremity fractures in childhood. Spine fractures may indicate a marked deficit in bone quality, quantity, or both, particularly if other risk factors such as chronic glucocorticoid exposure are present. Bone densitometry is warranted in these patients to assess bone mass at nonvertebral sites and to establish a baseline measure prior to treatment. BMD may be increased in areas of compression as an artifact of the collapsed vertebrae. For this reason, fracture sites should be excluded when analyzing a DXA scan of the spine.

Osteopenia on Conventional X-Ray

Standard radiographs are an insensitive tool for assessing bone mineral; an estimated decrease of 30–40% must occur before osteopenia is detected. For this reason, pediatric patients found to have low bone mass on standard radiograph may warrant a DXA scan if there are other identifiable risk factors for poor bone health. Osteopenia can be an incidental finding on a chest or abdominal x-ray taken for nonskeletal indications or reported on a radiograph ordered because of bone pain or trauma. Unfortunately, there is a poor correlation between osteopenia on conventional x-ray and DXA measures of bone mass.

TIMING OF INITIAL DXA STUDIES

Increased use of DXA for pediatric clinical research has led to the extensive list of conditions that are associated with low bone mass or fractures in childhood. Unfortunately, this research is not sufficient to establish evidence-based indications for performing pediatric DXA scans in clinical practice *(58–61)*. Without systematic screening of large numbers of children with the same diagnosis, the prevalence and severity of low bone density and fractures cannot be established. Little is known about the frequency of fragility fractures in these conditions because cohort size is often too small to determine

Table 3
Published Recommendations for Bone Density Testing for Specific Disorders

Disorder	Recommendation
Cystic fibrosis (62)	Baseline DXA by age 18
	DXA before age 18 if risk factors exist
	(i.e., malnutrition, delayed puberty, or glucocorticoids)
	If normal at baseline, repeat every 2–5 yr
	If low at baseline, repeat yearly
Survivor of childhood cancer (63)	Baseline DXA at age 18
	Consider earlier screening if clinically indicated
	Repeat as clinically indicated

DXA, dual-energy x-ray absorptiometry.

if fractures exceed the expected incidence for age. Larger studies are also needed to determine with certainty the clinical factors associated with greatest risk of poor bone health. Until further research is available, recommendations for who to screen by DXA and how frequently to repeat the studies represent expert opinion rather than evidence-based indications.

For a few disorders, subspecialty panels have developed recommendations for DXA examinations based on analysis of the available literature by assembled experts. For example, a consensus conference report on bone health in CF has recommended that all patients have a baseline DXA scan of the spine no later than age 18 (62). Densitometry was advised for younger patients with CF who have clinical risk factors such as evidence of undernutrition, delayed puberty, hypogonadism, or severe lung disease or with post-organ transplantation status. The guidelines recommended repeat DXA scans every 2–5 yr if the baseline was normal and yearly scans for patients with the identified risk factors. Table 3 summarizes the published guidelines for two chronic disorders (62,63).

For disorders in which specific recommendations have not been established, the decision to perform a DXA scan should be based on clinical judgment of risk. The lengthy list of disorders linked to low bone mass (Table 2) is derived from clinical research studies. Routine DXA screening in each of these conditions is not mandated. The decision to perform a DXA scan in an individual patient is influenced by disease severity, immobility, bone pain, skeletal deformity, malnutrition, or use of medications known to adversely affect bone. As with any test in clinical practice, bone density testing should be done only when it is likely to influence patient management. For example, a DXA would be indicated if results would modify the decision to initiate therapy. If treatment is initiated, a DXA is appropriate to establish a baseline measurement for monitoring the response to therapy.

The potential value of DXA must be weighed against impediments to obtaining useful information from the scan. If the child is too young to remain still or if normative data are not available for the age and gender of the child at specific skeletal sites, DXA may not be successful or useful. Children over the age of 5 yr can usually cooperate long enough to permit DXA studies using rapid fan beam DXA systems. For younger children, the lack of normative data and the need for sedation make densitometry more challenging and potentially less valuable. Immobilized patients and children with more severe forms of

OI may have skeletal deformities that prevent proper positioning. Performing densitometry in these children with special considerations is discussed in Chapter 9.

The information to be gained from DXA must also be weighed against the risk of misinterpretation. Bone densitometry in children requires specialized skill and attention to avoid errors in acquiring or interpreting densitometry data, as outlined in Chapters 3 and 5. The most serious errors involve reporting T-scores and the WHO criteria for osteoporosis and osteopenia in patients under age 20. Younger patients who have not yet reached peak bone mass are often identified as abnormal by these criteria, causing unwarranted concern and potentially exposing them to inappropriate treatment. Failure to adjust for delayed maturation or bone size and failure to use gender-specific normative data also contribute to the overdiagnosis of low bone mass (64). To avoid these diagnostic errors, the clinician should arrange for DXA studies to be performed in DXA centers with established expertise in pediatric densitometry. If that cannot be arranged, DXA results should be reviewed for accuracy by an experienced pediatric DXA consultant.

Panels of bone specialists in the United Kingdom (58,59), the United States (60), and Canada (61) have attempted to develop standardized indications for bone densitometry. The suggested indications for pediatric DXA included presence of a chronic condition (such as chronic inflammatory disorders, hypogonadism, immobilization, OI, or long-term systemic glucocorticoid use) in conjunction with "low-trauma or recurrent fractures, back pain, spinal deformity or loss of height, change in mobility status, or malnutrition" (58,59). In a consensus statement for men, women, and children, the International Society for Clinical Densitometry (60) recommended DXA scans in "any individual being considered for pharmacological therapy, any individual being treated in order to monitor treatment effect, or any individuals not receiving therapy in whom evidence of bone loss would lead to treatment." The Canadian standards suggest that "bone densitometry may be helpful in assessing skeletal health in children using glucocorticoids or those with chronic disease, radiographic evidence of osteopenia, or recurrent low-impact fractures" (61).

Selecting the skeletal region or regions to scan will depend on technical considerations and the clinical indications for the study. Careful positioning and consistent repositioning are required to complete scans for the spine, proximal hip, and whole body. In addition, scanning of more than one site will require increased time. Based on these limitations, it may not be appropriate or possible to study all three sites in younger children. Skeletal sites with permanent hardware such as a rod or pin should not be scanned. As discussed in Chapter 5, the lumbar spine and whole body are preferred sites in children because of the precision and published reference norms. The vertebrae contain considerable trabecular bone, which is selectively lost in response to glucocorticoid excess and hypogonadism. By contrast, the whole body is comprised largely of cortical bone, which is reduced in growth hormone deficiency, hyperthyroidism, and hyperparathyroidism.

As in adults, the primary goals of DXA for children and adolescents include monitoring the bone health of high-risk patients, identifying those at greatest risk for fracture, and assessing responses to therapy. Because a certain relationship between bone density and fracture has not been established in younger populations, the diagnosis of osteoporosis should not be made in children and adolescents solely on the basis of densitometric criteria alone. Conversely, a child with vertebral compression fractures or fractures with minimal trauma has evidence of osteoporosis and may not require bone densitometry for confirmation of low BMD by DXA.

OPTIMAL TIMING FOR FOLLOW-UP STUDIES

A key factor determining the timing of follow-up is the precision or reproducibility of the densitometry measurement *(65,66)*, discussed in detail in Chapter 3. Bone mass changes slowly, and the variability in repeated measures of bone density can exceed the rate of change in bone mass. Therefore, the precision of the measurement factors into the decision regarding timing of repeat DXA studies. Variability in repeated measurements can occur in the same individual on the same day. This reflects both the limitations of DXA machinery and software as well as differences in density that are due to errors in repositioning the patient.

Precision is routinely expressed in terms of the number of SDs by which repeated measurements vary from the mean of multiple measurements. Alternately, precision can be described in terms of the percent coefficient of variation (%CV). In the hands of a skilled technician, the %CV for repeated DXA measurements at spine and whole body is less than 1%. The more precise the measurement, the smaller the change in bone density that can be detected with certainty. Least-significant change (LSC) is a term describing the minimum increase or decrease between serial DXA measurements that exceeds the variability of the technique itself. This is typically defined as $2.8 \times \%CV$. The absolute or percent change in BMD meeting the definition of LSC varies both with the precision (i.e., the %CV) of the technique and with the level of statistical confidence desired (i.e., 80–95%). For most sites studied, a true change in bone density will have to be at least 3% to exceed the error of the technique.

In adults, the recommended interval between repeat DXA studies is long enough that the LSC is likely to have occurred. The monitoring time interval (MTI) is an estimate of the minimal time required to be able to detect a meaningful change in bone mineral using a particular densitometric technique *(65)*. The MTI is derived mathematically by factoring in both the LSC and the expected rate of change per year *(65)*.

Although estimates of MTI would be valuable in guiding pediatric DXA practice, establishing this parameter for pediatric patients is far more challenging than it is for adults. Yearly rates of bone mineral accrual vary considerably through childhood and adolescence, with the greatest gains occurring several months after peak height velocity *(67)*. Given the rapid changes in bone size and mineral during the adolescent growth spurt, the MTI would potentially be shortened, but this has not been established. In the absence of data, adult guidelines for the timing of repeat studies are applied to younger patients. To repeat a DXA study more frequently than every 12 mo is rarely warranted except for clinical research, to monitor response to new drug intervention, or to monitor rapidly worsening clinical status. However, a longer interval between repeat scans may be appropriate if the baseline DXA indicates normal bone mineral for age. Continued threats to bone health such as ongoing glucocorticoid therapy, immobilization, malnutrition, or organ transplantation may prompt a yearly follow-up study to monitor bones more closely and to assess the rate of bone gain or loss.

REFINING INDICATIONS FOR PEDIATRIC DXAS

The demand for densitometry in children is likely to increase in coming years. The US Surgeon General's Report on Osteoporosis and Bone Health underscores the importance of early skeletal health and outlines the causes of pediatric bone fragility. The increase in fracture rates among children over the past three decades has also raised awareness and concern about the bone health of today's youth. Finally, the growing number of long-term survivors of childhood malignancy or organ transplantation will add to the pool of candidates for bone densitometry.

Further research is needed to make pediatric densitometry a more valuable tool for the clinician. Standardized pediatric DXA reference data collected using current software and equipment would reduce variability in Z-scores. This would provide a more uniform definition of low bone mass. Studies are also needed to establish the best approach to adjust for bone size, maturity, body composition, and other clinical variables. Ideally, it will be possible for each of these methods to be evaluated against a gold standard of predicting clinical bone fragility.

SUMMARY POINTS

- Bone densitometry is performed to determine if deficits in bone mineral are present, to identify those at greatest risk for fracture, to help identify which patients warrant therapy, and to monitor response to treatment.
- Specific indications for bone densitometry in clinical pediatric practice remain controversial because there are insufficient data to derive evidence-based recommendations.
- Potential candidates for DXA include children with genetic disorders or chronic diseases associated with low bone mass; children with recurrent fractures, low-impact fractures, or vertebral compression fracture; and those identified as having osteopenia on a standard radiograph.
- For a few disorders, subspecialty panels have developed recommendations for DXA examinations based on the available literature and expert opinion.
- For disorders in which specific recommendations have not been established, the decision to perform an initial bone densitometry scan is based on clinical factors such disease severity, bone pain, skeletal deformity, or history of fragility fracture.
- Clinical DXA scans should be performed only if the results will influence patient management.
- A decision to perform a follow-up DXA depends on initial findings and interval risk factors. To perform a repeat DXA scan more frequently than every 12 mo is rarely warranted except in the setting of a research study, new drug intervention, or rapidly worsening clinical status.
- DXA studies should be performed in DXA centers with established expertise in pediatric densitometry to avoid misinterpretation of data.
- Potential impediments to obtaining useful information from DXA should be considered before ordering a scan. These include a child unable to cooperate without sedation, lack of normative data for the age group of the patient, or skeletal deformities that will prevent proper positioning.

REFERENCES

1. Soyka LA, Fairfield WP, Klibanski A. Hormonal determinants and disorders of peak bone mass in children. J Clin Endocrinol Metab 2000;85:3951–3963.
2. Heaney RP, Abrams S, Dawson-Hughes B, et al. Peak bone mass. Osteoporosis Int 2002;11:985–1009.
3. Mora S, Gilsanz V. Establishment of peak bone mass. Endocrinol Metab Clin N Am 2003;32:39–63.
4. Landin LA. Fracture patterns in children. Analysis of 8682 fractures with special reference to incidence, etiology and secular changes in a Swedish urban population 1950–1979. Acta Orthop Scand Suppl 1983;202:1–109.
5. Khosla S, Melton LJ III, Dekutoski MB, Achenbach SJ, Oberg AL, Riggs BL. Incidence of childhood distal forearm fractures over 30 years. A population-based study. JAMA 2003;290:1479–1485.

6. Chan GM, Hess M, Hollis J. Book LS. Bone mineral status in childhood accidental fractures. Amer J Dis Child 1984;138:569–570.

7. Goulding A, Jones IE, Taylor RW, Manning PJ, Williams SM. More broken bones: a 4-year double cohort study of young girls with and without distal forearm fractures. J Bone Miner Res 2000;15: 2011–2018.

8. Goulding A, Jones IE, Taylor RW, Williams SM, Manning PJ. Bone mineral density and body composition in boys with distal forearm fractures: a dual-energy x-ray absorptiometry study. J Pediatr 2001;139:509–515.

9. Ma DQ, Jones G. The association between bone mineral density, metacarpal morphometry, and upper limb fractures in children: a population-based case-control study. J Clin Endocrinol Metab 2003;88:1486–1491.

10. The Writing Group for the ISCD Position Development Conference. Diagnosis of osteoporosis in men, premenopausal women, and children. J Clin Densitom 2004;7:17–26.

11. Ward LM, Glorieux FH. The spectrum of pediatric osteoporosis. In Glorieux FH, Pettifor JM, Juppner H (eds) Pediatric Bone: Biology and Diseases. San Diego, CA: Academic 2003, pp. 401–442.

12. Whyte MP. Osteogenesis imperfecta, in Favus M. Primer on Metabolic Diseases and Disorders of Mineral Metabolism. Washington, DC: American Society for Bone and Mineral Research, 2003; pp. 470–473.

13. Collins MT, Bianco P. Fibrous dysplasia, in Favus M. Primer on Metabolic Diseases and Disorders of Mineral Metabolism. Washington, DC: American Society for Bone and Mineral Research, 2003;466–470.

14. Glorieux, FH, Pettifor, JM, Juppner H, eds. Pediatric Bone: Biology and Diseases. San Diego: Academic, 2003.

15. Lucas AR, Melton LJ 3rd, Crowson CS, O'Fallon WM. Long-term fracture risk among women with anorexia nervosa: A population-based cohort study. Mayo Clin Proc 1999;74:972–977.

16. Seeman E, Karlsson MK, Duan Y. On exposure to anorexia nervosa, the temporal variation in axial and appendicular skeletal development predisposes to site-specific deficits in bone size and density: a cross-sectional study. J Bone Miner Res 2000;15:2259–2265.

17. Zipfel S, Seibel MJ, Lowe B, Beumont PJ, Kasperk C, Herzog W. Osteoporosis in eating disorders: a follow-up study of patients with anorexia and bulimia nervosa. J Clin Endocrinol Metab 2001;86:5227–5233.

18. Soyka LA, Misra M, Frenchman A, et al. Abnormal bone mineral accrual in adolescent girls with anorexia nervosa. J Clin Endocrinol Metab 2002;87:4177–4185.

19. Leone FT, Fish JE, Szefler SJ, West SL. Systematic review of the evidence regarding potential complications of inhaled corticosteroid use in asthma. Chest 2003;124:2329–2340.

20. Kelly HW, Strunk RC, Donithan M, Bloomberg GR, McWilliams BC, Szefler S. Growth and bone density in children with mild-moderate asthma: a cross-sectional study in children entering the Childhood Asthma Management Program (CAMP) J Pediatr 2003;142:286–291.

21. Bayer M, Stepan JJ, Sedlackova M, Wergedal JE, Kutilek S. Spinal bone mineral density in children with celiac disease. J Clin Densitometry 1998;1:125–136.

22. Mora S, Barera G, Beccio S, et al. A prospective, longitudinal study of the long-term effect of treatment on bone density in children with celiac disease. J Pediatr 2001;139:516–521.

23. Bhudhikanok GS, Lim J, Marcus R, Harkins A, Moss RB, Bachrach LK. Correlates of osteopenia in patients with cystic fibrosis. Pediatrics 1996;97:103–111.

24. Tiosano D, Hochberg Z. Endocrine complications of thalassemia. J Endocrinol Invest. 2001;24:716–723.

25. Vestergaard P. Bone loss associated with gastrointestinal disease: prevalence and pathogenesis. Eur J Gastro Hep 2003;15:851–856.

26. Arikosko P, Komulainen J, Riikonen P, Voutilainen R, Knip M, Kroger H. Alterations in bone turnover and impaired development of bone mineral density in newly diagnosed children with cancer: a 1-year prospective study. J Clin Endocrinol Metab 1999;84:3174–3181.

27. van der Sluis IM, van den Heuvel-Eibrink MM, Hahlen K, Krenning EP, de Muinck Keizer-Schrama SMPF. Altered bone mineral density and body composition, and increased fracture risk in childhood acute lymphoblastic leukemia. J Pediatr 2002;141:204–210.

28. Rose SR. Endocrinopathies in childhood cancer survivors. Endocrinologist 2003;13:488–495.

29. Daniels MW, Wilson DM, Paguntalan HG, Hoffman AR, Bachrach LK. Bone mineral density in pediatric transplant recipients. Transplantation 2003;6:673–678.

30. Kuizon BD, Salusky IB. Renal osteodystrophy: pathogenesis, diagnosis and treatment. In: Glorieux FH, Pettifor JM, Juppner H, eds. Pediatric Bone—Biology and Diseases. Boston: Academic, 2003;679–701.

31. Kotaniemi A, Savolainen A, Kroger H, Kautiainen H, Isomaki H. Development of bone mineral density at the lumbar spine and femoral neck in juvenile chronic arthritis—a prospective one year followup study. J Rheumatology 1998;25:2450–2455.

32. Bianchi ML, Cimaz R, Bardare M, et al. Efficacy and safety of alendronate for the treatment of osteoporosis in diffuse connective tissue diseases in children. Arth Rheum 2000;43:1960–1966.
33. Mortensen LA, Chan GM, Alder SC, Marshall BC. Bone mineral status in prepubertal children with cystic fibrosis. J Pediatr 2000;136:648–652.
34. Rovner AJ, Zemel BS, Leonard MB, Schall JI, Stallings VA. Mild to moderate cystic fibrosis is not associate with increased fracture risk in children and adolescents. J Pediatr 2005;147:327–331.
35. Leong GM, Center JR, Henderson NK, Eisman JA. Glucocorticoid-induced osteoporosis, in Marcus R, Feldman D, Kelsey J, eds. Osteoporosis. San Diego: Academic, 2001;169–193.
36. Khanine V, Fournier JJ, Requeda E, Luton JP, Simon F, Crouzet J. Osteoporotic fractures at presentation of Cushing's disease: two case reports and a literature review. Joint Bone Spine 2000;67:341–345.
37. Baroncelli GI, Bertelloni S, Sondini F, Saggese G. Lumbar bone mineral density at final height and prevalence of fractures in treated children with GH deficiency. J Clin Endocrinol Metab 2002;87:3624–3631.
38. Lucidarme N, Ruiz JC, Czernichow P, Leger J. Reduced bone mineral density at diagnosis and bone mineral recovery during treatment in children with Graves' disease. J Pediatr 2000;137:56–62.
39. Boechat MMI, Westra SJ, Van Dop C, Kaufman F, Gilsanz V, Roe TF. Decreased cortical and increased cancellous bone in two children with primary hyperparathyroidism. Metabolism 1996;45:76–81.
40. Riggs LB, Khosla S, Melton LJ. Sex steroids and the construction and conservation of the adult skeleton. Endocrine Rev 2002;23:279–302.
41. Miller KK, Klibanski A. Amenorrheic bone loss. J Clin Endocrinol Metab 1999;84:1775–1783.
42. Moyer-Mileur LJ, Dixon SB, Quick JL, Askew EW, Murray MA. Bone mineral acquisition in adolescents with type I diabetes. J Pediatr 2004;145:662–669.
43. Brown SA, Sharpless JL. Osteoporosis: an under-appreciated complication of diabetes. Clin Diab 2004;22:10–20.
44. Leonard ML, Feldman HI, Shults J, Zemel BS, Foster BJ, Stallings VA. High-dose chronic glucocorticoids and bone mineral content in childhood steroid-sensitive nephrotic syndrome. N Engl J Med 2004;351:868–875.
45. Henderson RC, Lin PP, Greene WB. Bone-mineral density in children and adolescents who have spastic cerebral palsy. J Bone Joint Surg 1995;77A:1671–1681.
46. Bianchi ML, Mazzanti A, Galbiati E, et al. Bone mineral density and bone metabolism in Duchenne muscular dystrophy. Osteoporosis Int 2003;14:761–767.
47. Kiratli BJ. Immobilization osteopenia, in Marcus R, Feldman D, Kelsey J, eds. Osteoporosis. San Diego: Academic, 2001;207–227.
48. Krassas GE. Idiopathic juvenile osteoporosis. Ann N Y Acad Sci 2000;900:409–412.
49. Rauch F, Travers R, Norman ME, Taylor A, Parfitt AM, Glorieux FH. Deficient bone formation in idiopathic juvenile osteoporosis: a histomorphometric study of cancellous iliac bone. J Bone Miner Res 2000;15:957–963.
50. Cheng JCY, Qin L, Cheung CSK, et al. Generalized low areal and volumetric bone mineral density in adolescent idiopathic scoliosis. J Bone Miner Res 2000;15:1587–1595.
51. Harrison HE, Harrison HC. Disorders of Calcium and Phosphate Metabolism in Childhood and Adolescence. Philadelphia: W.B. Saunders, 1979.
52. Levine B-S, Carpenter TO. Evaluation and treatment of heritable forms of rickets. Endocrinologist 1999;9:358–365.
53. Malloy PJ, Pike JW, Feldman D. The vitamin D receptor and the syndrome of hereditary 1,25-dihydroxyvitamin D-resistant rickets. Endocrine Rev 1999;20:156–188.
54. Bailey DA, Wedge JH, McCulloch RG, Martin AD, Bernhardson SC. Epidemiology of fractures of the distal end of the radius in children as associated with growth. J Bone Joint Surg 1989;1A:1225–1231.
55. Blimkie CJR, Lefevre J, Beunen GP, Renson R, Dequeker J, Van Damme P. Fractures, physical activity and growth velocity in adolescent Belgian boys. Med Sci Sports Exerc 1992;25:801–808.
56. Cook SD, Harding AF, Morgan EL, et al. Association of bone mineral density and pediatric fractures. J Pediatr Orthoped 1987;7:424–477.
57. Skaggs DL, Loro ML, Pitukcheewanont P, Tolo V, Gilsanz V. Increased body weight and decreased radial cross-sectional dimensions in girls with forearm fractures. J Bone Miner Res 2001;16:1337–1342.
58. Adams J, Shaw N, eds. A Practical Guide to Bone Densitometry in Children. Camerton, Bath, UK: National Osteoporosis Society, 2004.
59. Fewtrell MS, British Paediatric & Adolescent Bone Group. Bone densitometry in children assessed by dual x-ray absorptiometry: uses and pitfalls. Arch Dis Child 2003;88:795–798.
60. The Writing Group for the ISCD Position Development Conference. Indications and reporting for dual-energy x-ray absorptiometry. J Clin Densitometry 2004;7:37–44.

61. Khan AA, Bachrach L, Brown JP, et al., Canadian Panel of the International Society of Clinical Densitometry. Standards and guidelines for performing central dual-energy x-ray absorptiometry in premenopausal women, men, and children. J Clin Densitometry 2004;7:51–63.
62. Cystic Fibrosis Foundation Consensus Conferences. Concepts in care: Guide to bone health and disease in cystic fibrosis, vol. X, sec. 4. Bethesda, MD: Cystic Fibrosis Foundation, 2002.
63. Hudson MM, Landier W, Eshelman D, et al. The COG Late Effects Committee and Nursing Discipline. Childhood cancer survivor long-term follow-up guidelines, version 1.1. Children's Oncology Group, September 2003. Available online at http://www.childrensoncologygroup.org/disc/le.
64. Leonard MB, Propert KJ, Zemel BS, Stallings VA, Feldman HI. Discrepancies in pediatric bone mineral density reference data: potential for misdiagnosis of osteopenia. J Pediatr 1999;135:182–188.
65. Stewart A, Reid DM. Precision of quantitative ultrasound: comparison of three commercial scanners. Bone 2000;27:139–143.
66. Bonnick SL, Johnston CC, Jr., Kleerekoper M, et al. Importance of precision in bone density measurements. J Clin Densitomtry 2001;4:105–110.
67. Bailey DA, McKay HA, Mirwald RL, Crocker PRE, Faulkner RA. A six-year longitudinal study of the relationship of physical activity to bone mineral accrual in growing children: The University of Saskatchewan Bone Mineral Accrual Study. J Bone Miner Res 1999;14:1672–1679.

5

Acquisition of DXA in Children and Adolescents

Nicola J. Crabtree, PhD, MSc, BSc(Hons), Kyla Kent, BS, and Babette S. Zemel, PhD

CONTENTS

INTRODUCTION
GENERAL
SKELETAL SITES TO BE STUDIED
SPINE SCANS
WHOLE-BODY SCANS
HIP SCANS
OTHER SITES
INTERFERENCE
SUMMARY POINTS
REFERENCES

INTRODUCTION

The aim of this chapter is to provide the operator with the basic information required to achieve a good-quality dual-energy x-ray absorptiometry (DXA) scan. Topics such as patient preparation, standard scan acquisition, and typical acquisition problems are discussed. This information is intended to supplement instructions provided in operator manuals and individual department protocols.

GENERAL

Information Prior to Scan

Essential to acquiring a good-quality DXA evaluation is the exchange of information prior to the scan. It is helpful to provide the child and guardian with adequate information about the risks and comfort level of the procedure. It can be helpful to include a picture or diagram of the machine in the appointment letter and also to clarify that no needles or injections are required and that radiation exposure is typically lower than daily exposure

From: *Current Clinical Practice: Bone Densitometry in Growing Patients: Guidelines for Clinical Practice*
Edited by: A. J. Sawyer, L. K. Bachrach, and E. B. Fung © Humana Press Inc., Totowa, NJ

from the environment (Chapter 3). This will help the parent or guardian explain the procedure and will also, hopefully, allay any fears the child or parent may have about the test.

It is equally important for the referring clinician to provide sufficient clinical history to the DXA operator. Specifically, the requisition for densitometry should include the reason for the test, relevant information about diseases or medications, and unusual aspects of the physical exam (e.g., short stature, delayed maturation, or metal implants). The ordering physician should also alert the operator to any potential problems such as mental or physical difficulties that may either prevent the scan being performed or require sedation or modification of standard practice (Chapter 9). A sample requisition questionnaire for collecting such clinical data is provided in Appendix D at the end of this volume.

Room Preparation

As with any investigation involving children, it is important to ensure that the environment is child-friendly. The use of colorful pictures and soft toys will make the scanning room more appealing to a young child and, hence, will make it easier for the child to relax and cooperate during the scan. Maintaining a low noise level and limiting the number of persons in the room also improves cooperation.

Patient Preparation

Prior to scanning, height and weight should be recorded in light indoor clothes after removal of shoes and any highly attenuating objects that may cause image artifacts such as clothing with metal zippers or buckles, bras with metal clasps or underwires, and body jewelry (e.g., umbilical rings) that would be in the scanning region. To achieve high-quality results, the child should be scanned in light indoor clothes or in a hospital gown. Multiple layers of clothing may lead to a poor-quality scan and may inhibit the operator from noticing possible artifacts underneath clothing layers.

The operator should put the child at ease by offering an explanation suitable to his or her level of understanding. The operator should also explain the procedure to the parent or guardian, as they are often in the best position to assist and to reassure the child. Throughout the scan, the operator should keep the child informed of what he or she is doing, of what the scanner will do, of the noises the scanner will make, and of how long each scan and the entire procedure will take.

Performing the Scan

The goal is to obtain a scan with the child in an ideal scanning position that can be easily reproduced at follow-up visit. However, this is not always possible. Younger children and those with special needs require adaptations to standard protocols (also discussed in Chapter 9). It is important to assess the child's cooperation prior to starting the scan to avoid any unnecessary radiation exposure caused by having to repeat unusable acquisitions.

YOUNGER INFANTS (0–9 MO)

Young infants are among the hardest patients to scan. However, some general guidelines are useful. Before scanning a baby, ask the caregiver to feed and settle the infant and to place him or her on the scanning table in a clean diaper (1). If necessary, the child can be wrapped in a thin cotton sheet to reduce any small involuntary movements. Room lighting should be subdued to help the baby relax. If it is possible to settle the child, he or she might sleep through the scan, therefore requiring little operator intervention, although some will startle with the movement of the machine. It is important to constantly watch the child for any involuntary movements. If the operator is unable to settle the infant, it is reasonable to reschedule the scan to avoid unnecessary radiation exposure.

OLDER INFANTS (AGED 9 –36 MO) AND TODDLERS

Older infants and toddlers are unlikely to settle easily or to be able to follow instructions. At this age, some children can be quieted by being allowed to watch television while they are being positioned on the table. Having a parent next to the child is also calming.

However, 9- to 36-mo-olds are difficult to scan because they are often frightened by the equipment and unfamiliar faces. Therefore, the easiest way to scan this group is with light sedation. This must be performed in departments with full resuscitation facilities. Different hospitals will have different sedation procedures, and local protocol should be used at all times. Once the child is sedated, scan acquisition should follow standard scanning procedures, taking extra care that any monitors or lines that are required for the sedation do not overlie the region of interest. Special consideration should be given to this age group to ensure that the benefit of the results from a DXA scan far outweigh the risks of sedation.

CHILDREN (3–12 YR)

Sedation is not usually necessary in children over the age of 3 yr; an explanation of the procedure is generally sufficient to reassure the child. The promise of a treat, such as a sticker or certificate, at the end of the scan may also help. Once the child is settled and acquisition has started, it is essential to continually remind him or her to stay still. If it is necessary to gently hold the child, the operator should be aware of where the x-ray tube is located and should keep his or her hands away from the x-ray path.

TEENAGERS (13–18 YR)

This age group is theoretically the easiest to scan as they have a greater understanding of the procedure and can usually follow instruction. However, there are some special considerations that should be noted. Teenagers may or may not wish their parent or guardian to be present. They are typically more modest and may be reluctant to undress and put on a hospital gown. Some may have body piercings, and if these were obtained recently, teenagers will be particularly reluctant to remove them for the scanning procedure. For females who have attained menarche, the possibility of pregnancy must be considered.

Many of these issues can be addressed with an appropriate information leaflet sent along with the appointment letter or provided just prior to the scan. Subjects can be advised to wear light indoor clothing without zippers or metal closures and to remove any jewelry within the region being scanned (such as an umbilical ring, if a spine scan is ordered). Local procedures should be applied regarding the potential for radiation exposure and pregnancy. Some facilities will require a negative serum or urine pregnancy test prior to the scan, whereas others will accept a written or oral statement from the patient that she is not pregnant.

After the Scan

After successful acquisition of the bone densitometry scan:

- If appropriate, reward the child for cooperating with a sticker or certificate.

- If possible, let the patient and parent see the acquired scan on the screen to help them understand the procedure. Providing a copy of the whole-body scan, without analysis, often delights children.
- Inform the parents or guardians of how the results of the scan will be transmitted.

SKELETAL SITES TO BE STUDIED

DXA can be used to measure many skeletal sites. In deciding which region or regions of interest to scan, it is important to consider the following:

- Availability of reference data for the acquired region;
- Reproducibility and precision of the site to be scanned, and any nonstandard sites or techniques;
- Clinical information to be gained;
- Radiation exposure (Chapter 3, Table 1);
- The clinical or research question to be addressed by the scan.

All DXA manufactures provide standard procedures for scan acquisition, and these should be followed as closely as possible. However, the operator also should be aware of the points addressed in the following subsections.

Patient Position

If possible, the child should be positioned according to standard manufacturer's guidelines, ensuring that he or she is comfortable and is able to maintain the position for the duration of the scan. Measurement precision will be affected by poor and nonreproducible positioning. In addition, several of the analysis programs, especially for whole body, require that lines marking the different regions are accurately placed. Incorrect positioning of the patient may result in the inability to correctly place the body part in the correct region for the analysis, thereby influencing the scan results. For example, if the arms are extended above the head for a whole-body scan, it is not possible to analyze the arms in the arm region of interest analysis, thus lowering the whole-body bone mineral content (BMC) measurements.

Scan Area

Most DXA software will automatically set the scan area according to the child's height or body size. However, if necessary, the area can be adjusted by the operator. Any deviation from the standard protocol should always be noted so that the scan area can be reproduced in a follow-up visit.

Scan Mode

Bone densitometers have different scan acquisition modes according to the subject's size or desired image resolution. As discussed in Chapter 3, low-density or pediatric whole-body software may be required to differentiate between bone and soft tissue in younger or sicker patients (2–4). If these programs are used to obtain the initial study, follow-up scans should be determined in this mode to allow for an accurate assessment of change. However, it may be appropriate to scan in both the low-density and standard modes to allow for flexibility through later growth.

The newest versions for the Hologic Discovery (version 12.1 and above) have an auto-low-density whole-body analysis. Use of the actual auto-low-density algorithm depends on body weight (it is recommended for children <40 kg) for the whole-body scan and poor bone mapping by the standard adult analysis for anteroposterior (AP) spine and hip scans. The pediatric reference data recently published by Zemel et al. *(5)* on Hologic instruments were obtained using the auto-low-density algorithms.

SPINE SCANS

The AP (or posteroanterior [PA]) lumbar spine is one of the preferred sites for measuring pediatric bone mass because of the speed and precision of measurements, the easily identified bony landmarks, and the increasing amount of pediatric normative data *(6–26)* (*see* Appendix C) The spine is a predominantly trabecular site and is therefore sensitive to metabolic changes in bone turnover. However, the spine may not be indicative of bone changes resulting from low calcium intake or other nutritional deficiencies *(27)*. It is easily accessible with adequate soft tissue on either side of the vertebrae to allow for bone quantification *(6)*. However, as with all bones in the child's skeleton, the vertebral bodies will change in size and shape during growth *(28)*. The problems associated with growth may be addressed by employing an estimate of volumetric bone mineral density (BMD) such as bone mineral apparent density (BMAD; g/cm^3; Chapters 3 and 10) or by inclusion of body parameters (i.e., height, weight, and bone area [BA]). Using curves for BMC by BA or height also will help in avoiding this potential problem.

Factors that may preclude a successful scan include severe scoliosis, vertebral collapse, and interference caused by high-attenuating materials such as metal rods, feeding tubes, umbilical rings, and radiographic contrast material

Positioning for the PA Lumbar Spine

In positioning the child for a PA lumbar spine scan, the following steps should be taken:

- Place the child centrally on the scanning table in the supine position, with the spine as straight as possible.
- For follow-up visits, review the scan from the previous visit ensure consistent positioning.
- Elevate the child's legs using foam pads appropriate for his or her size. Knees should be flexed at a 90° angle to allow the lower back to be pressed flat against the table. This should diminish any lordosis in the lower spine. It should be noted that the knee cushion provided by the manufacturer is generally too large for young children. Smaller cushions can be custom-made to meet the leg dimensions of young children.
- Place the child's arms down by his or her sides.
- Check that all removable objects have been moved away from the scan area.
- Feel for the patient's iliac crest and umbilicus (or, alternately, lift the shirt to visualize the umbilicus), and position the laser beam approximately 2 cm below this point, ensuring that the beam is centered over the patient and that the scan area has equal amounts of soft tissue on each side of the spine.
- Start acquisition, reminding the child to stay still and to breathe normally for the duration of the scan.
- Observe the emerging image to ensure that the spine is centrally positioned and is as straight as possible and that L5 is visible. Stop the scan, reposition, and start again if any of these points are incorrect. To minimize radiation exposure, restarting the scan should be kept to a minimum.
- Continue scanning until T12, usually identified by the ribs, is visible.
- Review the scan for movement, and repeat if necessary.

The acquired scan should include top of the iliac crest, the top of L5, and the bottom of T12 to aid vertebrae identification; it should also be centrally located in the scan field,

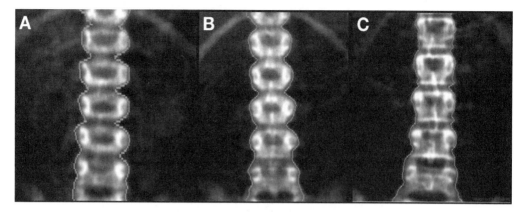

Fig. 1. Correctly acquired spine scans for children of different ages. **(A)** Child, aged 4 yr, with tyrosinaemia type I; **(B)** child, aged 11 yr, with Duchenne muscular dystrophy; **(C)** child, aged 16 yr, with galactosaemia.

with adequate soft tissue either side of the vertebrae (Fig. 1). If using a Hologic densitometer, it is important to use the iliac crest as a starting point. For some edge-detection algorithms, inclusion of the sacrum in the scan field can result in failure of the algorithm to locate the first and second lumbar vertebrae; this should be clarified with the manufacturer's operations manual.

Positioning Problems

It may not always be possible to achieve the ideal scan due to marked scoliosis or vertebral collapse.

Longitudinal Spine Studies

The spine is a useful site to monitor changes in bone mass. However, to achieve successful follow-up scans the operator must:

- Accurately reproduce the patient scan position, using the baseline scan as a guide;
- Use the same scan acquisition and analysis parameters (as much as possible).

If there have been significant weight changes between scans, these ideals may not be possible. For weight changes that result in scan mode variation, the mode change should be recorded so that any necessary corrections and other considerations can be made. When weight change places the child at the borderline between scan modes, scanning in both standard and low-density or pediatric modes is recommended. This creates a comparable scan for the previous measure and a new baseline scan for any future follow-up. When making these decisions, it is important to consider the additional radiation exposure from repeat scans.

Use of the auto-low-density analysis method (Hologic Discovery) will allow the results to be compared to a large pediatric reference database collected using this software *(5)*.

Figure 2 illustrates a successful series of measurements over a 2-yr period beginning at age 16 in a boy being monitored for the effects of three monthly intravenous bisphosphonate treatments.

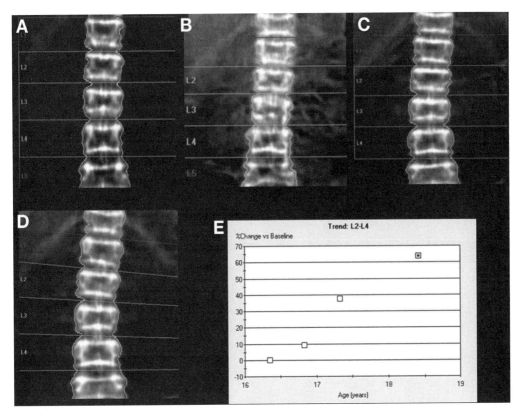

Fig.2. Serial scans over a 2-yr period of a child from age 16 to 18 following a bisphosphonate treatment regime.

WHOLE-BODY SCANS

The whole body is also a preferred site in children. This scan provides measurements of total and regional bone and body composition parameters, making it a useful site for both clinical and research purposes. Growth and disease may affect both bone and body composition values.

With older-generation pencil beam densitometers, whole-body scan times could be as long as 10–20 min. With newer fan beam and narrow fan beam machines, scan times have been reduced to a few minutes, thus making it far more reasonable to acquire a whole-body scan even on a young or fidgety child *(29)*.

Although analysis of specific skeletal regions can be performed from the whole-body scan, the precision is relatively low as a result of the positioning of defining specific regions. Precision is improved with the whole-body measurements *(30)*.

When acquiring a whole-body scan, it is important that the child is not wearing any high-attenuating objects. Ideally, the child should be scanned in a hospital gown or in light indoor clothing. The operator should be aware that thick elasticized waist bands and plastic buttons may also cause problems with image artifacts. Additionally if body composition is to be calculated, polyvinyl chloride (PVC) sheets or pillows, as well as sand bags used in positioning, will affect the calculations and should therefore be removed from the scanning table.

Whole-body scanning can be performed in children with internal high-attenuating objects (e.g., metal rods, pins, or plates) if they are likely to remain *in situ* for follow-up. However, special attention should be given to the analysis and interpretation of such scans, especially when attempting to compare them with normal data (Chapter 6).

Positioning for the Whole-Body Scan

In positioning a child for a whole-body scan, the following steps should be taken:

- Check the scanning table for any high-attenuating objects, and remove any pillows or pads from the scan area.
- Change the child into a hospital gown or check light indoor clothes for any objects that may interfere with the scan.
- For follow-up visits, review the scan from the previous visit to assure consistent positioning.
- Position the child in the center of the scanning table, with the head approximately 4 cm from the top of the scan region.
- Ensure that the child is lying flat and straight within the scan area, with arms placed alongside the body and the palms flat against the bed. (If the child is too large to place his or her hands in this position, rotate the hands so that they are flat alongside, not underneath, the thighs.)
- Ask the child to relax his or her shoulders. Stretch the child's hands toward the foot of the bed.
- Extend the legs on either side of the central line marked on the table, making them as straight as possible, and secure them together with a Velcro strap around the ankles or feet.
- Start the scan, reminding the child to lie still (but to not hold his or her breath). The child should be able to lie comfortably in this position for the duration of the scan. For younger children, it may be necessary to hold either arms or legs to help them maintain this position. If it is necessary to hold the child, be aware of where the x-ray tube is located and wear suitable protection from the radiation, keeping your hands away from the x-ray path.
- Once the scan is complete, remind the child to remain still until the scan arm returns to its home position, at which point it will be safe to get down from the scan table.

Figure 3 demonstrates acceptable scans of a 12-mo-old infant who is post–liver-transplantation (Fig. 3A), a 12-yr-old with a history of multiple low-trauma fractures (Fig. 3B), and a 16-yr-old with galactosemia (Fig. 3C).

For small children, the size of the scan field may be adjusted to reduce the scan time. However, this may become problematic when comparing scans at follow-up as the child grows larger. For very tall adolescents, it may not be possible to fit the entire body in the scan field; therefore, it is suggested to position the child with his or her head is just below the top of the table and with the feet flexed upward. If the child is still to long for the scan table, the scan should be acquired by excluding the feet from the scan area.

When performing scans on obese adolescents, it can be difficult to position them so that the entire body is in the scan field. Several techniques can be used in this situation, depending on the fat distribution. With centralized obesity, the elbows may be too close to the edge of the scan field. A folded cotton sheet can be wrapped tightly around the middle portion of the body to hold the elbows close to the body. In this case, care should be taken to keep the palms flat on the DXA table. When there is a large amount of soft tissue at the hips and the hands are too close to the edge of the scan field, the hands can be tucked under the buttocks, provided the bones of the hands and the proximal femur are not superimposed. If this modified positioning is used, however, it should be noted that

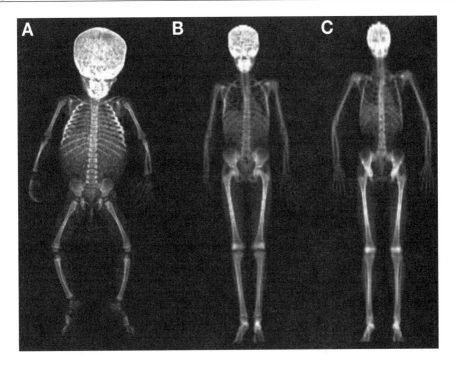

Fig. 3. Correctly acquired total-body scans. (**A**) Child aged 12 mo post liver transplantion; (**B**) child aged 12 yr with a history of multiple low trauma fractures; (**C**) child aged 16 yr with galactosemia.

the regional percent fat, and possibly the whole-body percent fat, measurements will not be correct.

When these techniques fail, an alternative approach is to perform two whole-body scans, one with the right side of the patient optimally positioned in the scan field and the other with the left side optimally positioned. The values for the right and left side are then combined and used as the whole-body measure. In all cases, scans should be monitored for movement and repeated if necessary.

HIP SCANS

The proximal hip and femoral neck are frequently measured sites in adults. Scanning the proximal hip in children, however, is more difficult because the skeletal landmarks may not be well developed and the femoral neck may be too small for the standard software. These factors contribute to poorer precision in this region. Additionally, there are few pediatric reference data for this site. The femoral neck region is not recommended in young children because its changing shape makes longitudinal studies difficult and unreliable.

Regardless, if a hip scan is warranted, the femoral neck box generated by standard DXA software for this region of interest may be too large for the anatomy of smaller subjects. The operator can customize the width and placement of the neck box for a better fit, but this introduces operator-related variability that can also complicate subsequent studies.

The advantage of scanning the proximal hip is that it is a predominately cortical site; therefore, it allows the evaluation of an alternative bone element. It is also well established that bone strength is not just a function of bone density but also of bone geometry and bone distribution. Models have been developed to assess femoral neck geometry and biomechanical bone strength in adults and adolescents *(32,33)*. To date, the evaluation of strength parameters has been calculated and validated primarily in adults, in whom hip fractures are clinically significant *(33–35)*.

Precision is lower at the proximal hip than at the spine. Studies in adults have shown that use of bilateral hip measurements improved precision *(36–38)*. A further problem for hip scans is caused by malrotation. External over rotation of the hip will cause an increase in BMD values, whereas an internal rotation will reduce the BMD *(39)*.

Positioning for the Proximal Hip Scan

In positioning a child for a proximal hip scan, the following steps should be taken:

- Place the child on the scanning table in the supine position, with the head supported by a small pillow if necessary.
- Rest the arms on the abdomen above the region to be scanned.
- Rotate the whole leg inward, ensuring that the leg rotates from the hip (to approximately 30°) and not from the knee.
- Attach the foot to the hip-positioning aid supplied by the manufacturer. (When performing dual hip measurements, position each hip separately to avoid overabduction by the adult hip positioner.) It should be noted that some hip-positioning aids are too large for young children, resulting in Plexiglas in the scan field. This can lead to uninterpretable results.
- Start the acquisition at the point recommended by the DXA manufacturer, reminding the child to stay still for the duration of the scan.
- Observe the emerging image. The femoral shaft should be parallel to the edge of the bed, the scan should start well below the lesser trochanter, and the image should include the total hip region.
- If the hip is either over- or underabducted, reposition and restart the scan.
- Stop the acquisition a short distance above the acetabulum.

The acquired scan should include a portion of the femoral shaft, the femoral neck, the whole of the acetabulum, and part of the pelvis. Figure 4 illustrates two correctly acquired hip scans. Figure 4A shows the immature hip of a 4-yr-old with OI. Figure 4B shows the mature hip of a 16-yr-old with anorexia nervosa.

Even a developed femur may be problematic to scan and analyze, as illustrated by Fig. 5. Figure 5A shows the shortened femoral neck of a 16-yr-old with Charcot-Marie-Tooth disease. The child in Fig. 5B is a wheelchair-bound 10-yr-old with OI. The unusual load on her femur and femoral neck has resulted in an increased angle between the femoral neck and shaft and, hence, an unusual femoral neck morphometry.

The greatest challenge in the use and interpretation of hip scans in children is in the analysis procedure. Especially in younger and smaller children, the software can fail to properly identify the midline and the border of the greater trochanter. Longitudinal comparisons are particularly challenging due to the changes in bone size as children grow. Guidelines for longitudinal analysis of scans are provided by McKay et al. *(40)* and are discussed in Chapter 6.

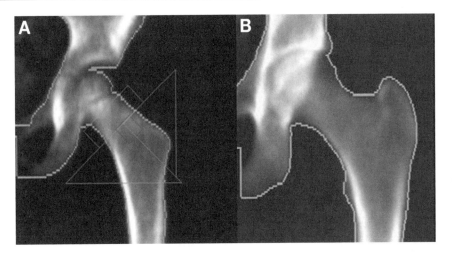

Fig. 4. Correctly acquired hip scans. (**A**) Child, aged 4 yr, with osteogenesis imperfecta; (**B**) child, aged 16 yr, with anorexia nervosa.

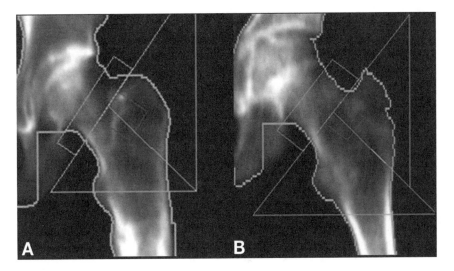

Fig. 5. Problems associated with hip morphometry of underloaded bones. (**A**) Child, aged 16 yr, with Charcot-Marie-Tooth disease (walks with crutches); (**B**) child, aged 10 yr, with osteogenesis imperfecta (mostly wheelchair-bound).

OTHER SITES

Distal Radius and Lateral Distal Femur

The distal radius and lateral distal femur are scanned less commonly in children, although they can provide useful information, particularly for those unable to lie still or who are too contracted for a whole-body exam and those who exceed the weight limitations for the table.

The radius can be scanned using either axial and peripheral devices *(41)*. It is usual to measure the nondominant arm at the ultradistal and distal third section. Within these two regions, it is possible to measure sections of predominantly trabecular (in the ultradistal radius) and cortical (in the distal third section) bone.

The forearm-positioning device should be used if the child is large enough to reach it while keeping the elbow at shoulder level and flexed at a 90° angle. For smaller children, cushions may be needed to achieve the proper position, or the child may need to sit on his or her parent's lap. When these positioning techniques fail, the child can be positioned prone on the table with the arm extended above the head and centered on the table (without the positioner).

In patients with joint contractures, it may be possible to perform a lateral distal femoral scan. This scan is achieved by placing the child on his or her side on the scanning table, with the femur to be imaged parallel to the edge of the bed (Chapter 9, Fig. 6). The leg is usually scanned using forearm software and is analyzed using the forearm subregional analysis software with an adapted technique *(42)*.

Calcaneum

The calcaneum can also be measured using an axial densitometer, but it is more commonly measured using a portable peripheral device. Note that reference data in children are sparse for this trabecula-rich site.

INTERFERENCE

Artifacts

Unfortunately, a frequent problem when scanning children is interference caused by metal artifacts and motion. Problems caused by artifacts should be limited to only those resulting from immovable objects such as pins, plates, rods, and feeding tubes. External highly attenuating objects such as leg braces, plaster casts, or monitors should be removed prior to scanning, or the scan should be rescheduled to when they are no longer required.

Figure 6 illustrates examples of both removable and immovable internal and external artifacts. Child A has bilateral hip and knee prostheses included in the scan field. Artifacts such as these may not cause too much interference for longitudinal scanning if they remain in place for the follow-up period, but they will affect the ability to compare the results to reference data (Chapter 6). Child B has a subclavian portocatheter *in situ* that could not be removed. Child C has a plaster cast on her left leg and the scan should have been delayed until the leg cast had been taken off. Finally, child D is a young child with quadriplegia who is on continual ventilation. The induction loops required for the child's ventilation could not be moved and, therefore, the best acquirable scan was achieved with them in place.

When it is not possible to remove the interfering object or to postpone the scan, data from the whole-body scan can be used by interpolating the values for the affected side based upon results from the unaffected side.

Not all artifacts are limited to the whole-body scan. Figure 7 illustrates a selection of spine scans affected by immovable internal artifacts. Excluding a specific region of interest during analysis may reduce the effect of such artifacts, but the exclusion makes comparison to a reference range difficult.

Unavoidable interferences may also occur as result of the child's clinical condition or treatment. Figure 8A illustrates a common pattern of high-density endplates associated with bisphosphonate treatment. Figure 8B illustrates a child with primary oxalosis type

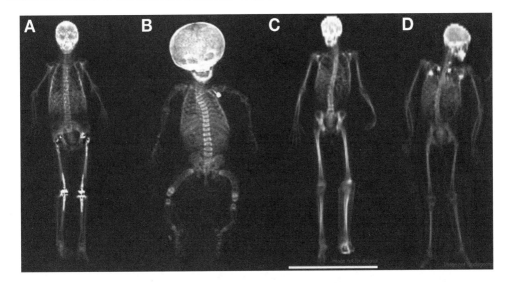

Fig. 6. Whole-body artifacts. (**A**) Bilateral hip and knee prostheses; (**B**) subclavian portocath; (**C**) lower leg plaster cast; (**D**) ventilator connectors.

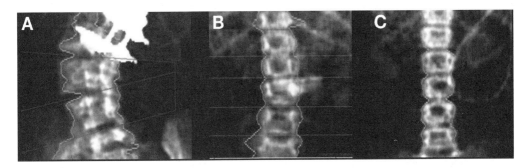

Fig. 7. Lumbar spine artifacts. (**A**) spinal rods; (**B**) feeding tube; (**C**) lymphatic shunt.

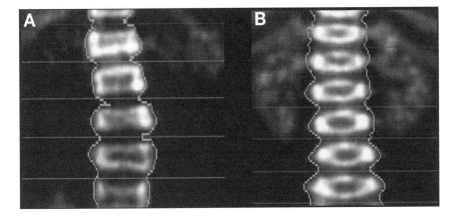

Fig. 8. Artifacts resulting from treatment or clinical conditions. (**A**) Infant, aged 3 yr, with osteogenesis imperfecta, after bisphosphonate treatment; (**B**) child, aged 4 yr, with primary oxalosis type I and calcium deposits in his kidneys.

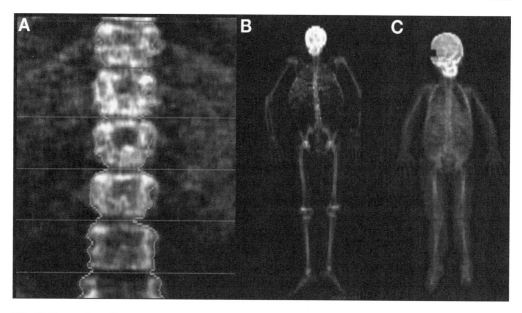

Fig. 9. Examples where poor edge detection has occurred. **(A)** 14-yr-old child with dermatomyositis and extremely low spine density and less than 4% body fat; **(B)** 16-yr-old child with brain tumor and associated obesity with more than 60% body fat; **(C)** 6-yr-old child with marked lymphedema and fluid overload.

I, in whom kidney calcium deposits may affect soft tissue estimation. For suggestions regarding analysis of these scans, *see* Chapter 6.

Poor Edge Detection

Poor edge detection may be a result of photon starvation (when not enough x-rays can pass through the body) at the detectors or poor tissue differentiation observed with extremely low density bone. Figure 9 illustrates three examples in which poor edge detection has occurred. Figure 9A is of a 14-yr-old with dermatomyositis who has extremely low spine density and less than 4% body fat. The 16-yr-old in Fig. 9B has a brain tumor and associated obesity: the child has more than 60% body fat. The 6-yr-old child in Fig. 9C has marked lymphedema and fluid overload.

In all of these examples, the densitometer had difficulty distinguishing between bone and soft tissue, which resulted in erroneous values being generated during the analysis. With densitometers that allow for modifications in the acquisition parameters, photon starvation can be overcome by rescanning the child in a different scan mode using an increased sample time. Poor tissue differentiation may be overcome at the analysis stage by analyzing the acquired image with a specific low-density analysis package.

For the spine, the low-density analysis mode available in the older QDR 2000 and QDR 4500 models results in values for BMD that are significantly different from the standard analysis mode *(43)*. The most recent version of the Hologic (Waltham, MA) software for the QDR Discovery includes an auto-low-density analysis. BMD values for this mode do not differ as greatly from standard analysis mode results as older low-density software versions. However, it is uncertain as to whether there is a significant bias

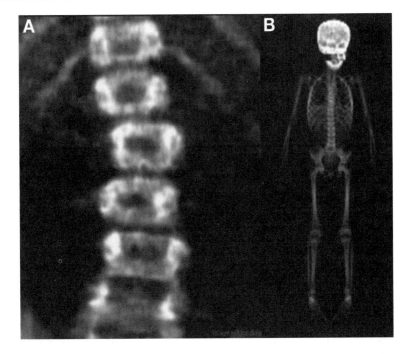

Fig. 10. (A) Lumbar spine with small lateral movements; **(B)** total-body scan with a small lateral movement of the head.

associated with this analysis mode *(44)*. Use of the new "auto-low-density" software will ensure that the scan results obtained are comparable to the pediatric reference data provided by the manufacturer, which were obtained from healthy children using this software *(5)*.

Similar changes have occurred in the pediatric whole-body analysis mode. Because the detection algorithm can have a significant impact on the results for BA, BMC, and BMD, it is of critical importance that the reference data used to interpret the results have been obtained using the same scan analysis procedures.

Movement

The most common problem when scanning young children is movement, which may result in as much as a 4% increase in BMD values *(46)*. Although most analysis techniques can cope with a small amount of movement (Fig. 10), any movement in the scan field will reduce the measurement precision and may produce unreliable results. If the child is unable to stay still for the duration of the scan, the following points must be considered.

- How urgent is the scan? Can it be delayed until the child is older and able to understand and cooperate better?
- Would practicing remaining still be helpful? Sometimes this can be done at home prior to scanning.
- Is sedation necessary? It is not always young children who require sedation; sometimes older children with learning difficulties may require sedation to achieve an analyzable scan (Fig. 11).

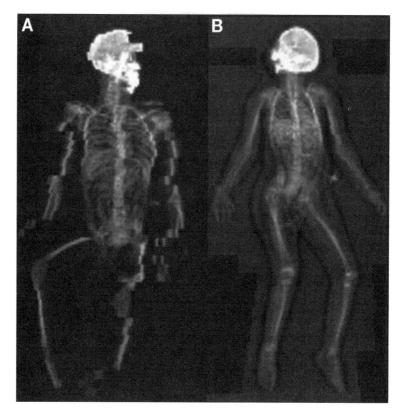

Fig. 11. Effect of sedation. (**A**) Unsedated 18-yr-old child with cerebral palsy; (**B**) sedated 11-yr-old girl with cerebral palsy.

The aim of this chapter has been to give general guidelines for scan acquisitions that are appropriate to most children scanned on most DXA machines. Obviously, each center will have different scan protocols, and these should be followed as closely as possible. The operator should always minimize radiation exposure by only performing clinically useful scans. By explaining the procedure to the child, the operator is likely to reduce fear, to maximize cooperation, and to obtain scans of the highest possible quality.

SUMMARY POINTS

- Different age groups require unique considerations with regard to obtaining the optimal scan.
- Every effort should be made to prepare the child and family prior to the procedure to avoid having to repeat scans.
- Specific details are provided for positioning patients for the three most frequently used scans: spine, total body, and proximal femur (i.e., hip).
- Spine scans can be performed on most pediatric patients Spine reference data for children ages 3 and older are provided in some software.
- Total-body scans can be performed on all pediatric patients who are able to remain still during the procedure without sedation. Gender-specific pediatric reference ranges for patients age 3 or older are provided in some software.

- Hip scans can be performed on older children, in whom the hip is more developed. Pediatric reference ranges for children ages 5 and older are provided in some software programs.
- Other scans such as the distal radius (i.e., the forearm), the lateral distal femur, and the calcaneum are currently used primarily for research purposes or in special populations (Chapter 9).
- Scan interference such as movement, attenuating artifacts, and excess fluid should be reduced as much as possible. This may require postponing scans if there are nonremovable artifacts or the child is unable to cooperate. If the scan is required urgently, selective skeletal sites may be analyzed or sedation may be needed (to avoid motion).

REFERENCES

1. Koo WWK, Massom LR, Walters J. Validation of accuracy and precision of dual energy x-ray absorptiometry for infants. J Bone Miner Res 1995;10:1111–1115.
2. Wang J, Thorton J, Horlick M, et al. Dual x-ray absorptiometry in pediatric studies. J Clin Densitom 1999;2:135–141.
3. Picaud J-C, Duboeuf F, Vey-Marty B, et al. First all-solid pediatric phantom for dual-x-ray absorptiometry measurements in infants. J Clin Densitom 2003;6:17–23.
4. Laskey MA. The influence of tissue depth and composition on the performance of the lunar dual-energy x-ray absorptiometer whole-body scanning mode. Eur J Clin Nutr 1992;46:39–45.
5. Zemel BS, Leonard MB, Kalkwarf HJ, et al. Reference data for the whole body, lumbar spine and proximal femur for American children relative to age, gender and body size. (Abstract). J Bone Miner Res 2004;19 (Suppl1):SU112.
6. Carrascosa A, Gussinye M, Yeste D, del Rio L, Audi L. Bone mass acquisition during infancy, childhood and adolescence. Acta Paediatr 1995;411:18–23.
7. Del Rio L, Carrascosa A, Pons F, Gussinye M, Yeste D, Domenech FM. Bone mineral density of the lumbar spine in white Mediterranean Spanish children and adolescents: changes related to age, sex, and puberty. Pediatr Res 1994;35:362–366.
8. Zanchetta JR, Plotkin H, Alvarez-Filgueira ML. Bone mass in children: normative values for the 2–20 year old population. Bone 1995;16:393S–99S.
9. Bonjour JP, Theintz G, Buchs B, Slosman D, Rizzoli R. Critical years and stages of puberty for spinal and femoral bone mass accumulation during adolescence. J Clin Endocrinol Metab 1991;73:555–563.
10. Boot AM, De Ridder MAJ, Pols HAP, Krenning EP, De Muinck Keizer-Schrama SMPF. Bone mineral density in children and adolescents: relation to puberty, calcium intake, and physical activity. J Clin Endocrinol Metab 1997;82:57–62.
11. Faulkner RA, Bailey DA, Drinkwater DT, Wilkinson AA, Houston CS, McKay HA. Regional and total body bone mineral content, bone mineral density and total body tissue composition in children 8–16 years of age. Calcif Tissue Int 1993;53:7–12.
12. Arikoski P, Komulainen J, Kroger L, Kroger H. Lumbar bone mineral density in normal subjects aged 3–6 years: a prospective study. Acta Paediatr 2002;91:287–291.
13. Bachrach LK, Hastie T, Wang M-C, Narasimhan B, Marcus R. Bone mineral acquisition in healthy Asian, Hispanic, black, and Caucasian youth: a longitudinal study. J Clin Endocrinol Metab 1999;84:4702–4712.
14. Bailey DA. The Saskatchewan pediatric bone mineral accrual study: bone mineral acquisition during the growing years. Int J Sports Med 1997;18:S191–194.
15. Binkley TL, Specker BL, Wittig TA. Centile curves for bone densitometry measurements in healthy males and females aged 5–22 years. J Clin Densitom 2002;5:343–353.
16. De Schepper J, Derde MP, Van den Broeck M, Piepsz A, Jonckheer MH. Normative data for lumbar spine bone mineral content in children: influence of age, height, weight, and pubertal stage. J Nucl Med 1991;32:216–220.
17. DePriester JA, Cole TJ, Bishop NJ. Bone growth and mineraliation in children aged 4 to 10 years. Bone Miner 1991;12:57–65.
18. Drake AJ, Armstrong DW, Shakir KMM. Bone mineral density and total body bone mineral content in 18- to 22-year-old women. Bone 2004;34:1037–1043.

19. Kroger H, Kotaniemi A, Kroger L, Alhava E. Development of bone mass and bone density of the spine and femoral neck. A prospective study of 65 children and adolescents. Bone Miner 1993;23:171–182.

20. Lazcano-Ponce E, Tamayo J, Cruz-Valdez A, et al. Peak bone mineral determinants among females aged 9 to 24 years in mexico. Osteoporos Int 2003;14:539–547.

21. Magarey AM, Boulton TJC, Chatterton BE, Schultz C, Nordin BEC, Cockington RA. Bone growth from 11–17 years: relationship to growth, gender and changes with pubertal status including timing of menarche. Acta Paediatr 1999;88:139–146.

22. Ponder SW, McCormick DP, Fawcett D, Palmer JL, McKernan MG. Spinal bone mineral density in children aged 5 through 11.99 years. Amer J Dis Children 1990;144:1346–1348.

23. Sabatier J-P, Guaydier-Souquieres G, Laroche D, et al. Bone mineral acquisition during adolescence and early adulthood: a study in 574 healthy 10–24 years of age. Osteoporos Int. 1996;6:141–148.

24. Unsi-Rasi K, Haapasalo H, Kannus P, et al. Determinants of bone mineralization in 8 to 20 year old Finnish females. Eur J Clin Nutr 1997;51:54–59.

25. van der Sluis IM, De Ridder MAJ, Boot AM, Krenning EP, De Muinck Keizer-Schrama SMPF. Reference data for bone mineral density and body composition measured with dual energy x-ray absorptiometry in white children and young adults. Arch Dis Child 2002;87:341–347.

26. Wen Lu P, Cowell CT, Lloyd-Jones SA, Briody JN, Howman-Giles R. Volumetric bone mineral density in normal subjects, aged 5–27 years. J Clin Endocrinol Metab 1996;81:1586–1590.

27. Specker B, Wosje K. A critical appraisal of the evidence relating calcium and dairy intake to bone health early in life, in Burkhardt P, Dawson-Hughes B, Heaney R, eds. *Nutritional Aspects of Osteoporosis*, San Diego: Academic, 2001;107–123.

28. Lu WP, Briody JN, Ogle GD, et al. Bone mineral density of total body: spine femoral neck in children and young adults: a cross-sectional and longitudinal study. J Bone Miner Res 1994;9:1451–1458.

29. Mazess RB, Barden HS. Evaluation of differences between fan-beam and pencil-beam densitometers. Calcif Tissue Int 2000;67:291–296.

30. Kiebzak GM, Leamy LJ, Pierson LM, Nord RH, Zhang ZY. Measurement precision of body composition variables using the Lunar DPX-l densitometer. J Clin Densitom 2000;3:35–41.

31. Lark RK, Henderson RC, Renner JB, et al. Dual energy x-ray absorptiometry assessment of body composition in children with altered body posture. J Clin Densitom 2001;4(4)325–335.

32. Van der Meulen CMH, Moro M, Kiratli BJ, Marcus R, Bachrach LK. Mechanobiology of femoral neck structure during adolescence. J Rehab Res Devel 2000;37:201–208.

33. Beck TJ, Ruff C, B, Warden KE, Scott WW, Rao G. Predicting femoral neck strength from bone mineral data. Invest Radiol 1990;25:6–18.

34. Beck TJ, Oreskovic TL, Stone KL, et al. Structural adaptation to changing skeletal load in the progression toward hip fragility: the study of osteoporotic fractures. J Bone Miner Res 2001;16:1108–1119.

35. Beck TJ, Looker A, Ruff C, B, Sievanen H, Wahner HW. Structural trends in the aging femoral neck and proximal shaft: analysis of the third national health and nutrition examination survey dual-energy x-ray absorptiometry. J Bone Miner Res 2000;15:2297–2304.

36. Mazess RB, Nord RH, Hanson JA, Barden HS. Bilateral measurement of femoral bone mineral density. J Clin Densitom 2000;3:133–140.

37. Faulkner KG. Improving femoral bone density measurements. J Clin Densitom 2003;6:353–358.

38. White J, Harris S, Dallal G, Dawson-Hughes B. Precision of single vs. bilateral hip bone mineral density scans. J Clin Densitom 2003;6:159–162.

39. Lekamwasam S, Lenora RSJ. Effect of leg rotation on hip bone mineral density measurements. J Clin Densitom 2003;6:331–336.

40. McKay HA, Petit MA. Analysis of proximal femur DXA scans in growing children: comparison of different protocols for cross-sectional 8-month and 7-year longitudinal data. J Bone Miner Res 2000;15:1181–1188.

41. Ellis KJ. Selected body composition methods can be used in field studies. J Nutr 2001;131:S1589–1595.

42. Henderson RC, Lark RK, Newman JE, et al. Pediatric reference data for dual x-ray absorptiometric measures of normal bone density in the distal femur. AJR 2002;178(2):439–443.

43. Leonard MB, Feldman HI, Zemel BS, Berlin JA, Barden EM, Stallings VA. Evaluation of low density spine software for the assessment of bone mineral density in children. J Bone Miner Res 1998;13:1687–1690.

44. Simpson DE, Dontu VS, Stephens SE, Archbold LJ, et al. Large variations occur in bone density measurements of children when using different software. Nucl Med Commun 2005;26:483–487.

45. Hangartner TN. Influence of fat on bone measurements with dual-energy absorptiometry. Bone Miner 1990;9:71–78
46. Pietrobelli A, Wang Z, Formica C, and Heymsfield SB. Dual-energy x-ray absorptiometry: fat estimation errors due to variation in soft tissue hydration. Am J Physiol 1998;274:E808–E816.
46. Koo WWK, Walters J, Bush AJ. Technical considerations of dual-energy x-ray absorptiometry-based bone mineral measurements for paediatric studies. J Bone Miner Res 1995;10:1998–2004.

6

Analysis

Moira Petit, PhD, *Kyla Kent,* BS,
Mary B. Leonard, MD, MSCE,
Heather McKay, PhD, *and Babette S. Zemel,* PhD

CONTENTS

INTRODUCTION
FUNDAMENTALS OF ANALYSIS
MANUFACTURER, MODEL, AND SOFTWARE DIFFERENCES
SPECIFIC PEDIATRIC SOFTWARE
ANALYSIS ISSUES AND RECOMMENDATIONS FOR SCAN ANALYSIS
FOLLOW-UP SCAN ANALYSIS
CONCLUSIONS
SUMMARY POINTS
REFERENCES

INTRODUCTION

Analysis is a key step between image acquisition and the interpretation required for clinical decision making. The technologist performing this step is responsible for making informed decisions to provide accurate baseline and serial measurements. Originally, software programs were designed to analyze the adult skeleton, that is, a skeleton that is fully mineralized with well-developed skeletal landmarks and regions of interest (ROIs) that do not change markedly in size or shape over time.

Numerous models of dual-energy x-ray absorptiometry (DXA) densitometers from each of the three manufacturers and several corresponding software versions are available (Chapter 3), which makes it essential to pay attention to the version of hardware and software used. Applying these standard adult programs and protocols when analyzing pediatric scans has posed several problems that have not been adequately addressed in instrumentation manuals.

Children's undermineralized bones and small bone size can make it difficult for standard software to differentiate bone from soft tissue and to identify skeletal landmarks that are used to determine the ROI. This is a problem for pediatric scan analyses for several

From: *Current Clinical Practice: Bone Densitometry in Growing Patients: Guidelines for Clinical Practice*
Edited by: A. J. Sawyer, L. K. Bachrach, and E. B. Fung © Humana Press Inc., Totowa, NJ

reasons: (1) untrained operators may have difficulty defining the ROI for the hip or spine when these are not fully developed; (2) the DXA software may not detect undermineralized regions, resulting in systematic bias; and (3) the US Food and Drug Administration (FDA)-approved auto-analysis software is currently not designed to handle changes in bone size over time.

This chapter will address (1) the fundamentals of analysis; (2) differences among manufacturers and models; (3) software differences regarding the analysis of pediatric scans, and how software can affect results and interpretation; and (4) analysis issues and recommendations for how to analyze each site. For many of these topics, there are no standard, established approaches, so decisions will have to be made by individual technologists, clinicians, and researchers, who must have full awareness of the implications of these decisions.

Issues inherent to differences in DXA manufacturer, model, and software are relevant both to baseline interpretation of clinical scans and to follow-up measures. For clinical interpretation to be meaningful, patient scan acquisition and analysis modes should be equivalent to the normative data to which they are to be compared. If differences exist, clinical assessment should be made with caution and with full awareness of the population from which the normative data were collected. Furthermore, with changes in the DXA hardware or software version, comparison of sequential results in clinical patients or research subjects (enrolled in longitudinal trials or multicenter research centers) may be jeopardized.

FUNDAMENTALS OF ANALYSIS

The accuracy of analysis depends largely on the quality of the scans obtained. Correct patient positioning during scan acquisition is critically important for appropriate scan analysis. Scans with poor patient positioning are unacceptable and should not be analyzed because the result may be significantly affected by poor positioning. (Details regarding correct positioning for pediatric patients are provided in Chapter 5.)

With high-quality scans, analysis is fairly routine given the current auto-analysis software for most instrument models. However, the growing skeleton provides unique challenges that standard software may be ill-equipped to automatically handle. For example, low mineralization and changing skeletal size and shape often mean the automatic analyses will misplace the ROIs.

Analysis of spine, whole-body, and proximal femur scans is typically a four-step process: (1) identifying and choosing among the available software for the DXA machine, (2) confirming or correcting the global ROI, (3) confirming or editing the bone map, and (4) confirming or modifying subregional landmarks.

Spine Analysis

For spine scans in particular, Hologic densitometers have several analysis programs including a basic lumbar spine analysis, the Legacy low-density software (LDS), a subregional analysis program, and the recently introduced auto-low-density software. The lumbar spine software is chosen for most analyses; the LDS and auto-LDS options will be discussed under "Specific Pediatric Software: Spine" and "Specific Pediatric Software: New Software Versions," respectively.

The spinal global ROI has a defined pixel width and adjustable top and bottom lines. The global ROI may be adjusted to the left or right so that it can be centered around the vertebral column; however, the box width is not adjustable. The top line for ROI must be positioned within the intervertebral space between T12 and L1. The bottom line of the ROI must be positioned within the intervertebral space between L4 and L5. These lines may be angled slightly if necessary to account for alterations in spine physiology such as scoliosis.

Once the global ROI is adjusted, the bone map is either confirmed or edited. Then, the three horizontal intervertebral lines are placed between L1 and L2, L2 and L3, and L3 and L4. These lines should be adjusted up or down so that placement is between each of the defined vertebrae. There may be instances in which the software is unable to discern intervertebral spaces and does not automatically provide lines (e.g., if the global ROI is altered considerably with follow-up using the "compare" mode*). In this case, one or more lines must be inserted to complete the analysis. Once the lines are placed, confirm that the vertebral body labels are correctly assigned. Then, finally, results can be generated. Of note, some centers use only L2–L4, whereas others use L1–L4. Either approach is valid; however, consistency among individuals within clinical centers is important.

For Norland densitometers, point resolution can be set a priori by the operator when conducting scans on smaller patients; however, the system automatically regulates photon flux for the patient's body size. Therefore, it is unnecessary to vary scanner settings. There are no major differences in the final assessment of spine scans for children as compared to adults.

Whole-Body Analysis

Several software programs are available for the analysis of whole-body scans, including whole-body fan beam software, pediatric whole-body software, and auto-whole-body software. Specific software versions are discussed under "Specific Pediatric Software: Whole Body." In general, the total-body scan is always analyzed in subregions that must be defined by the technologist during analysis. There are 10 subregions: the head, the left and right arms, the left and right ribs, the thoracic and lumbar spine, the pelvis, and the right and left legs. Once again, the quality of the scan is important as poor patient positioning or movement will affect the accuracy of the analysis.

Subregions are first defined by adjusting the three horizontal lines provided. The first is placed just below the patient's jaw, the second is placed between T12 and L1, and the third line is placed just above the iliac crest. Next, the vertical lines are adjusted. Two lines are placed on either side of the spine; two lines are placed between the arm and chest regions, running through the glenoid fossa; two lines are placed on the outside of the leg regions; and the last line is adjusted to separate the legs and feet. When necessary, the lines surrounding the pelvis may need to be adjusted so that the femoral neck is bisected on both sides. Once the lines are correctly placed, confirm that the subregions of interest are correctly assigned. Then, finally, results can be generated.

---

*The "compare" mode allows baseline and follow-up scans (for spine, hip, or the whole body) to be viewed on the screen at the same time. This is useful even in growing patients, allowing technologists to place ROIs using similar bony landmarks and to identify any changes in positioning that may influence results.

The analysis approach is similar for General Electric (GE) Lunar and Norland densitometers. Again, the auto-analysis program identifies where the bone edges appear to be and places the global ROI and intervertebral lines appropriately. Neither Lunar nor Hologic densitometers bend lines or angle the ROI in the auto-analysis mode, so technologists will have to assess whether the ROI and lines need to be adjusted and whether the software placed the ROI over the correct vertebral bodies.

Again, the analysis approach is similar for GE Lunar densitometers, although GE Lunar also has an extended subregional analysis reporting (for gynoid and android regions) and, in addition, allows easy exclusion of the head region from the calculated totals. (It is also possible to manually subtract the head region from totals with Hologic software.)

For Norland densitometers, finer resolutions may be preselected by the operator, but the analysis approach for a pediatric patient is similar to that for an adult patient.

Proximal Femur (i.e., Hip) Analysis

The proximal femur only has one method of analysis but slightly different guides, depending on whether you have disk operating system (DOS) or Windows software. Understanding the DOS analysis parameters provides a greater understanding to the Windows version.

For analysis within a DOS system, once the scan has been acquired, the global ROI is defined. For Hologic, the distal side of the ROI is placed 5 pixels out from the most prominent portion of the greater trochanter. The bottom side is placed 10 pixels below the bottom of the lesser trochanter. If no lesser trochanter is visible, the bottom line is placed at a point two times the height of the greater trochanter, measuring down from the top of the trochanteric region. The top and medial sides of the box are placed 5–10 pixels out from the acetabulum.

Once the global ROI is set, the bone is mapped. At this step, there are two ways that the analysis may need to be adjusted. If the map is very poor, the global ROI may be enlarged by moving the upper inner corner a greater distance away from the head of the femur, giving the software more soft tissue to use in differentiation from bone. The system may have also identified some of the tendon as bone. If this is the case, the tendon may need to be deleted away from the bone.

Once the map is complete, the next step is to let the software determine the midline, Ward's triangle,* the base of the greater trochanter, and the neck box placement. If the midline is not running perpendicular to the narrowest part of the neck region, the analysis must be adjusted. A misplaced midline can be caused by very low density or by unusual proportions in a growing child. By increasing the global ROI upward and in so that there is additional soft tissue to compare to bone, the software may find the midline more accurately. If the midline is still off, it can be manually adjusted. However, it can be difficult to reproduce the analysis if adjustments to the midline are made, so it is best to use auto-analysis for the midline when possible.

The next step is to place the neck box on the neck region. It will come up at a default width that should not be changed unless the top of the box is in the head of the femur or the bottom is overlapping the ischium. If either of these is the case, the box should be moved or, possibly, narrowed the smallest amount possible. Any changes in the size or location of the neck box should be noted on the report. It is not recommended that this region be narrowed lower that 12 pixels. In addition, if the width of the box is adjusted, it will not be possible to apply bone mineral apparent density (BMAD) equations because the equations assume this region is at the default box size.

---

*We do not recommend using Ward's triangle region in children. This region is defined as the region of least density within the femoral neck. Therefore, the region is in a different location for each child and may change locations over time, making interpretation somewhat meaningless.

Arrow keys are used to place the femoral neck ROI so that the lower outer corner is just touching the bone in the neck region at the point where the curve of the greater trochanter meets the curve of the neck region. The other three corners must be in soft tissue. If the patient is very small or has a very short hip axis length, it may not be possible to place the neck box without overlapping the ischium region. In this case, go back to the mapping step and manually delete bone away from the neck region by carefully following along the neck with the delete function and then drawing straight in from the head of the femur to the edge of the global ROI. Once this region is deleted, place the neck box appropriately.

The last thing to check is the placement of the base of the greater trochanter. If it is not resting at the correct anatomical location, it also can be adjusted. Once all of the lines are placed correctly, press "end."

Windows versions have a preset dual-lined edge for setting the global ROI. The ROI is set by resting the innermost of the two lines at the distal side against the edge of the greater trochanter, the innermost of the two bottom lines at the base of the lesser trochanter, or the bottommost line at two times the height of the greater trochanter. The upper and medial sides' innermost lines are placed at the edge of the acetabulum. These dual lines already have the aforementioned 5- and 10-pixel spacing. Navigation between steps is done by clicking on the desired step.

GE Lunar has a slightly different ROI, which uses the midline placement and triangulation to place the lower edge of the global ROI; it may or may not be able to calculate a total hip value. The neck region for Lunar is still perpendicular to the midline but is located in the center of the whole neck region.

For Norland densitometers, the femoral neck region is typically adjusted from the routine 1.5 cm used for adult patients to something smaller, depending on the size of the child. Similarly to the other two systems, all four regions are reported after analysis: the femoral neck, the trochanter, Ward's triangle, and the total.

MANUFACTURER, MODEL, AND SOFTWARE DIFFERENCES

Bone mineral density (BMD) results for the same person measured on instruments from different manufacturers can differ by as much as 20% (1). These clinically significant differences may be due to unique software and acquisition methods; for example, GE Lunar instruments use different scan modes based on patient weight to enhance bone detection, whereas Hologic scanner software is typically weight-independent (with the exception of a new software version discussed under "Specific Pediatric Software: New Software Versions"). These differences are most notable in the unique placement of the neck box and in the location of the hip region, in which, depending on the software used, varying amounts of femoral shaft are included in the ROI. As a result of these discrepancies, it is recommended that, if possible, the same instrument, model, and software version be used to assess an individual patient over time.

Although ideal, it is not always feasible to conduct serial measurements on identical instruments, as would be the case for a patient who receives care at multiple clinics or for clinics that have upgraded their DXA technology over time. In an attempt to allow comparisons among manufacturers and to reduce the range of error among systems, the three most common instrument manufacturers (Hologic, GE Lunar, and Norland) established cross-calibration factors through the International Standardization Committee (2).

The standardized BMD (sBMD) score permits comparison of results obtained on different instruments. The sBMD is expressed in mg/cm^2 to avoid confusion with manufacturer-specific BMDs, which are expressed in g/cm^2 *(2–4)* (*see* Appendix B at the end of the volume for conversion equations) Essentially, the BMD result obtained on each manufacturer's densitometer can be converted to an sBMD score.

This method may not be suitable for all clinical or research purposes, particularly if the ROI captured is not comparable. Furthermore, data used to develop algorithms for the sBMD were gathered only in adults, and, to our knowledge, no studies have assessed their applicability in pediatric scans. Therefore, caution should be used when applying the formulae to pediatric scans. Regardless, it does improve the overall comparability of BMD data collected on different instruments.

Of note, even different densitometer models produced by the same manufacturer may yield different results *(5)*. The older Hologic QDR-1000W densitometer used a single-beam (i.e., pencil beam) x-ray mode, whereas newer Hologic densitometers have either both single beam and the more rapid fan beam capabilities (i.e., QDR-2000) or fan beam-only capabilities (i.e., QDR-4500, Delphi, and Discovery). Results obtained from the QDR-2000 using the single beam mode correlate better with the QDR-1000W than do results obtained using the fan beam mode *(2,5)*. Most recently, narrow fan beam technology has been introduced into the latest GE Lunar models (Chapter 3).

The measurement of soft tissue composition by DXA is also instrument- and software-dependent. Body composition results may vary substantially (up to 20%) among different densitometer models from the same manufacturer *(5)* and even among different versions of software *(6)*. Standardized conversion equations are available in the literature for body composition values *(7,8)*. Despite the availability of these equations, the differences among models can be sizable.

Although manufacturers are reasonably careful to calibrate new software versions to make the BMD comparable to previous versions, it is important to be aware that software changes can, and do, alter results when comparing scans in a single patient over time. Of particular relevance for children is the Hologic pediatric total-body software, which presents substantially different values for body composition than the standard software for young patients (*see* "Specific Pediatric Software: New Software Versions").

If equipment must be upgraded or replaced, the effects on results must be considered. If only software analysis versions are upgraded, it is usually possible to reanalyze all prior scans using the new software so that follow-up values will be less divergent. If the instrument is replaced, it is ideal to determine differences between densitometer models by in vivo testing. If the clinic has the ability to maintain both instruments concurrently, at least a subset of subjects can be scanned on both instruments on the same day, and their values can be compared. If this is not possible, the change in instrument manufacturer, model, or software should be noted on the clinical report.

SPECIFIC PEDIATRIC SOFTWARE

Spine

The standard adult spine software may not be able to distinguish between bone and soft tissue when scanning very young subjects or those with very low bone mass. An estimated 40% of chronically ill children under age 12, and even healthy children under age 8, may have inaccurate spine scan results due to failure of the standard bone-edge-

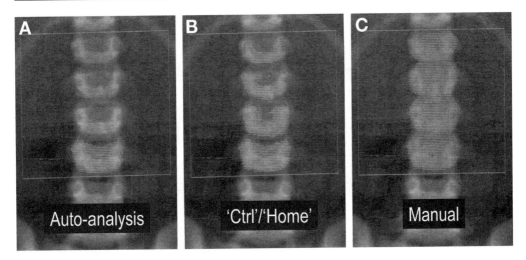

Fig. 1. (A) Standard analysis of the lumbar spine using an early version of the adult software (Hologic, version 8.20a:5) in an 8-yr-old boy. This illustrates that the auto-analysis software does not detect all the vertebrae; only the lowest lumbar vertebrae (L4) is completely detectable. **(B)** The "ctrl/home" function improves the amount of bone detected, and L1 and L3 are now partially detectable. **(C)** However, the operator is still required to manually "paint" in other areas within vertebrae as bone.

detection algorithm to identify and measure completely all four vertebrae *(9)*. For example, the automatic analysis using Hologic software (version 8.20A:5) for the spine scan of an 8-yr-old boy identified only one complete vertebrae (L4) as bone (Fig. 1A); it partially recognized the other three vertebrae (L1–L3) as bone (Fig. 1B). This occurs because the software makes the assumption that a spine should be continuous. If islands of bone are identified, then they are assumed to be nonspine artifact and are removed by the standard software.

Prior to the addition of the auto-paint function, the technologist was required to manually fill in, or hand-paint, the bone that was not detected, directing the system to identify material in the area that represented bone (Fig. 1C). The addition of auto-paint and fill-in functions reduced the manual process to outlining the bone region. Any of these manual processes introduces error because they are dependent on the technologist's perception of what is and is not bone, and they result in loss of the systematic algorithm's threshold definition of the bone edge *(9)*.

In an effort to address this limitation, Hologic introduced low-density software in 1993 to improve detection of low-density bone in children and severely osteopenic adults. The option can be installed on all Hologic densitometers. If the bone map is incomplete using the adult mode of analysis, LDS is recommended by manufacturers. The LDS option lowers the threshold density value to allow identification of pixels as bone that would be classified as soft tissue or would go undetected using the standard adult analysis software. LDS improves the detection of the bone edge and reduces the likelihood of manual intervention by the technologist (Fig. 2) *(9)*.

As this is an operator-selected mode chosen at the time of scan analysis, it is possible to analyze the same scan in both the LDS and the standard adult mode for comparison. The bone values acquired with standard and LDS modes differ considerably, making it

Standard Software   ## Low Density Option

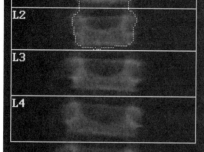
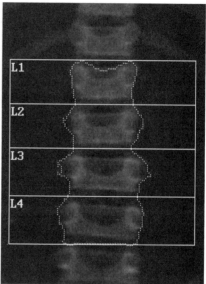

Fig. 2. Low-density software (Hologic software version 7.20 and LDS version 4.74A:1) improves the automatic detection of bone in pediatric spine analysis, as shown by the increased number of vertebrae identified. Technologists should be aware of the drastic difference in values using the low density software. (*See* text for full explanation.)

critical to be aware of which software is being used. The LDS mode increases the detection of low-density bone in children and reduces technologist intervention; however, there are systematic changes in bone values caused by this change in sensitivity. The algorithm increases the area of bone detected, and values for both bone area (BA) and bone mineral content (BMC) increase substantially. The LDS analysis includes regions at the margins of bone that are relatively undermineralized (compared with the regions detected by the standard mode software). This results in BMD values that are substantially lower (~9% on average) with the LDS option (using standard software version 7.20 and LDS version 4.74A:1; Fig. 3) *(9)*.

When compared with manufacturer normative data not analyzed using LDS, a clinically significant reduction in spine Z-score of 0.7 standard deviations (SDs) resulted. To account for this effect, the manufacturer has recommended that Z-scores be increased by a 0.7 SD when comparing to reference data not collected using LDS. As Leonard et al. *(9)* described, LDS is able to accurately predict standard BMD; however, given the range in Z-scores observed, one single correction factor may not be sufficient.

Obesity may further complicate the LDS analysis as the greater tissue thickness modifies the relationship between the LDS and the standard software. LDS has been shown to predict BMD slightly higher in obese vs nonobese children ($p = 0.07$) *(9)*.

Because of the large magnitude of differences, LDS and standard software modes should not be used interchangeably. Scans analyzed with the LDS mode should not be compared with published reference data obtained with the standard software *(9)*. There are currently no published normative data using LDS. This software discrepancy is not

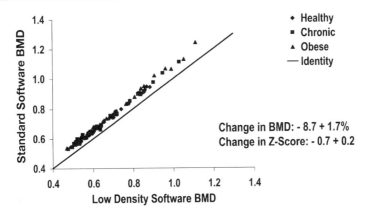

Fig. 3. Comparison of bone mineral density (BMD results between the standard and low-density software (LDS). BMD values were 8.7% lower using LDS. Diamonds, healthy children; squares, chronically ill children; triangles, obese children. (Reproduced from ref. 9, with permission.)

an issue for GE Lunar users because the same algorithm is used to detect bone edge across all age groups.

Other complications that arise during the analysis of spine scans are related to the auto-analyze software. This software may fail to correctly identify the lumbar spine vertebrae, may misplace the global ROI, or may misplace or fail to insert intervertebral lines. These problems arise frequently in pediatric undermineralized lumbar vertebrae. Additionally, auto-analysis software is unable to accurately analyze more complex anatomy such as scoliotic spines. Technologists must be trained to recognize the anatomy of the lumbar spine and to override the auto-analysis mode when necessary. Some recommendations on how to analyze scans of patients with altered body postures are provided in Chapter 9.

Whole Body

Adult versions of software for whole-body scan analysis often fail to identify the small bones of the hand and other undermineralized skeletal areas.

Algorithms used to quantify composition of the head may not be applicable in children. Furthermore, children have a disproportionally large head in comparison to body size. The combination of these two facts may lead to inaccuracy in the calculation of total-body BMC and BMD. This inaccuracy may be increased when applied to longitudinal measures because as a child grows, the skeletal portion below the neck increases in bone mineral content. However, the total-body BMC or BMD may not be sensitive enough to detect these changes given the disproportional contribution of the head region. For this reason, it is recommended that the head region be deleted from total-body analyses. To better identify the small or undermineralized bones, pediatric analysis modes have been developed for both Hologic and GE Lunar instruments. GE Lunar has also modified their analysis software to allow for selective inclusion or exclusion of the head region.

The Hologic pediatric mode was designed for analysis of whole-body scans to assist in the identification in small or young children of regions such as the hands and feet, which may go undetected with standard software. The principles of the pediatric mode for the whole body are the same as for LDS for the spine. The pediatric mode differs from the standard adult option by lowering the attenuation threshold for pixels identified as containing bone. The pediatric option alters only the analysis and does not require any changes in data acquisition or scanning procedures. For this reason, researchers and clinicians have the option of analyzing the scan using both standard software and the pediatric mode. There are few scientific publications that use the pediatric analysis mode for whole-body scans as this software is relatively new.

Hologic has now incorporated this pediatric software option into the standard software package for all fan beam instruments (i.e., the 4500A, Delphi, and Discovery). Importantly, the Hologic Discovery system does an automatic adjustment for children under 40 kg (i.e., 88 lbs; *see* "Specific Pediatric Software: New Software Versions"). This has serious implications for longitudinal scans, and clinicians must be aware of which software was used in analyses for accurate interpretation.

As with the LDS software for the spine, the pediatric whole-body software reassigns pixels from the soft tissue classification to bone classification, which causes more pixels to be identified as containing bone, thus increasing BA. The additional pixels tend to be along the bone edge; thus, they do not contain as much mineral as other pixels. Therefore, BMC will increase, but proportionately less than BA, so resulting BMD values are lower. In addition, the number of pixels identified as lean and fat tissue change dramatically (Leonard MB, unpublished observation). The extent of these changes has not been established, but at this point, it appears that using the pediatric whole-body analysis mode will increase the fat-to-lean ratio, resulting in higher values for the percentage of fat.

Whole-body BA, BMC, and BMD obtained from scans analyzed using the pediatric whole-body mode correlate well with the standard adult software ($r^2 > 0.94$; Fig. 4), but the absolute difference in results is dramatic. In 352 boys ($n = 175$) and girls ($n = 177$) aged 10–13 yr, BA was 25% greater and BMC was 18% greater (Fig. 5), but BMD was 13% lower when using the pediatric mode compared to the standard software (McKay HA, unpublished data). In a group of healthy children and children with chronic disease, BA increased an average of 38–45%, BMC increased 34–40%, and BMD decreased 3–5% when using the LDS software *(10)*. In addition, differences varied across disease groups *(10)*.

Equally important, the distinct software versions result in marked apparent differences in longitudinal change in BA, BMC, and BMD. Correlation for 1-yr change in BA, BMC, and BMD were moderate ($R^2 < 0.79$, Fig. 6), and values for change were –9%, –2%, and +6% different for BA, BMC, and BMD, respectively, using the pediatric mode (McKay HA, unpublished data). A 6% difference in change in BMD is equivalent to at least a 0.5 SD and would affect the apparent Z-score for the child. Thus, it is critical that all DXA users are aware of these important differences and that they use the same mode for analyses when assessing change in whole-body bone mineral or body composition over time. If the same mode cannot be used for technical reasons, the change in mode must be stressed, with warnings about potential inaccuracies of interpretation.

Proximal Femur

As analysis and positioning of the proximal femur (i.e., hip) in children are particularly complex, it is often recommended that the total hip and femoral neck not be used for clinical purposes in children. For DXA centers that opt to perform proximal femur scans, it is important to understand the challenges that are inherent to their analysis.

First, skeletal landmarks such as the lesser and greater trochanter that are used to place regions of interest are less visible (or nonexistent) in many children. The visibility and prominence of the lesser trochanter is important because operators use this anatomical

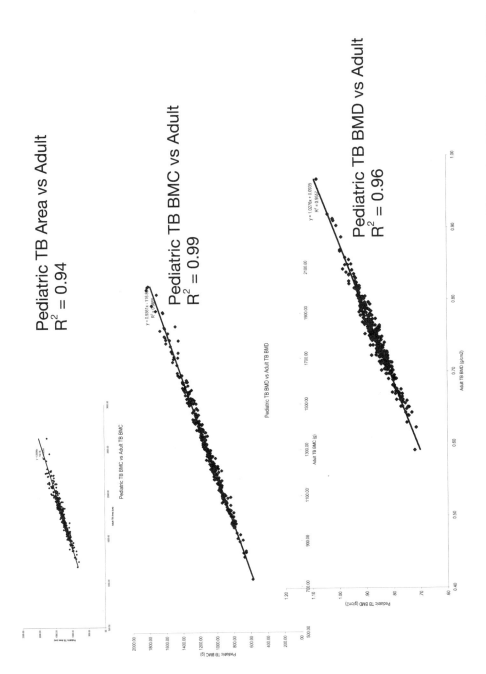

Fig. 4. Correlation between pediatric whole-body and adult whole-body software in 352 boys ($n = 175$) and girls ($n = 177$), aged 10–13 yr. Although correlation coefficients are high, actual values differ dramatically (McKay H, unpublished data)

103

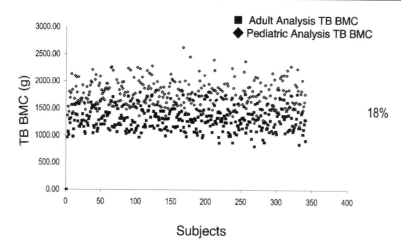

Fig. 5. Difference in total-body bone mineral content between pediatric whole-body (open diamonds) and adult (filled-in squares) whole-body software in 352 boys ($n = 175$) and girls ($n = 177$), aged 10–13 yr (McKay H, unpublished data).

structure to determine the degree of rotation of the femur during positioning and to define the bottom border of the proximal femur ROI. As a result of ill-defined skeletal landmarks, auto-analyze modes of standard proximal femur software often incorrectly place anatomical markers such as the trochanteric border (Fig. 7) or the midline, which are used to position other regions in the proximal femur analysis. The software has certain expectations regarding the general anatomy of a hip and may not place subregions correctly if the hip is a strange shape due to differing growth patterns or disease state. Changes to the size of the ROI (i.e., global or femoral neck) can influence algorithms and outcomes. The specifics of proximal femur analysis issues are discussed under "Analysis Issues and Recommendations for Scan Analysis: Total Hip and Femoral Neck Analysis."

New Software Versions

Both GE Lunar and Hologic have recently upgraded their software used to analyze pediatric spine, proximal femur, and whole-body scans. Hologic's Delphi and Discovery systems now have auto-low-density spine, hip, and auto-whole-body analysis capabilities, and the 4500 models may also be upgraded to this software change as well. These software changes were in response to the concern of imprecise assignment of bone and soft tissue using the LDS and standard whole-body software. Auto-whole-body analysis is only possible if the system is also configured for body composition analysis because the mass measurement is used to make adjustments in the bone detection threshold. The system will automatically use this analysis mode in patients measuring between 8 and 40 kg.

These new software modes have the potential to cause much confusion for the unaware user, especially if a patient changes weight and is within the weight range (8–40 kg; 17.6–88 lbs) at one visit and above the range for the next. The system uses the software based

Fig. 6. (*opposite page*) Correlations for change in (**A**) total-body bone area; (**B**) bone content; and (**C**) bone mineral density for pediatric total-body and adult software in 352 boys ($n = 175$) and girls ($n = 177$), aged 10–13 years. R^2 values are substantially lower for change compared to cross-sectional comparisons. Values for change also differed substantially (*see* details in text) (McKay H, unpublished data)

A $R^2=0.35$

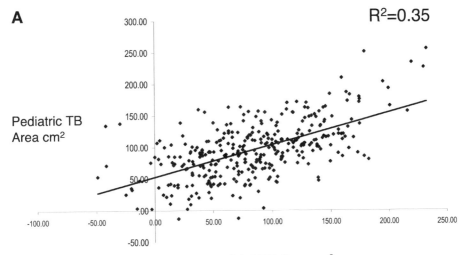

Pediatric TB
Area cm^2

Adult TB Area cm^2

B $R^2=0.79$

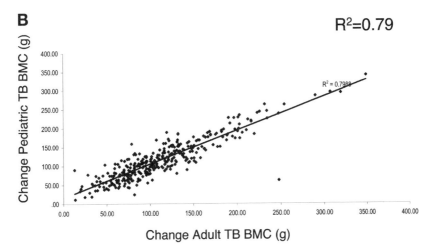

Change Pediatric TB BMC (g)

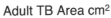

Change Adult TB BMC (g)

C $R^2=0.62$

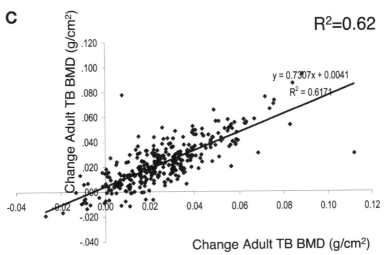

Change Adult TB BMD (g/cm^2)

Change Adult TB BMD (g/cm^2)

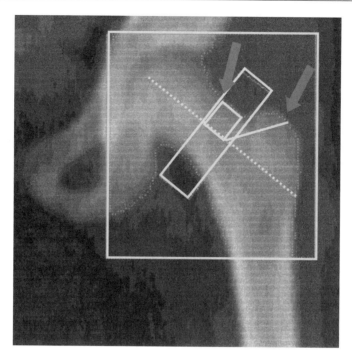

Fig. 7. Automatic placement of the proximal femur region of interest on a young child using the Hologic auto-analyze mode. Arrows point to misplacement of the trochanteric region of interest and Ward's triangle on the proximal femur scan.

not on the entered weight, but on the weight measured by the system. DXA technologists must be aware of which software was used and whether a change in software occurs, as it is important to take into account how this will affect the results.

In both the auto-low-density spine and proximal femur analysis software, changes to the older algorithms were made so that it is no longer based on a bone threshold concept. For example, the spine software uses anatomical assumptions to refine the bone mapping process; the skeleton is assumed to be articulated, the center of mass of the vertebral bodies are assumed to lie near the center of the image, and the adjacent vertebral bodies are assumed to lie within a certain distance of one another.

One concern is that most of the currently available pediatric reference data were generated using adult analysis software. Hologic has recently compiled data collected from pediatric subjects measured on Hologic 4500 instruments from five centers. Normative data curves were generated for age 3–20 yr for the spine, proximal femur, and whole body, but these are published only in abstract form *(11,12)*. These reference data are currently available for the newer Hologic models (i.e., Discovery) and as a software upgrade for older models (i.e., version 12.3).

GE Lunar has also responded to the need for normative data that can be applied to their pediatric software, but at present they have only spine and whole-body curves *(13)*. These data were collected from more than 2000 healthy children between 5 and 20 yr of age and were measured on either DPX or Prodigy series scanners (spine: 1135 females, 924 males; total body: 821 females; 673 males) *(13)*. GE Lunar is currently extending data collection to children as young as 3 yr and is including proximal femur scans (GE Lunar, personal communication).

GE Lunar makes the additional effort to adjust for frame size by comparing height for age, BMC for BA, and BA for height. Some of these alternative strategies such as BMC for BA are considered in greater detail in Chapter 10. Future studies are needed to evaluate the use of these new approaches in longitudinal studies and in children with altered body composition. These changes illustrate the rapidly evolving nature of the field.

Normative data available for Norland densitometers was gathered in 1995 from 433 females and 345 males between the ages of 2 and 20 yr. Similar to GE Lunar software, only data for spine and whole-body scans are currently available (14).

ANALYSIS ISSUES AND RECOMMENDATIONS FOR SCAN ANALYSIS

There is a clear need to standardize analysis protocols for clinical and research use in growing children. It is important to bear in mind, however, that the protocol of choice will depend on the clinical or research question being asked.

Several challenges exist when analyzing scans in the growing skeleton. These include general issues such as poor identification of skeletal landmarks, giving rise to incorrect placement of the ROI; a paucity of general guidelines for proceeding with adapting analysis as the skeleton changes size; and undertrained technologists. There are also manufacturer-specific software and hardware issues such as poor mapping of bone related to either scan mode or edge detection algorithms and auto-analyze features that continue to require technologist intervention.

Prior to the most recent release, the Hologic user's guide suggested that the pediatric mode be used for children aged 4–12 yr. There is no clear justification provided for the suggested upper age limit.

It may be more appropriate to base the criteria for selecting the pediatric analysis mode on patient height or body weight. It has been suggested by some that 30 or 40 kg (i.e., 66 or 88 lb) be used for a cutoff and that, below these weights, the pediatric software should be used (opinion). However, the pediatric analysis mode may be required to analyze scans of children who weigh more than 40 kg if they have markedly reduced bone mineral content.

There are currently no standard guidelines, and most published pediatric normative data have used the standard adult analysis modes, making interpretation of results from pediatric analysis difficult. The newest versions of analysis for the whole body from Hologic automatically choose auto-low density analysis based on the weight assessed by the body composition analysis software. The operator must use clinical judgment regarding selection of the mode (pediatric vs standard) for analysis in cases that are dependent upon the ability of the standard adult software to detect bone margins. It may also be useful to analyze the scan in both modes to maximize available data for comparison at the time of future scans.

Spine

Analysis of spine scans in pediatric patients is similar in some respects to adult osteoporotic patients. Prior to the most recent software release, it was often necessary to manually define the ROI if a vertebra did not have connectivity to the rest of the spine. In addition, auto-analyze software often incorrectly identifies vertebral levels and is not equipped to automatically bend the intervertebral lines of scoliotic spines. The technologist must be familiar with spine anatomy and should be prepared to reanalyze these scans as needed, either by moving the global ROI to cover the correct levels, by adding a bridge to create connectivity, or by manually determining where the intervertebral line should be placed to adjust the line for curvature. The newest software is more effective at identifying bone within the vertebrae; however, scoliotic spines may still require intervention during analysis. If significant adjustment is required during the analysis, it should be noted on the patient's report.

Whole Body

As with the spine analysis modes, it is important for technologists to be aware of the whole-body analysis mode currently in use for their scanner and to be familiar with its limitations. There are institutions that routinely perform whole-body scans in infants and young children for research and clinical purposes (Chapter 9). The GE Lunar Prodigy scanner will soon be able to assess whole-body BMD in infants who weigh as little as 2 kg (i.e., 4.4 lb; personal communication); however, this software is not currently commercially available. Of particular interest is the latest analysis versions available on GE Lunar instruments, which allow for exclusion of the head region *(13)*. Hologic has also stated that removing the head subregion may give a more accurate assessment of the total-body BMD, but they do not currently offer this option in the auto-analysis package; the subtotal results represent BMC, BA, and BMD for the whole body including the head. Pediatric normative data is currently only available for scans collected with the head subregion included in the analysis.

At this time, it is not recommend to scan young children who weigh less than 8 kg (17.6 lb) for clinical purposes.

Total Hip and Femoral Neck Analysis

As mentioned previously, assessment of total hip scans in children is fraught with complexity. Analysis becomes particularly complicated during the assessment and interpretation of serial scans because, in children, the proximal femur changes in both size and shape (Fig. 8). These issues have been examined in a longitudinal study of children scanned using standard Hologic software *(15)*. Several approaches were employed to analyze longitudinal data, and these gave differing results. In analyzing longitudinal changes in total hip scans in 40 healthy children over an 8-mo period, if the global ROI was increased over time (as the hip region grew), BA increased by 3.2% and BMC increased by 3.7% more than if the regions were analyzed using an unchanging global ROI (Fig. 9). This difference is substantial, approximating the magnitude of change in proximal femur BMC over an entire year's growth during prepuberty (3–4%) *(16,17)*.

When differing methods of analysis for the femoral neck box (Fig. 10) were applied to scans collected from 10 healthy children over a 7-yr period, the magnitude of change in BA and BMC varied depending on the method used. Most importantly, however, BMD values were fairly robust and did not change significantly with different analyses as BMC and BA changed in similar magnitude and direction (Fig. 11).

Historically, analysis of the femoral neck box was operator-dependent; all aspects of the ROI size and placement were controlled by the operator. Manufacturer recommendations have changed over time; because there are, to our knowledge, no published recommendations as to how pediatric hip scans should be analyzed, operators have often narrowed or shortened the femoral neck ROI depending on the size of the child being measured.

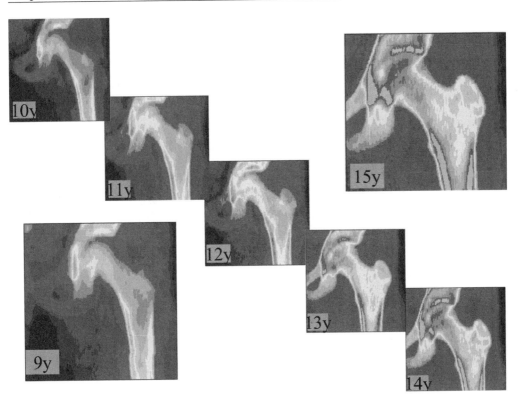

Fig. 8. Hip scans from one child measured annually from age 9 to 15 yr. Clear changes in the size and shape of the hip occur with normal growth.

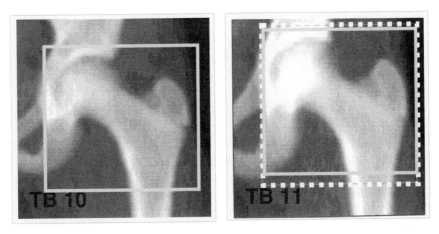

Fig. 9. Illustration of how the size and position of the global region of interest can change significantly for a proximal femur scan as a child grows. Time 1, solid lines; Time 2, broken lines. (Reproduced from ref. *15*, with permission.)

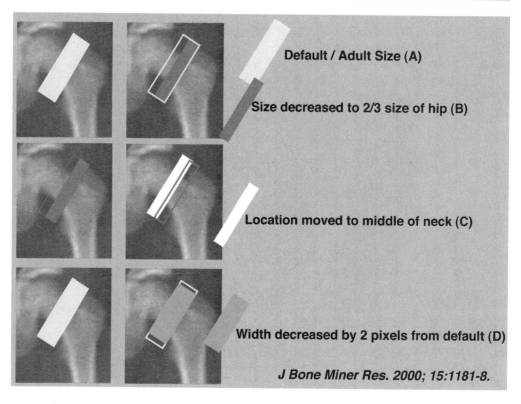

Fig. 10. Schematic illustration of differences in the size and positioning of the femoral neck (FN) subregion of interest among **(A)** default, **(B)** decreased width, **(C)** decreased length, and **(D)** changed location of analyses. (Reproduced from ref. *15*, with permission.)

This decision presents potential problems both for clinical assessment and research studies. If the neck box is reduced from the standard width, certain equations to adjust for size (e.g., BMAD) are no longer applicable, and comparison with normative data may be invalid. In a research setting, if the femoral neck ROI size is reduced for smaller children as compared to larger children within the same study, the BA and BMC will vary considerably among children; values may change for an individual child simply because technologists choose different analysis methods. For example, if a narrower femoral neck ROI were selected, BMD values may be similar but BMC and BA values could be 13% less than those for same-aged children whose scans were analyzed using the system default *(15)*.

BMD values for both the proximal femur and femoral neck appear to be more robust, but the association to fracture risk and BMD is not clear. Similarly, the location of the femoral neck ROI may also influence study outcomes. If the femoral neck ROI is moved to the center of the femoral neck and away from the medial border of the greater trochanter, BA and BMC increase by approximately 3% *(18)*.

GE Lunar has recently released a version of software that will take into consideration the size of the bone being analyzed, although it is currently not approved by the FDA and is only available with Institutional Review Board (IRB) approval (personal communication). Studies examining the reliability of pediatric scan analysis using other DXA systems are needed.

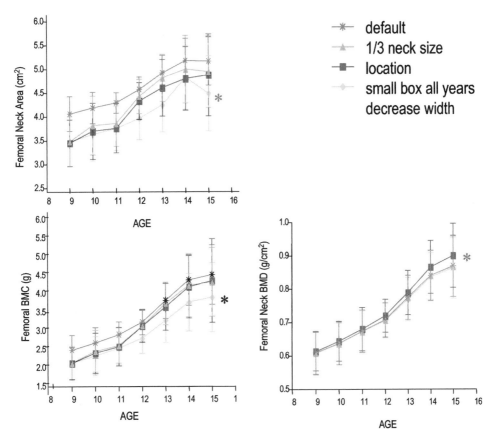

Fig. 11. Results of trend analysis comparing regression slopes for bone area, bone mineral content (BMC), and bone mineral density (BMD) at the femoral neck across 7 yr. Scans were analyzed by four methods (Fig. 10), with no significant differences observed in areal BMD among methods as BMC and bone area changed in similar magnitude and direction. (Reproduced from ref. *15*, with permission.)

If biologically feasible, the system-derived ROI should be used when possible for both the global ROI and, especially, for the femoral neck ROI. Maintaining the size of this ROI is ideal but may be difficult in studies of children younger than 8 yr. The global ROI will increase as a child grows, but clinicians and researchers should be aware that the apparent effect of an intervention may be confounded when changes in global ROI are required. It is recommended (and insisted, by reviewers) that all clinical reports and research manuscripts include a description of how pediatric scans are analyzed if a protocol other than the system default is utilized. Clinicians should determine a standard protocol for use within their clinics and should ensure that all technologists consistently use the same analysis protocols.

FOLLOW-UP SCAN ANALYSIS

Analysis of longitudinal changes in hip and spine DXA data in growing children can prove to be difficult. Although no one approach has been shown to be best, some suggestions can minimize error. When possible, one operator should acquire and analyze all scans (baseline and follow-up) for an individual patient so that consistency of procedures will be optimized. When that is not possible, protocols should be standardized among technologists. Changes from the default analysis software should be minimized, and any changes to the default mode must be stated in detail in the DXA reports or in scientific publications. Documentation of manufacturer, model, and software should be noted on all clinical reports, and particular comments should be included on serial reports when there have been changes made to the model or software used.

Manufacturers recommend that the compare mode of analysis be used to analyze all adult follow-up scans. It may not be possible to employ the compare mode and maintain the same-sized global ROI in longitudinal exams of children who are growing rapidly. The compare function can and should be used, however, to ensure a similar positioning of the regions of interest between time points, to help the operator identify positioning errors *(19)* and to minimize changes in the ROI. Regardless of the method used, it is important that technologists in the same clinic agree on a consistent protocol for all children and at all examinations and that researchers report details of scan analyses in manuscripts.

CONCLUSIONS

We concur with the International Society for Clinical Densitometry (ISCD) *(20),* which recommends that, for children, "serial BMD studies should be done on the same machine using the same scanning mode, software, and analysis when appropriate. Changes may be required with growth of the child.... Any deviation from standard adult acquisition protocols, such as use of auto-low density software and manual adjustment of the region of interest, should be stated in the report."

SUMMARY POINTS

- Most DXA software has been developed for adults, which leads to difficulties in the analysis of pediatric scans.
- Basic analysis of pediatric spine, hip, and whole-body scans differ slightly among densitometer manufacturers (i.e., Hologic, Lunar, and Norland) and instrument models.
- Manufacturers will likely support their most current versions of any software and equipment packages including the pediatric analysis software. DXA centers must be aware of the impact of changing software and hardware on results so as to avoid erroneous interpretations of longitudinal data.
- Standard, low-density, auto-low-density, and pediatric whole-body software (Hologic-specific) give different results. Low-density software and pediatric whole-body software give substantially higher BMC and BA values and lower BMD compared to standard software. Body composition values also change with variable effects on lean mass, fat mass, and percentage of body fat. As the child approaches 40 kg (i.e., 88 lb), the new Hologic software will revert to adult analysis.
- For Lunar instruments, the mode of scan acquisition will likely need to be changed from thin to standard when a child approaches 40 kg (i.e., 88 lb).
- Standard criteria for when to implement pediatric analyses have not been established. Recommendations are usually based first on the weight of the patient, and then on age. Analyze data in both the standard and low density modes whenever possible to allow for more accurate interpretations of change at subsequent follow-up scans.
- For analysis of pediatric whole-body scans, it is recommended that the head region be deleted during analysis when this software option is available and corresponding normative data exist.

- As a result of the complexities of positioning and scan analyses in the proximal femur, it is suggested that the femoral neck or total hip scans be used with caution for clinical purposes when working with children.
- Ideally, the same instrument model and software mode should be used for repeat scans on individual patients. However, if the same mode or software cannot be used, the change must be documented, with warnings about potential inaccuracies of interpretation.
- Regardless of the method used, thoughtful analysis and standardized protocols within a clinic or research study are crucial.

REFERENCES

1. Genant HK, Block JE, Steiger P, Glueer CC, Ettinger B, Harris ST. Appropriate use of bone densitometry. Radiology 1989;170:817–822.
2. Genant HK, Grampp S, Gluer CC, et al. Universal standardization for dual x-ray absorptiometry: patient and phantom cross-calibration results. J Bone Miner Res 1994;9:1503–1510.
3. Hanson J. Standardization of femur BMD. J Bone Miner Res 1997;12:1316–1317.
4. Steiger P. Standardization of postero-anterior (PA) spine BMD measurements by DXA. Committee for standards in DXA. Bone 1995;17:435.
5. Abrahamsen B, Gram J, Hansen TB, Beck-Nielsen H. Cross calibration of QDR-2000 and QDR-1000 dual-energy x-ray densitometers for bone mineral and soft tissue measurements. Bone 1995;16:385–390.
6. Van Loan M, Keim N, Berg K, Mayclin P. Evaluation of body composition by dual energy x-ray absorptiometry and two different software packages. Med Sci Sports Exerc 1995;27:587–591.
7. Hui SL, Gao S, Zhou XH, et al. Universal standardization of bone density measurements: a method with optimal properties for calibration among several instruments. J Bone Miner Res 1997;12:1463–1470.
8. Ellis KJ, Shypailo RJ, Pratt JA, Pond WG. Accuracy of dual-energy x-ray absorptiometry for body-composition measurements in children. Am J Clin Nutr 1994;60:660–665.
9. Leonard MB, Feldman HI, Zemel BS, Berlin JA, Barden EM, Stallings VA. Evaluation of low density spine software for the assessment of bone mineral density in children. J Bone Miner Res 1998;13:1687–1690.
10. Zemel BS, Leonard MB, Stallings VA. Evaluation of the Hologic experimental pediatric whole body analysis software in health: children with chronic disease (Abstract). J Bone Miner Res 2000;15(Suppl 1):S400.
11. Zemel BS, Leonard MB, Kalkwarf HJ, et al. Reference data for the whole body, lumbar spine and proximal femur for American children relative to age, gender and body size. J Bone Miner Res 2004;19(Suppl 1):S231.
12. Kelly TL, Zemel BS, Leonard MB, et al. Gender-specific BMD reference values for U.S. white children. ISCD 11th Annual Meeting, 2005.
13. Barden HS, Wacker WK, Faulkner KG. Pediatric enhancements to Prodigy software: variable standard deviations and subcranial total body results. ISCD 11th Annual Meeting; Poster #4, 2005.
14. Zanchetta JR, Plotkin H, Alvarez Filgueira ML. Bone mass in children: normative values for the 2–20-year-old population. Bone 1995;16:393S–399S.
15. McKay HA, Petit MA, Bailey DA, Wallace WM, Schutz RW, Khan KM. Analysis of proximal femur DXA scans in growing children: comparisons of different protocols for cross-sectional 8-month and 7-year longitudinal data. J Bone Miner Res 2000;15:1181–1188.
16. Bailey DA. The Saskatchewan Pediatric Bone Mineral Accrual Study: bone mineral acquisition during the growing years. Int J Sports Med 1997;18:S191–S194.
17. Bonjour JP, Theintz G, Buchs B, Slosman D, Rizzoli R. Critical years and stages of puberty for spinal and femoral bone mass accumulation during adolescence. J Clin Endocrinol Metab 1991;73:555–563.
18. Kuiper JW, Van Kuijk C, Grashuis JL. Distribution of trabecular and cortical bone related to geometry: a quantitative computed tomography study of the femoral neck. Invest Radiol 1997;32:83–89.
19. Fulkerson JA, Himes JH, French SA, et al. Bone outcomes and technical measurement issues of bone health among children and adolescents: considerations for nutrition and physical activity intervention trials. Osteoporos Int 2004;15:929–941.
20. The International Society for Clinical Densitometry. Official positions, http://www.iscd.org/visitors/positions/official.cfm. Accessed March 2006.

7 Evaluation

Babette S. Zemel, PhD and Moira Petit, PhD

CONTENTS

INTRODUCTION
NORMATIVE DATA
INTERPRETING SCANS
CONCLUSIONS
SUMMARY POINTS
REFERENCES

INTRODUCTION

As with scan acquisition and analysis, interpretation of pediatric dual-energy x-ray absorptiometry (DXA) scans presents a myriad of challenges. Historically, DXA was developed predominantly for the diagnosis and management of postmenopausal osteoporosis. For older adults, the amount of bone mineral mass is a reasonable surrogate of bone strength because adult bone does not change much in size or shape,* and low bone mineral density (BMD) measured by DXA is predictive of fragility fractures.

However, children are not small adults. In children, bone mineral mass and areal BMD are strongly related to growth attained, and bone fragility may be the result of many other factors. In contrast to adults, the size, shape, and mineralization of a child's bones change rapidly over time due to growth and maturation changes (see Chapter 6, Fig. 8). The pace of growth and maturation is variable, especially surrounding the ages when peak height velocity and sexual maturation usually occur. During this age range, it is possible to have two children of the same age with considerable differences in body size and physical maturity (Fig. 1) or two children of the same body size and maturity who are of very

---

*Even this concept must be qualified. Long bones (such as the proximal femur) continue to expand throughout life to compensate for the loss of bone mass. This expansion causes DXA BMD values to decrease even though bone bending strength may remain stable (1,2).

From: *Current Clinical Practice: Bone Densitometry in Growing Patients: Guidelines for Clinical Practice*
Edited by: A. J. Sawyer, L. K. Bachrach, and E. B. Fung © Humana Press Inc., Totowa, NJ

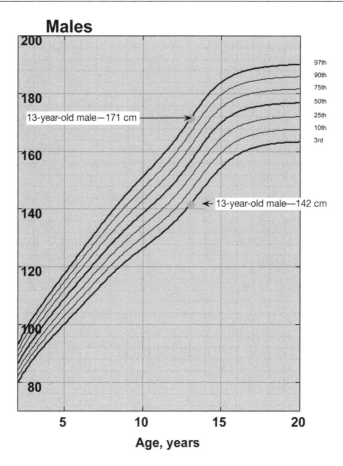

Fig. 1. Children of the same age can have pronounced differences in body size. For example, among normal healthy 13-yr-old boys, stature can range from 142 to 171 cm (i.e., 4'8" to 5'7").

different ages. Consequently, it is difficult to categorize a DXA BMD measurement as normal or abnormal for an individual child without consideration of additional factors.

As discussed in Chapter 3, bone mineral content (BMC) and BMD are very much size dependent. DXA systematically underestimates BMD in a smaller individual because it is an areal (g/cm^2), not a volumetric (g/cm^3), measure. This limitation of DXA is particularly important in pediatric evaluations. Children with chronic diseases that place them at risk for poor bone mineral accrual because of malabsorption, poor dietary intake, inflammation, reduced physical activity, or medications are also likely to have delayed growth and maturation relative to same-age peers. In order to assess whether a child has inadequate bone mineral accrual, it is important to consider whether low BMC or BMD is the result of short stature or delayed maturation vs a primary abnormality in bone metabolism. As part of a growth assessment, pediatricians will take into account the stage of maturity, gender, and ethnicity of the child. Similar considerations need to be applied in the evaluation of bone health, and a DXA measurement should be one of several components of a medical evaluation.

NORMATIVE DATA

Ideal Characteristics of Reference Data

The first important step in the interpretation of DXA measurements in pediatric patients is the appropriate selection of reference data. Reference data should have several characteristics, especially if used proscriptively (i.e., to define healthy bone mineral status) *(3)*. The reference data should be derived from a sample of healthy children who are representative of the overall population. Healthy children can be defined as those who are free of chronic diseases, medication use, and physical limitations that might affect bone mineral accrual. They should also be of normal nutritional, growth, and developmental status because these are also known to affect bone mineral status. Because of the possibility of regional differences in lifestyle, ethnic composition, sunlight exposure, and so forth, a multiregional sample is optimal. The sample must be of sufficient size to adequately characterize the variability in bone measures for each gender. Because the variability in bone measures increases with age, it is important to assure a reasonable distribution of the sample by age so that the age-dependent differences in variability are also fully characterized in the data set.

Handling of the reference data, once collected, is important. Use of a mean and a standard deviation (SD) is the most common approach to the use of reference data. However, because the distribution of bone measures is sometimes skewed, more sophisticated biostatistical techniques are required. A variety of these sophisticated statistical models have been proposed, including parametric regression modeling *(4,5)* and the LMS method *(6)*. The LMS method uses a power transformation to normalize data. The optimal power to obtain normality is calculated for a series of age groups, and the trend is summarized by a smooth (L) curve. Smoothed curves for the mean (M) and coefficient of variation (S) are also acquired, and these three measures, L, M, and S, are used to describe the data distribution.

Presently, there are no reference data sets for bone mineral measures in children that meet all of these criteria. As described below, development of a pediatric reference data set that meets most of these criteria is in progress.

Calculation of the Z-Score

Ultimately, reference data are used to calculate a Z-score or an SD score that is used as an indicator of bone mineral status. When using the mean and SD to calculate a Z-score, the following formula is employed:

$$Z\text{-score} = (\text{observed} - \text{mean}) / SD$$

When the LMS method is applied, a more complex equation is required, using the L (skewness), M (median), and S (coefficient of variation) values:

$$Z\text{-score} = ([(\text{Observed value} / M)^L] - 1) / (L \times S)$$

A BMC or BMD Z-score is used as an indicator of bone mineral status, just as a height Z-score is used as an indicator of growth status. Children whose BMC or BMD is close to the median for their age and gender will have a Z-score of zero. A Z-score of 2 corresponds to the 97th percentile, and a Z-score of –2 corresponds to the 3rd percentile. An advantage of Z-scores over percentile values is that very low or very high values that are outside the reference population distribution (i.e., >100th percentile or <0th percentile) can be quantified. This is especially important for longitudinal follow-up of children with low BMD, as it allows for quantifying the changes in BMD relative to the expected values for age and gender.

Selection of Reference Data

Options for selecting pediatric reference data include (1) using the manufacturer's database, (2) comparing your data to published data, or (3) using locally collected normative values. Each approach has its benefits and limitations. As with all decisions related to acquiring, analyzing, and interpreting DXA scans, the most important point is for the clinician to be aware of the method used and the limitations involved.

As noted in Chapter 3, DXA results obtained with machines from different manufacturers and, in some instances, different software versions by the same manufacturer are not always comparable. Thus, selecting a database established with the same software version and hardware version by the same manufacturer is ideal. The selection of a reference database from the same manufacturer is absolutely essential, because the conversion equations between manufacturers are based on adults *(7)* and have not been validated for children. Using the manufacturer's dataset is appealing because of the ease of availability and the fact that data were collected on instruments by the same manufacturer. However, reference data may have been collected using differing versions of DXA software from those currently employed. Furthermore, details related to the size and demographics of the population studied are not typically provided. The advantage of using published normative data is that details of the population are described in the manuscript. Unfortunately, many of the normative data studies of bone development in children suffer from a sample size inadequate to provide sufficient normative values for children across various maturational stages and ethnic and gender groups. Most pediatric BMD reference data sets used to calculate Z-scores contain small numbers of participants within each age category and may not adequately characterize normal variability in BMC or BMD.

An earlier comparison of published pediatric DXA normative data revealed differences in the age-specific means and SDs for BMD and BMC that will alter the calculated Z-score. Age-adjusted SD scores (Z-scores) varied by as much as 1 SD, depending upon the normative data used to calculated them *(8)* (Fig. 2). Use of reference data that were not gender-specific resulted in significantly greater misclassification of males as having BMD values below –2 SDs *(8)*.

Some DXA centers have collected their own normative data by scanning otherwise healthy children from the clinics and the community populations. Use of local reference data may be advantageous since the cohort may be more similar in ethnicity and lifestyle to the patient and because the same acquisition and analysis protocols will have been used for DXA studies. The costs in time and dollars to collect normative data are too great for all but the largest centers.

In 2001, the US National Institutes of Health initiated the Bone Mineral Density in Childhood Study (BMDCS). This study aims to develop longitudinal reference data in a multiethnic sample of more than 1500 children nationwide using carefully standardized data-collection techniques. Whole-body, lumbar spine, proximal femur, and forearm data are being collected, along with skeletal age, puberty status, dietary intake, and physical activity information. Data collection began in 2002 at five medical centers and

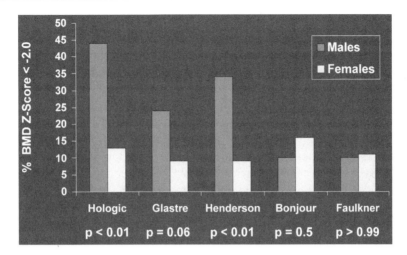

Fig. 2. Using five different reference data sources, large differences in the estimated prevalence of osteopenia were observed. Use of reference data that was not gender-specific resulted in overestimation of the prevalence of osteopenia in males *(9)*. (Reprinted from ref. *8*, with permission from Elsevier.)

is ongoing. Healthy children, ages 6–17 yr, were recruited and will be followed for 5 yr. The BMDCS has the advantage of being designed specifically for the purpose of providing reference data representative of American children *(9–11)*.

While the results of this study are pending, a separate initiative was undertaken by numerous pediatric researchers in collaboration with Hologic, Inc. The goal was to develop a large pediatric database for whole-body, spine, and proximal femur scan data and to make it available for users of Hologic DXA devices *(12,13)*. The sample consisted of data on healthy children from six centers around the United States engaged in pediatric research programs collecting data on healthy children. Although the recruitment criteria were variable, all scans were obtained on Hologic 4500 or Delphi devices and were centrally analyzed using the latest generation of pediatric software and the LMS statistical technique *(6)*. These reference data are used to calculate Z-scores for pediatric subjects in software version 12.3 or higher.

Ethnicity

A final consideration in the selection of reference data is the problem of ethnic differences in bone mineral accrual *(5,14–19)*. In particular, African Americans are noted to have significantly greater BMD than other ethnic groups. Differences in growth, body composition, skeletal maturation, and the timing of puberty only partly explain these ethnic differences. There is no consensus on how to address these ethnic differences in evaluating DXA results among pediatric patients, nor are there evidence-based studies relating to outcomes such as fracture risk to provide guidance. Additionally, few studies of ethnic minorities are of sufficient size to adequately serve as reference data.

For adults, the International Society of Clinical Densitometry (ISCD) has recommended that Z-scores and T-scores be derived from reference data based on the Caucasian population *(20)*. The rationale for this recommendation, in part, relates to the difficulty in defining and identifying patient ethnicity, especially for those of mixed ethnicity, and the lack of data relating fracture risk to BMD in many ethnic groups. In addition, when African Americans are compared to a Caucasian reference population, the comparison results in a lower prevalence of osteoporosis, which corresponds to their lower rate of fracture.

For children, the correspondence between DXA Z-score and fracture risk is not defined, and ethnic differences in fracture rates among children are not well characterized. Thus, it is not possible to use the relationship between Z-score and fracture risk as a guide in the use of ethnicity-specific reference data in children. The emphasis on promoting good bone mineral accrual during childhood to attain optimal peak bone mass would point to the importance for African American children to attain a peak bone mass appropriate to their ethnic group. However, this is more of a theoretically based consideration than an evidence-based one. In the absence of evidence-based guidelines for the use of ethnic-specific reference data, the rationale chosen by the ISCD may reasonably be applied to children. Alternatively, if ethnic-specific or multiethnic reference data are used, it is important that this factor be explicitly stated in the reporting of results.

INTERPRETING SCANS

The Z-score is the central element in interpreting the DXA results. Although it cannot be used for diagnostic classification (as the T-score is used in adults), it is an indicator of how an individual child's DXA result compares to his or her peers. For example, 3% of the population of healthy children will have a Z-score less than –2. When evaluating an individual child with a Z-score less than –2, one must consider whether the child is a member of the 3% of children in this segment of the population distribution or whether the child is failing to accrue bone appropriately. This question can never be answered on the basis of a DXA result alone, and additional risk factors such as multiple fractures, bone pain, small body size, delayed maturation, physical activity level, medical history, and nutritional status must be considered. As with a height or weight measurement, a BMC or BMD Z-score may be an indicator of an underlying problem. A low (<–1) or very low (<–2) Z-score should trigger a set of additional diagnostic evaluations to better identify the nature of the abnormality.

A child with a BMC or BMD Z-score that is not in the "low" or "very low" range may still be failing to achieve his or her genetic potential for bone mass. Twin studies and parent–offspring comparisons have shown that BMD has a high heritable component (21–24). However, at present, there is no way to estimate this genetic potential. In a growth evaluation, parental height is used to estimate the genetic potential for linear growth, and a target height range can be identified. Unfortunately, at this point, we are far from being able to estimate a comparable measure for target range for the genetic potential for height. A somewhat analogous concept is that of optimal peak bone mass, or the maximum bone mass that a child can attain in young adulthood under ideal conditions such as good health, adequate intake of calcium, and weight-bearing physical activity (25). Particularly in the presence of risk factors for low BMD, monitoring bone mineral accrual and adjusting modifiable factors such as diet and physical activity may serve the purpose of taking steps toward achieving optimal peak bone mass in a child at risk for poor bone mineral accrual and suboptimal peak bone mass.

In the clinical care setting, a number of approaches have been used to adjust for factors associated with low bone density. Because BMD is influenced by skeletal maturation, some clinicians use bone age in the BMD evaluation. Bone age is determined by comparison of a left hand and wrist radiograph to an atlas or standard showing typical stages of development in healthy children. In the United States, the Greulich and Pyle atlas *(26)* is most commonly used. This atlas was based on 1000 radiographs obtained from Caucasian children participating in the Brush Foundation study between 1931 and 1942 in Cleveland, Ohio. The atlas consists of a series of plates (hand–wrist x-rays) that represent the typical bone development of children at various ages: from birth to 18 yr in girls, and from birth to 19 yr in boys. The children were evaluated within a few days of their birthday, so the bone ages are age-centered, meaning the standardized image representing bone age at 10 yr for boys represents boys who are 10.0 yr of age. The atlas includes a table with the SD in months for each bone age.

Outside the United States, the Tanner-Whitehouse III method is commonly used *(27)*. This scoring system differs from the Greulich and Pyle method in that the 13 bones (the radius, the ulna; the first, third, and fifth metacarpal; and the proximal, middle, and distal phalanx) are compared to reference radiographs and pictograms and are assigned a rating. The corresponding score from these ratings are referred to as the radius, ulna, short bone (RUS) score. An independent scoring system is also provided for the carpal bones. Because the bones are rated individually, this scoring system allows for uneven maturation of the bones in the hand and wrist. The total score is used to calculate bone age. The bone ages assigned are based on longitudinal data from the Harpenden study, conducted in the United Kingdom in the 1950s and 1960s (number of radiographs [n] = 3000), with additional data from studies of children from Belgium in the 1970s (n = 30,872), Spain in the 1980s (n = 5266), Japan in 1985 (n = 1075), Italy in the 1990s (n = 1831), Argentina in 1972 (n = 775), and the United States from 1985 to 1995 (n = 1090).

Presently, there are no published BMC or BMD reference data relative to bone age using either bone-age scoring system. However, in healthy children, bone age has been found to be a good predictor of BMD *(28)*, and delayed bone age is associated with fracture *(29)*. In addition, as shown by Mora et al. *(30)* in a large, multiethnic sample of healthy children in the United States, with bone age assessed by the Greulich and Pyle method, the variability in the difference between skeletal and chronological ages was quite large and varied significantly by ethnic group. Jones and Ma *(29)* also found large deviations between skeletal and chronological age in healthy Australian children. Bone age is often advanced in obese children *(31)*, so the increasing prevalence of overweight and obese children may contribute to the differences between bone age and chronological age. Therefore, it is not likely that the distribution of BMC or BMD for bone age is the same as the distribution of BMC or BMD for chronological age. However, in the absence of an alternative, some clinicians substitute the bone age for a chronological age in using age-based reference data to calculate a BMD for age Z-score. In one study of children with Crohn's disease, it was shown that this approach only had a significant effect on the findings when bone age was more than 2 yr less than chronological age *(32)*. Because bone age corresponds generally to pubertal maturation and is closely linked to the timing of the adolescent growth spurt, this approach has the advantage of taking into account biological maturation in the assessment of BMC or BMD.

Another approach that is sometimes used clinically is the substitution of height age for chronological age in the calculation of a BMD Z-score. Height age is calculated by identifying the age at which the child's height is the median height. This approach has two problems. For children with growth abnormalities, the use of height age has the potential to force a comparison with an age group that is developmentally inappropriate. In other words, this technique is likely to result in the comparison of a short pubertal child to reference values for children within a prepubertal age range. Because of the profound effects of puberty on bone mineral accrual, this technique is particularly inappropriate and is not recommended.

Although there are no established guidelines on how to account for pubertal status in the evaluation of DXA results, advanced or delayed puberty is an important consideration in the overall interpretation. Pubertal status is categorized according to the stages described by Tanner (33) for breast development in girls, genital development in boys, and pubic hair development for both sexes. Testicular volume may also be assessed and used in defining pubertal status. When it is not possible to obtain information about pubertal status by physical exam, a self-assessment pictorial questionnaire can be used (34).

Even if a child's BMC or BMD falls within a normative reference range, there may be additional factors that place the child at risk for fracture. As an example, a severely obese child may have a normal or increased BMC for chronological age (35,36); however, the load to the skeleton places the child at increased risk for fracture (37,38). Although this is a theoretical concept at present, current studies investigating bone quality in addition to quantity may provide understanding of these complex issues of bone strength (25).

As described in the Chapter 10, researchers have been developing and testing a variety of other approaches to account for factors associated with bone mineral accrual in the calculation of Z-scores, such as height, lean body mass, and ethnicity. However, few are feasible for use in a clinical setting. The reference data currently under development by Hologic and the BMDCS will ultimately provide BMC and BMD values relative to height and bone age, overcoming the limitations of the approaches discussed previously.

Longitudinal Follow-Up

As noted in Chapter 4, the rate of increase in bone mass during growth and development is variable, and, generally, DXA exams are rarely repeated more frequently than every 12 mo. Occasionally, evaluations made at shorter time intervals are warranted to monitor response to new drug intervention or to monitor rapidly worsening clinical status if they will influence therapeutic decision-making. Longer intervals (i.e., >12 mo) may also be appropriate. Changes in DXA results should be evaluated in the context of the growth that has occurred in that interval.

Generally, children who are increasing in height (i.e., are increasing the size of their skeleton) should increase in BMC. However, it is possible for BMC to increase while BMD remains the same or decreases. This can occur because bone area does not increase at the same rate as BMC. Because BMD is the ratio of BMC to bone area, the disproportionate changes in BMC and bone area can make it appear as if BMD is declining when, in fact, BMC and bone area are both increasing. For this reason, longitudinal follow-up evaluations should consider the changes in all three measures.

In adults, bone loss is likely to be the main cause for a decline in T-score. In children, failure to gain bone at the rate expected for age and sex is the more likely cause of a declining Z-score. However, bone loss may also occur in childhood, as is likely, for example, in the case of a child with acute lymphoblastic leukemia (ALL) who begins glucocorticoid therapy or a child affected by Duchenne's muscular dystrophy (39). Again, this is where inspection of growth status, BMC, bone area, BMD, and associated Z-scores is helpful in interpreting the findings. A child whose growth percentile is declining is not likely to be accruing bone at a rate that is similar to his or her peers. Thus, that child's bone Z-scores are likely to decline, reflecting a failure to accrue bone at the appropriate rate rather than an actual loss of bone.

Presently, there are no reference data for bone mineral accrual to assist in the interpretation of longitudinal follow-up results. The National Institutes of Health (NIH)-sponsored BMDCS is collecting longitudinal data, and interval data will be forthcoming. Results from the Saskatchewan Longitudinal Study showed that peak bone mineral accrual occurs after the peak in the adolescent growth spurt in height *(40)*. Thus, although skeletal growth and bone mineral accrual are closely linked, they do not correspond exactly, and continued accrual of bone mineral occurs after the session of linear growth.

CONCLUSIONS

As shown in healthy children, DXA BMD is predictive of future fractures; it is estimated that the risk of fracture increases 1.5- to 2-fold for every 1-SD decrease in total body, spine, or hip BMD *(37,41)*. These findings speak to the importance of DXA in evaluating bone health in children at risk for poor bone mineral accrual, fractures, and osteoporosis later in life, especially within the context of its wide availability, relatively low cost, and minimal radiation exposure. Although DXA technology has several limitations, as outlined in previous chapters, it remains a useful tool in the context of these limitations.

Substantial efforts are underway to develop appropriate DXA reference data for children and to identify the best approaches to account for important related factors such as growth, body composition, ethnicity, and skeletal and sexual maturation. DXA evaluation in children will certainly improve over the coming decades; yet, it is still a useful tool when used along with other clinical data to evaluate bone health in children. Great care should be taken in the selection of appropriate reference data that most closely match the device and software version used in the evaluation. Important additional considerations include the history, the clinical exam (including growth status, bone age, and pubertal status), the presence of other risk factors (including bone pain and fracture history), and laboratory values.

SUMMARY POINTS

- Optimal reference data are based on the same software and hardware version used, with adequate numbers of healthy children within age and gender groupings and appropriate statistical techniques to adequately capture the normal variability in DXA measures of bone mineral.
- Reference data should be selected based on (1) data collected from the same instrument manufacturer and a similar software version as the clinical scan of interest, (2) provision of gender-specific reference curves, and (3) a large sample size used to generate the curves.
- For children, the age- and gender-specific reference values are used to calculate a Z-score. The T-score should never be used for children.
- BMD or BMC Z-scores cannot be used for diagnostic classification, but they are an indicator of how a child's DXA result compares to his or her peers. Low or very low scores should trigger additional evaluations; however, even children without scores in these low ranges may be not be achieving their genetic potential for bone mass.

- Interpretation of DXA scan results should be done within the context of other relevant clinical information such as patient history, growth assessment, clinical exam, presence of other risk factors, and laboratory values.
- Bone age, particularly if delayed by 2 yr or more, may be a useful aid in interpreting DXA Z-scores. However, at present, there are no universally available reference data for BMD in relation to bone age. Height–age adjustment can lead to erroneous interpretation and should not be applied to DXA Z-scores.
- Failure to accrue bone mineral at an age-appropriate rate, rather than bone loss, is more likely to occur in children and to cause a decline in Z-score with longitudinal follow-up.

REFERENCES

1. Beck TJ, Looker AC, Ruff CB, Sievanen H, Wahner HW. Structural trends in the aging femoral neck and proximal shaft: analysis of the Third National Health and Nutrition Examination Survey dual-energy x-ray absorptiometry data. J Bone Miner Res 2000;15:2297–2304.
2. Ahlborg HG, Johnell O, Turner CH, Rannevik G, Karlsson MK. Bone loss and bone size after menopause. N Engl J Med 2003;349:327–334.
3. Cameron N. The use and abuse of growth charts, in Eveleth P, ed. *Human Growth in Context*. London: Smith Gordon, 1999.
4. Hastie T, Tibshirani R. *Generalized Additive Models*. New York: Chapman and Hall, 1990.
5. Bachrach LK, Hastie T, Wang MC, Narasimhan B, Marcus R. Bone mineral acquisition in healthy Asian, Hispanic, black, and Caucasian youth: a longitudinal study. J Clin Endocrinol Metab 1999;84:4702–4712.
6. Cole TJ, Green PJ. Smoothing reference centile curves: the LMS method and penalized likelihood. Stat Med 1992;11:1305–1319.
7. Hui SL, Gao S, Zhou XH, et al. Universal standardization of bone density measurements: a method with optimal properties for calibration among several instruments. J Bone Miner Res 1997;12:1463–1470.
8. Leonard MB, Propert KJ, Zemel BS, Stallings VA, Feldman HI. Discrepancies in pediatric bone mineral density reference data: potential for misdiagnosis of osteopenia. J Pediatr 1999;135:182–188.
9. Shepherd J, Fan B, Sherman M, et al. Pediatric DXA precision varies with age. J Bone Min Res 2004;19(Suppl 1):234, abstract#SU124.
10. Wren TAL, Gilsanz V, Pitukcheewanont P, et al. The Bone Mineral Density in Childhood Study (BMDCS): Substudy comparing DXA and CT vertebral bone measurements in healthy children and adolescents. J Bone Min Res 2004;19(Suppl 1):567, abstract#F102.
11. Horlick M, Lappe J, Gilsanz V, et al. The Bone Mineral Density in Childhood Study (BMDCS): baseline results for 1554 healthy pediatric volunteers. J Bone Min Res 2004; 19(Suppl 1):14, abstract #1048.
12. Zemel BS, Leonard MB, Kalkwarf HJ, et al. Reference data for the whole body, lumbar spine and proximal femur for American children relative to age, gender and body size. J Bone Miner Res (Abstract) 2004;19(Suppl 1):S231.
13. Kelly T, Specker B, Binkley T, et al. Pediatric BMD Reference Database for U.S. White Children. Bone, 2005;36(Suppl 1):S30, abstract#O-15.
14. Nelson DA, Simpson PM, Johnson CC, Barondess DA, Kleerekoper M. The accumulation of whole body skeletal mass in third- and fourth-grade children: effects of age, gender, ethnicity, and body composition. Bone 1997;20:73–78.
15. Ellis KJ. Body composition of a young, multiethnic, male population. Am J Clin Nutr 1997;66:1323–1331.
16. Ellis KJ, Abrams SA, Wong WW. Body composition of a young, multiethnic female population. Am J Clin Nutr 1997;65:724–731.
17. Wang MC, Aguirre M, Bhudhikanok GS, et al. Bone mass and hip axis length in healthy Asian, black, Hispanic, and white American youths. J Bone Miner Res 1997;12:1922–1935.
18. Gilsanz V, Roe TF, Mora S, Costin G, Goodman WG. Changes in vertebral bone density in black girls and white girls during childhood and puberty. N Engl J Med 1991;325:1597–1600.
19. Gilsanz V, Skaggs DL, Kovanlikaya A, et al. Differential effect of race on the axial and appendicular skeletons of children. J Clin Endocrinol Metab 1998;83:1420–1427.
20. Leib ES, Lewiecki EM, Binkley N, Hamdy RC. Official positions of the International Society for Clinical Densitometry. J Clin Densitom 2004;7:1–6.

21. Arden NK, Spector TD. Genetic influences on muscle strength, lean body mass, and bone mineral density: a twin study. J Bone Miner Res 1997;12:2076–2081.

22. Davies JH, Evans BA, Gregory JW. Bone mass acquisition in healthy children. Arch Dis Child 2005;90:373–378.

23. Jones G, Nguyen TV. Associations between maternal peak bone mass and bone mass in prepubertal male and female children. J Bone Miner Res 2000;15:1998–2004.

24. Hopper JL, Green RM, Nowson CA, et al. Genetic, common environment, and individual specific components of variance for bone mineral density in 10- to 26-year-old females: a twin study. Am J Epidemiol 1998;147:17–29.

25. Heaney RP, Abrams S, Dawson-Hughes B, et al. Peak bone mass. Osteoporosis Int 2000;11:985–1009.

26. Greulich WW, Pyle SI. *Radiographic Atlas of Skeletal Development of the Hand and Wrist.* Stanford University Press, 1950.

27. Tanner J, Healy M, Goldstein H, Cameron N. *Assessment of Skeletal Maturity and Prediction of Adult Height (TW3) Method.* London: W.B. Saunders, 2001.

28. Glastre C, Braillon P, David L, Cochat P, Meunier PJ, Delmas PD. Measurement of bone mineral content of the lumbar spine by dual energy x-ray absorptiometry in normal children: correlations with growth parameters. J Clin Endocrinol Metab 1990;0:1330–1333.

29. Jones G, Ma D. Skeletal age deviation assessed by the Tanner-Whitehouse 2 method is associated with bone mass and fracture risk in children. Bone 2005;36:352–357.

30. Mora S, Boechat MI, Pietka E, Huang HK, Gilsanz V. Skeletal age determinations in children of European and African descent: applicability of the Greulich and Pyle standards. Pediatr Res 2001;50:624–628.

31. Beunen GP, Malina RM, Lefevre JA, Claessens AL, Renson R, Vanreusel B. Adiposity and biological maturity in girls 6–16 years of age. Int J Obes Relat Metab Disord 1994;18:542–546.

32. Semeao EJ, Jawad AF, Zemel BS, Neiswender KM, Piccoli DA, Stallings VA. Bone mineral density in children and young adults with Crohn's disease. Inflamm Bowel Dis 1999;5:161–166.

33. Tanner JM. *Growth at Adolescence.* Oxford: Blackwell Scientific Publication, 1962.

34. Morris NM, Udry JR. Validation of a self-administered instrument to assess stage of adolescent development. J Youth and Adolesc 1980;9:271–280.

35. Leonard MB, Shults J, Wilson BA, Tershakovec AM, Zemel BS. Obesity during childhood and adolescence augments bone mass and bone dimensions. Am J Clin Nutr 2004;80:514–523.

36. Petit MA, Beck TJ, Shults J, Zemel BS, Foster BJ, Leonard MB. Proximal femur bone geometry is appropriately adapted to lean mass in overweight children and adolescents. Bone 2005;36:568–576.

37. Goulding A, Jones IE, Taylor RW, Williams SM, Manning PJ. Bone mineral density and body composition in boys with distal forearm fractures: a dual-energy x-ray absorptiometry study. J Pediatr 2001;139:509–515.

38. Goulding A, Cannan R, Williams SM, Gold EJ, Taylor RW, Lewis-Barned NJ. Bone mineral density in girls with forearm fractures. J Bone Miner Res 1998;13:143–148.

39. Bianchi ML, Mazzanti A, Galbiati E, et al. Bone mineral density and bone metabolism in Duchenne muscular dystrophy. Osteoporosis International 2003;14:9:761–767.

40. McKay HA, Bailey DA, Mirwald RL, Davison KS, Faulkner RA. Peak bone mineral accrual and age at menarche in adolescent girls: a 6-year longitudinal study. J Pediatr 1998;133:682–687.

41. Goulding A, Jones IE, Taylor RW, Manning PJ, Williams SM. More broken bones: a 4-year double cohort study of young girls with and without distal forearm fractures. J Bone Miner Res 2000;15:2011–2018.

8   Reporting DXA Results

Ellen B. Fung, PhD, RD,
Laura K. Bachrach, MD, Julie N. Briody, PhD,
and Christopher T. Cowell, MD

CONTENTS

INTRODUCTION
THE DXA REPORT: PURPOSE AND AUDIENCE
REPORT ELEMENTS
SUMMARY POINTS
REFERENCES

INTRODUCTION

Acquisition and accurate interpretation of bone densitometry scans in the pediatric patient are necessary first steps toward any clinical assessment process. The dual-energy x-ray absorptiometry (DXA) report fulfills the role of transmitting data clearly to the clinician. A timely, concise, and informative report is essential to relay the DXA findings and to avoid costly and potentially dangerous misinterpretations by physicians unfamiliar with pediatric densitometry data.

Reports generated using the DXA manufacturer's proprietary software have advanced significantly since x-ray-based bone densitometers were widely marketed in the late 1980s. Typically, these reports provide basic patient demographic data and a graphical image of the skeletal scan, as well as numeric data for bone area (BA), bone mineral content (BMC), and bone mineral density (BMD) for each region (and subregions). Additionally, the patient's BMD data are compared with reference data derived from healthy controls to generate standard deviation scores: Z-scores represent comparisons with age-matched norms, and T-scores, comparisons with young adults.

Regardless of the age of the subject, most of the standard software provided by the manufacturer automatically reports both the T-scores and the resulting diagnoses of osteopenia or osteoporosis, as established by the World Health Organization (WHO) (1). The software-generated reports appear to provide a comprehensive clinical evaluation of the results sufficient to estimate risk for osteoporosis. However, interpretation based

From: *Current Clinical Practice: Bone Densitometry in Growing Patients: Guidelines for Clinical Practice*
Edited by: A. J. Sawyer, L. K. Bachrach, and E. B. Fung © Humana Press Inc., Totowa, NJ

solely on these computer-generated reports is inappropriate and often misleading when interpreting the DXA results of children and adolescents. It is crucial that the software-generated report be modified and supplemented by a formal written report provided by an expert experienced in interpreting pediatric densitometry.

There are numerous guidelines for diagnosis and assessment of osteoporosis in adults *(2–5)*. However, guidelines for the reporting of DXA scan results are less common. General guidelines have been provided for the reporting of adult DXA scan results in the recent text *Bone Densitometry in Clinical Practice: Application and Interpretation (6)*. The United Kingdom National Osteoporosis Society published a position statement on *"Reporting of DXA bone mineral density scans"* in August, 2002 *(7)*, and, in 2004, the International Society for Clinical Densitometry (ISCD) published practice guidelines for standardization of DXA scanning and interpretation *(8)*.

To our knowledge, there are no similar guidelines for the reporting of pediatric clinical DXA results. This chapter offers guidelines specifically tailored to the pediatric patient. Examples of reporting formats used at pediatric clinical centers in the United States and Australia are provided in Appendix D at the end of this volume.

THE DXA REPORT: PURPOSE AND AUDIENCE

The clinical DXA report has three main purposes: (1) to present the numeric data in a concise, organized, and easily understood fashion to the referring physician; (2) to provide enough technical information to allow for comparison to subsequent DXA studies or to those studies done at other sites; and (3) to provide a preliminary interpretation of the findings in a clinical context. The report may also include recommendations to the patient or physician based on the findings. Typically, the report is sent only to the referring physician. However, some knowledgeable families may also request a copy of the report; therefore, it is best to provide definitions of all technical and clinical terminology used and to provide an objective, nonjudgmental review.

The technical DXA report, similarly to other clinical reports, typically has five basic elements: (1) patient demographics, (2) a brief medical history, (3) test results, (4) technical comments, and (5) interpretation and recommendations. Each element will be described in detail below, and data that are typically included in each section are elucidated.

The formal report may be written by any qualified, knowledgeable expert in the field. However, in several regions of the United States, the report must be signed or co-signed by a board-certified physician in order to receive insurance reimbursement. For details regarding training and educational courses available for both technologists and physicians who seek basic knowledge in bone densitometry acquisition and reporting procedures, please *see* Appendix A.

REPORT ELEMENTS

There is no formal consensus as to the elements that should be provided in every pediatric clinical DXA report. Tables 1 and 2 list the relevant recommended content for pediatric patient reports. These elements are provided as guidelines and should not be considered standard for all institutions. A more abbreviated version of the DXA report may be used, particularly when the referring physician is familiar with the procedure and the resulting data obtained.

Table 1
Suggested Elements of the DXA Report

I. Patient and provider information

Patient name
Medical record number
Date of birth
Gender
Measured weight, height
Calculated BMI, height, weight % or Z-scores
Primary diagnosis, indications for test
List of current relevant medications
Bone age or pubertal stage
Inclusion of possible risk factors, including documentation of nontraumatic fractures
Calcium intake or use of calcium supplements

II. Test results

Skeletal sites scanned
BMD, BMC, bone area for each site
BMD Z-scores for each site by chronological age
Z-scores for each site by bone age (if available)

III. Technical comments

Manufacturer, model of instrument used
Software version (Standard, pediatric, low-density software)
Technical quality of the scans obtained
Limitations of the study (e.g., artifacts, scoliosis)
Pediatric reference source(s) used

IV. Interpretation and recommendations

Qualitative assessment of BMD Z-score results
Recommendations for necessity and timing of follow-up DXA scan studies

Note. The elements in plain print are considered standard at most densitometry centers. Those in *italics* are provided as suggestions. DXA, dual-energy x-ray absorptiometry; BMI, body mass index; BMD, bone mineral density; BMC, bone mineral content. (Modified from refs. *8,21.*)

Patient Demographics

Typically, the report includes basic patient demographics (i.e., age, gender, and ethnicity or race) and anthropometrics. Weight and height taken at the time of the DXA scan should always be included in the report. It is very important to document patient height and weight because DXA measures areal, and not true volumetric, BMD. As mentioned previously in this text, bone density is underestimated in small patients as a result of the two-dimensional nature of the instrumentation *(9)*. Documentation of patient size will be important for interpretation of the scans during the evaluation phase (*see* Chapter 7).

Body mass index (kg/m^2), growth percentiles, and standard deviation Z-scores for growth should be calculated using current growth charts. In the United States and Aus-

Table 2
Additional Elements of the Follow-Up DXA Report *(8)*

I. Patient and provider information

Indication for follow-up DXA scan
Interval fractures, change in clinical status, medications

II. Test results

Skeletal sites scanned
BMD, BMC, bone area for each site
Annualized change in BMC, BMD
Change in Z-scores

III. Technical comments

Which previous scans are being used for comparison?
*Statement regarding what denotes statistical significance for change in BMD at the
   center, or "Least Significant Change" (LSC)*
Recommendation for necessity and timing of follow-up DXA Scan

Note. The elements in plain print are considered standard at most densitometry centers. Those in *italics* are provided as suggestions. For abbreviations, *see* Table 1. (Modified from ref. *21*.)

tralia, these growth charts include those developed by the Centers for Disease Control in 2002 *(10)*, whereas in the United Kingdom, these are referred to as the UK90 *(11,12)*. Examples of these growth charts are provided in Appendix.

The demographic and anthropometric data are helpful in determining if body size is sufficiently above or below the expected range to warrant adjusting DXA results. If warranted, there are a number of recommendations for how to attempt to correct BMD for the size effects *(13)*. These are explained in detail in Chapters 6, 7, and 10. One possible scenario is to provide a derivation of volumetric bone density, calculated from BA and BMC (*see* Chapter 10).

Medical History

The report should include a brief summary of the clinical history relevant to the interpretation of the scan. This might include the primary medical diagnosis, the use of medications known to affect BMD (e.g., growth hormone and glucocorticoid therapy), fracture history, mobility status, endocrine abnormalities, pubertal status, bone age, and family history of osteoporosis. Physical activity level, dietary history, and use of vitamin or mineral supplements may also be useful.

As discussed in Chapter 5, clinical information obtained prior to the scan improves both the acquisition and the interpretation of bone densitometry. Ideally, the patient's medical history should be obtained directly from the referring physician. This type of information is typically gathered with a Referral or Request for Procedure form. However, patients referred for bone densitometry assessment will come from a variety of clinical departments not familiar with the request form, and, therefore, complete medical history may not be readily available.

If the referring physician has not relayed the indications for the scan and the relevant medical history, it is possible to ask the patient, parent, or both to complete a brief registration questionnaire at the time of the DXA procedure. Examples of pediatric DXA registration questionnaires and request for procedure forms are provided in Appendix D.

The technologist should review the questionnaire with the parent, giving particular attention to details surrounding fracture history, endocrine or growth abnormalities, orthopedic surgeries, medication and supplement usage, and family history of osteoporosis. If, for some reason, the questionnaire can not be adequately completed at the time of examination (e.g., because of a language barrier or because the child is not accompanied by a parent), the form can be faxed to the referring clinic for completion by a qualified staff member familiar with the patient after the DXA procedure is completed.

Test Results

For each skeletal site that is assessed, BMD, BMC, and BA should be included, as should the corresponding BMD Z-score, to enable the clinician to determine if the measured values are within the expected range for age. BMC and BAs are used to calculate estimates of volumetric BMD (i.e., bone mineral apparent density [BMAD]) and should be included in the report. Reporting BMC and BA also allows the clinician to examine subsequent changes due to bone growth.

Comparing changes in BMD requires thoughtful consideration in pediatric patients. Many experts believe that it is more informative to follow change in BMC, rather than BMD, in pediatric patients because of the variable of growth (for more details, *see* Chapter 7) *(14)*. In adult patients, the size of the skeleton remains relatively constant, making longitudinal comparisons of BMD appropriate. In pediatric patients, bone growth leads to changes in BA as well as BMC. These parameters may not increase in parallel. In fact, Bailey et al. *(15)* have shown that peak height velocity precedes the periods of peak bone mineral accrual by several months in teens. Unfortunately, there is a paucity of pediatric-specific BMC reference data sets from which BMC Z-scores can be calculated. For this reason, the BMD Z-score is typically reported.

Providing an appropriate BMD Z-score, however, can also be challenging because there is currently no universal pediatric reference data set. Many centers utilize the normative data in the manufacturer's software program, whereas others use published or locally collected reference values. The source of the reference data used to calculate the Z-score should always be cited in the report because the Z-score will vary if a different reference data set is used *(16)*.

There are also important limitations to the pediatric reference data currently provided in the manufacturer's programs. In some early Hologic software versions, the pediatric spine BMD reference data were derived from a study that did not provide gender-specific norms. Leonard et al. *(16)* have shown that the use of these reference data can result in the overdiagnosis of low bone mass, particularly in adolescent males. More frequently, the manufacturer's reference database will lack complete data for sites such as the proximal femur and the whole body, or it may not provide reference norms below a certain age (e.g., for infants and young children). The printout from the DXA instrument will not list Z-scores in these situations, or it may delineate them as "N.A.," leading the inexperienced operator or clinician to conclude that reference data do not exist.

In this situation, it is important to search for alternative published reference data to calculate Z-scores. Chapter 3 and Appendix C provide citations for published normative

Table 3
International Society for Clinical Densitometry (ISCD) Guidelines for DXA
Reporting Nomenclature

Measure	Decimal places	Example
BMD (g/cm^2)	3	0.655
Z-score	1	−1.5
BMC, spine or hip scan (g)	2	28.52
BMC, whole body scan (g)	0	1652
Bone area, spine or hip scan (cm^2)	2	44.66
Bone area, whole body scan (cm^2)	0	1850

For abbreviations, see Table 1. (Modified from ref. 23.)

studies in pediatrics. In 2002, data collection began on the Bone Mineral Density in Childhood Study (BMDCS), funded by the US National Institutes of Health. This study aims to develop longitudinal reference data in a multiethnic sample of more than 1500 children from the United States. Whole-body, lumbar spine, proximal femur, and forearm data are being collected, along with skeletal age, pubertal status, dietary intake, and physical activity information. While results of this study are pending, a separate initiative was undertaken by pediatric investigators in collaboration with Hologic, Inc. Portions of these data have recently been incorporated into Hologic DXA software computations (Hologic Discovery, software version 12.3) *(17)*.

Finally, the units for reporting DXA results have become more standardized. The ISCD has published guidelines for nomenclature and has standardized of numeric data frequently reported (*see* Table 3).

Technical Comments

The report should include sufficient detail regarding how the DXA was performed and interpreted to allow comparisons with previous and future densitometry studies. Given the intrinsic differences between densitometers and the software used for bone densitometry assessment, the manufacturer and model of the instrument should be specified (e.g., Hologic Delphi A) (*see* Table 1, and further discussion in Chapter 3). Similarly, the software mode used to acquire and analyze the scan should also be provided (e.g., auto-low-density, low-density spine [LDS] software). If reference data are used in the calculation of Z-scores that are different from the manufacturer's normative data, it is important that this also be documented.

Prior to the preparation of the report, careful visual review of each scan must be made to ensure that artifacts do not affect data obtained. The report should outline any technical difficulties encountered with obtaining the scan. Documentation is important, both for the initial interpretation of the DXA scan and to alert the DXA technologist to these effects for future scan acquisitions. These might include noticeable scoliosis, degenerative disease, vertebral compression fractures, or nonremovable metal artifacts (*see* Table 4). Scans with motion artifacts or removable metal objects (e.g., metal from the underwire or clasp of a bra, a belt buckle, a pant zipper, or a belly button ring) should not be reported. These scans should be repeated before the patient leaves the clinic.

Table 4
Examples of Technical Problems Noted on Reports

I. Appropriate technical comments

Spine scan	Scoliosis noted in lumbar region
	Compression fracture in L1, L2–4 used for analysis
	Osteoarthritis noted in L1, L2–4 used for analysis
Proximal femur scan	Left hip replacement, right proximal femur scanned
	Incomplete hip rotation, prominent lesser trochanter
Whole-body scan	Permanent pins in right wrist secondary to fracture
	Gold crowns on molar teeth

II. Avoidable artifacts

Spine scan	Pant zipper artifact in L3, L4
Proximal femur scan	Metal coin artifact in pocket, interferes with femoral neck
Whole-body scan	Bracelet on left forearm
	Underwire bra in upper left and right quadrants

Interpretation and Recommendations

The most challenging and controversial elements of the pediatric DXA report are "Interpretation" and "Recommendations." For postmenopausal women, the interpretation of DXA results are fairly straightforward, based on universally accepted WHO criteria for osteopenia and osteoporosis (1). However, diagnostic categories for men and premenopausal women remain controversial (18,19). Guidelines for the interpretation of pediatric DXA results have been proposed but are not universally accepted (20).

In addition to the BMD Z-score, results can also be reported in qualitative terms. As has been suggested by the ISCD, a label such as "low BMD for chronological age" may be reasonable for pediatric patients with Z-scores less than –2.0 (21). In patients with delayed growth or puberty, it may also be appropriate to adjust for bone size and maturation; BMD or BMAD Z-scores corrected for age, bone age, or pubertal stage, or a combination thereof, may be provided in these cases. The limitations of these adjustments are described in detail in Chapter 7. If corrections are made, these must be included in the report. For example, separate Z-scores in a 12-yr-old boy with a bone age of 10 yr may be calculated based on reference data for healthy males with chronological ages 12 and 10.

An assessment of fracture risk in children should not be reported based on DXA data. In addition, the terms "osteopenia" and "osteoporosis" should not be used in pediatric DXA reports because they refer specifically to WHO fracture risk criteria developed for postmenopausal women. There are no similar criteria for osteoporosis based on BMD for children, adolescents, or premenopausal women (22).

Interpretation of follow-up scans should include a discussion on changes in BMC, BA, BMD, and BMD Z-scores. In follow-up scans, most pediatric patients would be expected to have an increase in BMC, BA, and BMD. It is important not to confuse an increase in BMD or BMC with an improvement in bone mineral status. In order for the change to be an improvement, the BMD Z-score of the follow-up scan should be greater than the previous BMD Z-score. If there has been a fall in BMD, examination of changes in BMC and BA will help explain the reason for the change in BMD (i.e., the loss of mineral or an increase in BA). Some investigators have advocated for not including BMD in studies of growing children *(14)*. For centers with access to locally acquired reference data that provide age- and gender-specific BMC Z-scores, these data are preferable. Unfortunately, given the current paucity in the literature of robust pediatric reference data for BMC by chronological age, the BMD Z-score for each scan is typically reported.

Interpretation of repeat scans also requires attention to physical changes that have occurred in the growing patient as well as any new pertinent medical findings. These findings may not be realistic to follow at all bone densitometry clinics; however, a comprehensive follow-up examination should highlight important physical changes in the patient. Specifically, observations of delay in growth or pubertal development of the child should be acknowledged because these alterations may also affect bone growth. Significant dietary changes (e.g., the resolution of anorexia nervosa or the initiation of calcium supplementation) might influence bone health and may be noted. If physical activity has increased or decreased significantly since the last examination or if the patient was confined to bedrest as a result of illness for a significant time period, this too may be noted. Detailing fractures that have occurred is critical, as is documentation of pertinent medical findings since the last examination, for example, bone age assessments or initiation or cessation of corticosteroid therapy.

Typically, if subsequent scans are to be arranged, they will be completed every 1 to 2 yr, and the time since the last examination should be included. Scans may be repeated in as little as 6 mo if a patient has a significant change in therapy or has had a worsening in clinical status that might render a greater change in BMC.

However, in order to assess biologically relevant change, calculations must be made a priori for what is commonly referred to as the least significant change (LSC). The LSC takes into account both the instrument's and the technologist's precision estimates, as well as the level of statistical confidence that is thought to be clinically relevant. Details for performing these precision studies and guidelines for how to calculate the LSC have been provided elsewhere *(6)* (*see* Chapter 3). The LSC should be included in any densitometry report that presents follow-up data. Only changes in the region of interest that are equal to or greater than the LSC can be considered significant, that is, greater than the noise of repeat studies.

Other Elements

Other elements that are ideally included in a formal DXA report are a header identifying the name of the clinic and the location at which the scan studies were performed, a signature line for the author of the report, and a footer that defines all key terminology.

There are advantages and disadvantages to including a copy of the DXA proprietary software report. These reports provide the raw data on which the report is based and the scan images in which acquisition errors may be observed. Unfortunately, these reports may also contain the T-scores and the WHO classification guidelines, which are inappropriate for use in pediatric subjects. Therefore, if included, the finalized report from the DXA center must caution against the use of the T-score. When the DXA software proprietary reports are provided to the referring physician, the summary report should still include BMC, BA, and BMD, and also the complete information on the DXA equipment used, in case the propriety and summary reports get separated in the medical record. For clinics that transmit reports by fax, be aware that color images do not reproduce well in facsimile.

SUMMARY POINTS

- A timely, concise, and informative DXA report is essential to relay densitometry findings and to avoid costly and potentially dangerous misinterpretations by referring physicians unfamiliar with interpreting pediatric densitometry data.
- Enough information should be provided in the report to allow for comparison to previous and subsequent DXA studies.
- The technical DXA report typically has five basic elements: (1) patient demographics, (2) a brief medical history, (3) test results, (4) technical comments, and (5) interpretation and recommendations.
- Medical history information should be obtained ideally from the referring physician, or otherwise from the patient or parent. Key information to include in the report are: primary medical diagnosis, use of medications known to affect bone, fracture history and when available, pubertal status, bone age, focused dietary and physical activity histories.
- Careful review of the DXA scan images must be made prior to reporting of results to avoid misinterpretation of the findings based on artifacts in the scan field.
- Inclusion of the model and software used for scan acquisition, as well as the reference data used in the interpretation of the data, is crucial to the pediatric report.
- Reporting densitometry data in pediatrics is unique and different than for adult patients—the most challenging and controversial elements are interpretation and recommendations.
- Although controversies persist regarding the choice of reference norms or methods to adjust for bone size or maturity, experts agree that WHO criteria relating BMD to fracture risk and the terms "osteopenia" and "osteoporosis" should not be included in pediatric DXA reports.
- Sample intake questionnaires and reporting forms are provided in Appendix D.

REFERENCES

1. World Health Organization. Assessment of fracture risk and its application to screening for post-menopausal osteoporosis. WHO technical report series. World Health Organ Tech Rep Ser 1994;843:1–129.
2. Brown JP, Josse RG, Scientific Advisory Council of the Osteoporosis Society of Canada. 2002 Clinical Practice Guidelines for the diagnosis and management of osteoporosis in Canada. CMAJ 2002;167:(10 Suppl)S1–S34.
3. Cadarette SM, Jaglal SB, Murray TM, McIsaac WJ, Brown JL. Evaluation of decision rules for referring women for bone densitometry by dual energy x-ray absorptiometry. JAMA 2001;286:1:57–63.
4. Diez F. Guidelines for the diagnosis of osteoporosis by densitometric methods. J Manipulative Physiol Ther 2002;25:403–415.
5. Kanis JA, Gluer CC. An update on the diagnosis and assessment of osteoporosis with densitometry. Osteoporos Int 2000;11:192–202.
6. Bonnick SL. *Bone Densitometry in Clinical Practice: Application and Interpretation*, 2nd ed. Totowa, NJ: Humana, 2004:287–300.
7. National Osteoporosis Society. Position statement on the reporting of dual energy x-ray absorptiometry (DXA) bone mineral density scans. Bath, UK: National Osteoporosis Society, 2002.
8. Writing Group for the ISCD Position Development Conference. Indications and reporting for dual-energy x-ray absorptiometry. J Clin Densitom 2004;7:1:37–44.
9. Fewtrell MS, British Paediatric & Adolescent Bone Group. Bone densitometry in children assessed by dual x-ray absorptiometry: uses and pitfalls. Arch Dis Child 2003;88:795–798.
10. Kuczmarski RJ, Ogden CL, Guo SS, et al. 2000 CDC growth charts for the United States: Methods and development. Vital Health Stat 2002;11:1–190.
11. Chinn S, Cole TJ, Preece MA, Rona RJ. Growth charts for ethnic populations in UK. Lancet 1996;347:839–40.
12. Wright CM, Booth IW, Buckler JM, et al. Growth reference charts for use in the United Kingdom. Arch Dis Child 2002;86:11–14.

13. Fewtrell MS, Gordon I, Biassoni L, Cole TJ. Dual x-ray absorptiometry (DXA) of the lumbar spine in a clinical pediatric setting: does the method of size adjustment matter? Bone 2005;37:413–419.
14. Heaney RP. BMD: The problem. Osteoporos Int 2005;16:1013–1015.
15. Bailey DA, McKay HA, Mirwald RL, Crocker PRE, Faulkner RA. A six-year longitudinal study of the relationship of physical activity to bone mineral accrual in growing children: The University of Saskatchewan Bone Mineral Accrual Study. J Bone Miner Res 1999;14:1672–1679.
16. Leonard MB, Propert KJ, Zemel BS, Stallings VA, Feldman HI. Discrepancies in pediatric bone mineral density reference data: potential for misdiagnosis of osteopenia. J Pediatr 1999;135:182–188.
17. Zemel BS, Leonard MB, Kalkwarf HJ, et al. Reference data for the whole body, lumbar spine, and proximal femur for American children relative to age, gender, and body size. J Bone Mineral Research 2004;19:suppl 1:SU112 abst.
18. Kanis JA, Seeman E, Johnell O, Rizzoli R, Delmas P. The perspective of the International Osteoporosis Foundation on the official positions of the International Society for Clinical Densitometry. J Clin Densitom 2005;8:145–147.
19. Lewiecki EM, Miller PD, Leib ES, Bilezikian JP. Response to the "Perspective of the International Osteoporosis Foundation on the official positions of the International Society for Clinical Densitometry" by John A. Kanis et al. J Clin Densitom 2005;8:143–144.
20. Khan AA, Bachrach L, Brown JP, et al., Canadian Panel of the International Society of Clinical Densitometry. Standards and guidelines for performing central dual energy x-ray absorptiometry in premenopausal women, men, and children. J Clin Densitom 2004;7:51–64.
21. Khan AA, Brown J, Faulkner K, et al., International Society for Clinical Densitometry. Standards and guidelines for performing central dual x-ray densitometry from the Canadian Panel of International Society for Clinical Densitometry. J Clin Densitom 2002;5:247–257.
22. Writing Group for the ISCD Position Development Conference. Diagnosis of osteoporosis in men, premenopausal women, and children. J Clin Densitom 2004;7:17–26.
23. Writing Group for the ISCD Position Development Conference. Nomenclature and decimal places in bone densitometry. J Clin Densitom 2004;7:45–49.

9

Children With Special Considerations

Laurie J. Moyer-Mileur, PhD, RD,
Zulf Mughal, MBChB, Ellen B. Fung, PhD, RD

CONTENTS

INTRODUCTION
INFANTS
CHILDREN WITH SPECIAL NEEDS
DXA IN THE ASSESSMENT OF MULTIPLE UNEXPLAINED FRACTURES
SUMMARY POINTS
REFERENCES

INTRODUCTION

A number of physical disabilities and medical conditions may adversely affect the growth and development of the immature skeleton, including cerebral palsy, muscular dystrophy, juvenile rheumatoid arthritis, acute lymphoblastic leukemia, cystic fibrosis, Prader-Willi syndrome, and various hematological disorders *(1–8)*. In these pediatric patients at risk for osteoporosis, bone mineral density (BMD) findings at one skeletal site cannot be reliably generalized to other areas of the skeleton *(9)*. Although BMD of the lumbar spine and hip regions are strongly related in healthy children, considerable anatomic differences between the two sites may become apparent as BMD decreases *(10)*.

Some pediatric conditions associated with low bone mass may also prevent or limit the use of standard measurement sites or positioning for densitometry evaluation *(11)*. Children with conditions like scoliosis, cerebral palsy, juvenile rheumatoid arthritis, or muscular dystrophy may have altered body postures or muscular contractures that prevent them from lying flat in a supine position for optimal measurement of the spine or hip. Children with cognitive delays, spastic movements, or seizure activity also present unique challenges for densitometry measurements because of their inability to lie still unassisted during the acquisition of the scan *(1)*. Medical instability in premature or seriously ill infants may preclude their movement to the scanner site *(12)*.

This chapter provides an overview of strategies used for bone mineral evaluation in infants and children with physical and cognitive disabilities.

From: *Current Clinical Practice: Bone Densitometry in Growing Patients: Guidelines for Clinical Practice*
Edited by: A. J. Sawyer, L. K. Bachrach, and E. B. Fung © Humana Press Inc., Totowa, NJ

INFANTS

Densitometry measurements of infants are generally considered a noninvasive *research* method to assess bone mass and body composition, and there is an extensive body of literature on preterm and term infants *(12–22)*. The whole body and lumbar spine are the most common sites of measurement by dual-energy x-ray absorptiometry (DXA) in these babies. Analysis of the whole body provides information on bone mineral content (BMC), bone area (BA), and lean and fat mass. Measurements of either the whole body or the lumbar spine in infants are fast and precise, with low radiation exposure *(19,22)*. Reference data for preterm and term neonates, however are limited to gestational ages greater than 27 wk and body weights of 1.2 kg or greater *(23)*. In addition, the risk of moving a medically unstable hospitalized infant to the scanner site often limits the use of DXA.

Measurement of the distal forearm and the forearm shaft by DXA has been shown in small studies to provide a reliable measure of BMC and BMD. Highly linear relationships between actual and measured BMC and BMD ($r = 0.94$ and 0.97, respectively) has been reported from in vitro precision studies using K_2HPO_4 phantoms with low BMC (simulating an infant forearm) *(24)*. As expected, in vivo precision was lower and significantly affected by patient movement *(24)*. BMC and BMD could be evaluated in all 25 term and preterm infants studied when a lower bone detection threshold was chosen (0.040 g/cm^2; Norland XR-26, pencil beam mode). However, systematic differences of 10 to 20% were observed between forearms analyzed using the standard vs lower bone threshold *(24)*.

Portable units such as peripheral DXA (pDXA) or quantitative ultrasound (QUS) devices allow measurements at the infant's bedside, although they can be used only to measure peripheral skeletal sites such as the forearm or tibia *(12,25)*. Fairly robust correlations between forearm bone and soft tissue measurements by pDXA and whole-body measurements by DXA ($r = 0.73$–0.84) have been reported *(26)*.

Examples of whole-body and forearm scans of preterm infants at body weights of 1.3 and 2.0 kg are shown in Fig.1. Currently, there are no published infant reference data for pDXA.

Despite the extensive use of DXA in infants, discrepancies exist among studies in the reported normative values for bone mass and body composition. These discrepancies may be as high as 18% for bone mass, 15% for fat mass, and 8% for lean mass in healthy infants *(27)*. They are likely the result of differences in the analysis software among DXA models and manufacturers (Fig. 2) *(26,28)*. Standard DXA software packages are not specific for infants or children, and, typically, pediatric software must be ordered separately from the manufacturer. Body size has also been shown to correlate with infant bone and soft tissue mass *(29)*; therefore, BMC, lean mass, and fat mass values should be adjusted for body weight and length.

Performing the Measurement

Infants are among the most challenging patients to measure. General guidelines for scanning are discussed in more detail in Chapter 5. Before measuring a term or older infant, it is helpful to feed and calm the child and to place the infant on the scanning table in a clean diaper. If necessary, the child should be swaddled in a thin cotton sheet or blanket to reduce small involuntary movements. Examples of whole-body infant scans (Fig. 3A,B) and infant forearm scans (Fig. 4A,B) are provided.

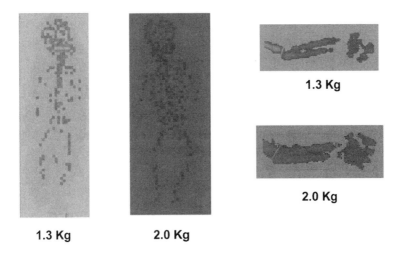

Fig.1. Whole-body dual-energy x-ray absorptiometry (DXA) and forearm peripheral DXA in preterm infants weighing 1.3 kg and 2.0 kg. The whole-body image includes the cotton blanket used to swaddle the infant, contributing to scan acquisition artifact and soft tissue variability. Forearm peripheral DXA scans were obtained without covering and clearly delineate bone and soft tissue. (From Moyer-Mileur, personal files, not previously published.)

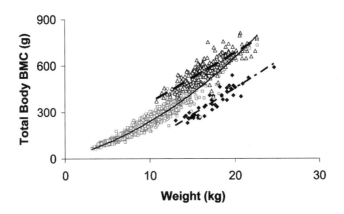

Fig.2. Measurement of total-body bone mineral content by body weight for pediatric subjects using different pediatric software (Hologic 1000W [squares, solid line] vs Hologic 4500A [triangles, upper dashed line]) and adult software (Hologic 1000W [solid diamonds, lower dashed line]). (Reproduced from ref. *26*, with permission.)

Subdued room lighting may also help the infant relax. Very young infants (i.e., <3 mo of age) will usually sleep through the measurement and will require limited operator intervention. However, it is important to constantly watch the infant for any involuntary movement *(30)*. General guidelines to minimize practical or technical situations that may affect densitometry measurements in infants are provided in Table 1.

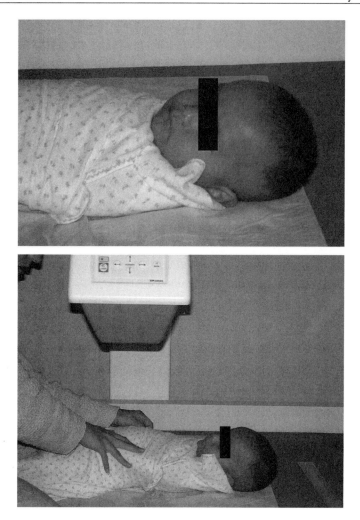

Fig.3. (A) Swaddling and positioning of an infant prior to whole-body dual-energy x-ray absorptiometry (DXA) measurement. **(B)** Correct holding of an infant in position to minimize movement as the DXA arm scans the upper body.

CHILDREN WITH SPECIAL NEEDS

Altered Posture

For children with conditions such as scoliosis, muscular dystrophy, cerebral palsy, juvenile rheumatoid arthritis, contractures or deformities often prevent positioning the patient in a fully supine position. Lark et al. *(11)* reported that for positions that simulated children with contractures, the mean errors for whole-body measurements were 4–6% for BMC, 1–3% for lean body mass, and 5–11% for fat mass. Comparisons of the correct fully supine position and the contracted positions were highly correlated; however, this study was conducted in healthy controls and did not consider movement artifact, which would increase measurement variability. These data suggest that for the majority of children with altered postures, precise and reasonably accurate measures of bone and body composition can be obtained if care is taken during scan acquisition.

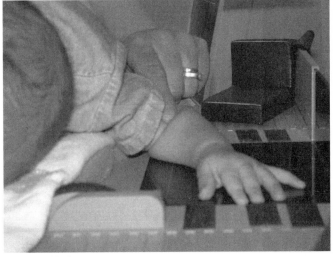

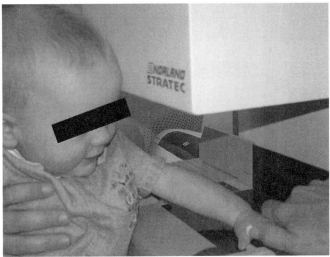

Fig. 4. (A) Alternate positioning for peripheral dual-energy x-ray absorptiometry (pDXA) measurement of infant forearm: infant lies on stomach on platform, with face turned away from scanner and arm extended. **(B)** Alternate positing for pDXA measurement of infant forearm: infant sits on caregiver's lap with arm extended and held in position.

Concerns regarding whether the lumbar spine accurately reflects other regions of the skeleton have led to the study of alternative sites for bone assessment by DXA. Additionally, for many pediatric conditions, the spine is an uncommon site for fracture and may not accurately predict risk. In adults, the proximal femur BMD is commonly measured because this provides the best prediction of osteoporotic hip fracture. In physically handicapped children, the distal femur is one of the more common sites of osteoporotic fracture (31–35). In a study of 339 young patients (2.2–17.0 yr) with an assortment of underlying conditions (cerebral palsy, cystic fibrosis, milk allergy, muscular dystrophy, and treated malignancies), the proximal femur BMD and lumbar spine BMD assessed by DXA were highly correlated ($r = 0.73, p = 0.0001$) (9). However, for individual patients, differences

Table 1

Sources of Variability in Densitometry Evaluation of Bone and Body Mass in Infants

Source of variability	Considerations	Recommendations
Software	**Dual-energy x-ray absoptiometry (DXA)**	
	Earlier prototypes of Infant Whole Body (IWB) software and scan acquisition on pencil beam systems without aluminum infant platform are unreliable for the study of small subjects (26).	Avoid using earlier prototypes of IWB with pencil beam systems without aluminum infant platforms.
	Pediatric software use in neonates weighing 2.0 kg underestimates bone mineral content (BMC) by three- to fivefold. At 6 wk of age (and ~4.0 kg), this difference is no longer evident.	Use Infant software for infants < 4.0 kg. (Note: check with specific manufacturer for availability.)
	Measurement in infants weighing >4.0 kg could result in overestimation of bone mineral acquisition if Pediatric software is used for two successive measurements (29).	
	Peripheral DXA	
	Adult software will provide inaccurate measures of bone and body mass (29).	Use manufacturer's small-subject software.
Platforms	**DXA**	
	Pencil beam systems require the infant platform to improve system linearity during scan acquisition and to allow a lower detection threshold for bone.	For pencil beam systems, avoid using the foam platform. Limit padding and covering the platform.
	The type of platform (aluminum vs foam) can result in differences in fat mass (up to 40%) and lean mass (5%). Use of padding or covering over the aluminum platform will also effect fat and lean mass measurements (26,29).	
	Fan beam systems do not require the infant platform for scan acquisition.	
	Peripheral DXA	
	Infants <5.0 kg: measurements taken at bedside require a customized platform and may require an overhead warmer to maintain body temperature.	Use an appropriate platform. (**Note:** use the platform for infants weighing <5.0 kg; infants >5.0 kg should sit on the caregiver's lap.)
Operator	**DXA**	
	When using pencil beam systems, placement of the external calibration standard during scan acquisition or its delineation during analysis must be consistent (26). This is not necessary for the newer fan beam systems.	Use consistent placement of external calibration standard. Do not allow obstruction by padding or covering (i.e., a blanket).

142

Subject		
Peripheral DXA	Incorrect forearm placement (e.g., allowing the arm to twist and not lay flat) will influence tissue values (*30*).	The extended forearm should be flat, with the palm down. Velcro straps may be used to hold the arm in the desired position.
DXA	*Covering*: in preterm infants, light covering is required to maintain body temperature; however, light cotton blankets and diapers have been shown to increase soft tissue mass, specifically lean mass (*26*).	Limit covering to a light cotton blanket and a diaper. Be consistent with covering for longitudinal studies. Document the type, amount, and weight of covering used for each subject.
	Movement artifacts: these can increase quantitative values for both fat and lean mass (*26*).	Obtain the scan while the infant is sleeping or swaddled. Use a nonmetallic pacifier. (Crying will not effect results.) Avoid sedation.
	Feeding artifacts (i.e., IV or enteral): a recent bolus can impact lean mass values (*26*).	Perform the scan acquisition > 30 minutes after feeding.
	Radiographic contrast artifacts: these can effect bone and body mass values (*26*).	Schedule DXA measurements prior to radiographic contrast studies.
	Tubing artifacts (i.e., IV lines, feeding tubes, nasal cannula, or monitor leads): these can increase bone and body mass values (*26*).	Remove tubing if possible; adjust the region of interest to exclude the tubing artifact.
Peripheral DXA	*Covering*: covering forearm area during scan typically not required even in preterm infants.	Measure the forearm without covering.
	Movement artifacts: these can increase quantitative values for both fat and lean mass.	Position the forearm correctly and use Velcro straps for restraint.
	Tubing artifacts: intravenous lines can increase bone and body mass values.	Measure opposite arm if it has no IV.

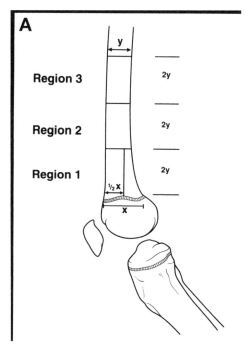

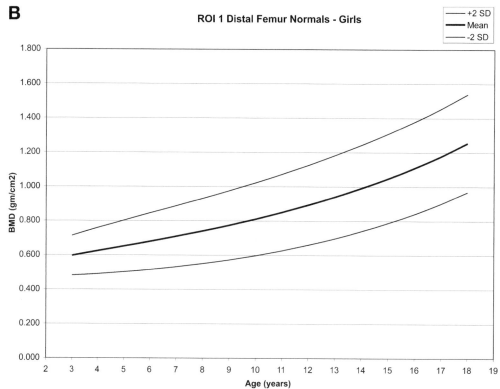

Fig. 5.

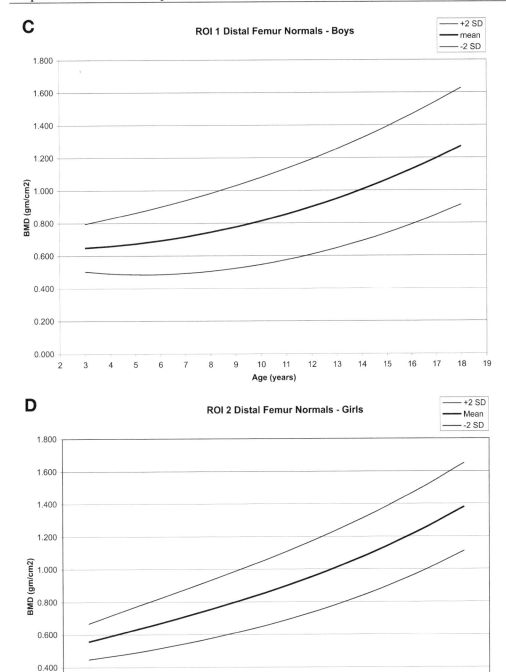

Fig. 5. *(continued)*

E

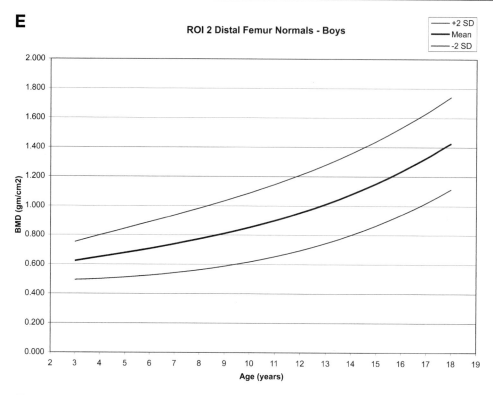

F

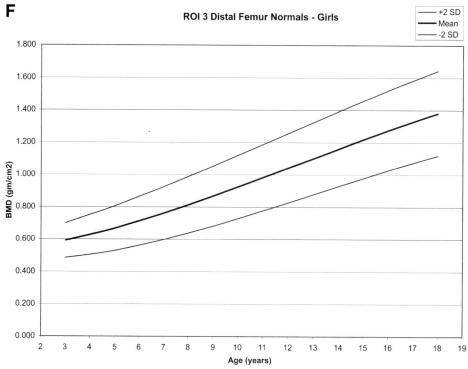

Fig. 5. *(continued)*

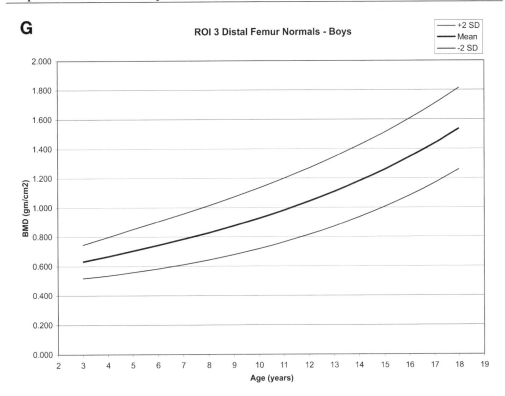

Fig. 5. Drawing showing the three separate regions in the distal femur that are independently analyzed using subregional analysis with Hologic forearm software. Region 1 is predominately cancellous bone; region 3 is predominately cortical bone. Regional analysis is an important aspect of the distal femur technique because the metabolism often differs between cancellous and cortical bone. (Reprinted from ref. *10*, with permission from the American Journal of Roentgenology.)

in Z-scores at these two sites were often significant, and they increased as BMD deviated further from normal *(9)*.

In children with cerebral palsy, whole-body, proximal femur, or spine BMD assessment by DXA may not be reliably or easily measured because of joint contractures or orthopedic fixation devices at the spine and hip. The distal femur in the lateral projection has been found to be a reliable peripheral site for children with cerebral palsy when whole-body, hip, and spine sites are not practical *(36)* (Fig. 5). Even children with significant contractures can usually be comfortably placed in the lateral position to obtain an accurate distal femur scan. An example of correct positioning for the distal femur measurement is found in Fig. 6 *(37)*.

Henderson et al. *(37)* recently published pediatric reference data for the distal femur derived from 256 healthy children and adolescents aged 3–18 yr. The distal femur correlated highly with bone density in the proximal femur ($r > 0.90$) and slightly less strongly with the lumbar spine ($r = 0.83$). To date, only pencil beam scanners have been utilized to measure the distal femur site; thus, there is not a validated reference for distal femur measurements using fan beam scanners and software. Given the limitations and the level of expertise required for interpretation of the scan, at most institutions, this measurement site should be used for research purposes only.

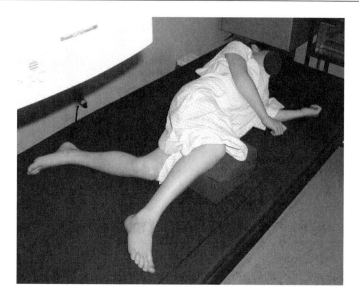

Fig. 6. Correct patient positioning for left proximal femur scan. The child is placed on his left side so that the left femur is centered on the table and is parallel to the table edge. The right hip and knee are flexed forward in front of the left distal femur and are supported by foam pads. (Reprinted from ref. 10, with permission from the American Journal of Roentgenology.)

Artifacts

A frequent problem when measuring children with special needs is interference caused by metal artifacts and motion as discussed in detail in Chapter 5. Problems caused by artifacts should be limited to those resulting from immovable objects such as pins, plates, rods, or feeding tubes. External, highly attenuating objects such as braces, plaster casts, or monitors should be removed prior to performing the measurement, or the measurement should be rescheduled to a time when the external object is no longer required.

Figure 9 in Chapter 5 illustrates examples of removable and permanent internal and external artifacts. The child in Fig. 9A has intermedullary rods in both the right and left femur included in the measurement. Artifacts such as these may not cause significant interference for longitudinal measurements if they remain in place for the follow-up period, but they will affect comparison of the results to reference data (Chapter 6).

The child in Fig. 9B in Chapter 5 has multiple intravenous catheters and a pulse-oximetry probe attached to the left foot. Because the child was sedated, it was necessary for the pulse-oximetry probe to remain in place. However, the other artifacts should have been removed prior to the measurement.

The child in Fig. 9C in Chapter 5 has an internal metal plate in the left arm and a plaster cast on the right leg. Although the metal plate in the left arm could not be removed, the measurement should have been delayed until the leg cast was removed.

In Chapter 5, Fig 9D, the child has quadriplegia requiring continuous ventilation. Because the ventilation equipment could not be removed; the best measurement was achieved with the ventilator artifacts in place. When it is not possible to remove the artifact or to reschedule the measurement, data from the whole-body measurement can be used by interpolating the values for the affected side based on the values determined for the unaffected side.

Artifacts are not limited to whole-body measurements. Figure 10 in Chapter 5 illustrates a selection of lumbar spine measurements affected by immovable internal artifacts. Excluding a specific region of interest during analysis may reduce the effect of such artifacts on the results.

Unavoidable interference may also result from the child's clinical condition or treatment. Figure 11A in Chapter 5 illustrates a common pattern of high-density endplates associated with bisphosphonate treatment. Figure 11B shows a child with primary oxalosis type I for whom calcium deposits in the kidney may affect soft tissue estimation.

Practical situations and technical issues may also confound DXA results in children with physical or cognitive limitations. Table 2 provides a summary of general guidelines to minimize the effect of these factors on densitometry measurements in children with special needs.

DXA IN THE ASSESSMENT OF MULTIPLE UNEXPLAINED FRACTURES

The possibility of nonaccidental injury (NAI) must be considered whenever an infant presents with multiple fractures at different skeletal sites and in various stages of healing. However, clinicians also have a duty to exclude an underlying medical disorder associated with diminished bone strength that can lead to pathological fractures during routine day-to-day handling. This section provides a brief review of some bone disorders that must be considered in the differential diagnosis of NAI in a young child, as well as the role of bone densitometry in discriminating between healthy infants (with likely NAI) from those with an underlying bone disorder.

Fractures Caused by Nonaccidental Injury

NAI is a common cause of fractures in infants. In one study, up to 82% of long bone fractures in infants less than 1 yr of age were considered to be the result of NAI *(38)*. Unexplained fractures in a nonambulant infant, especially if the fractures are multiple and of differing ages, are highly suspicious of inflicted injury. Suspicion of NAI is also aroused when the history of an injury, provided by parents or caregivers, is not consistent with physical findings; when there is variation in the histories of the injury given to health professionals; when there is delay in seeking medical attention; and when the given mechanism of injury is not consistent with development of the child. The affected infant may also have other features of physical, emotional, or sexual abuse.

Identification of skeletal and nonskeletal features of NAI is critically important because there is a risk of the child suffering further abuse, which could be fatal. Therefore, any suspicion of nonaccidental fractures should lead to a multidisciplinary assessment with social services and other child protection agencies. In the majority of cases, the diagnosis of NAI can be reached through a careful appraisal of detailed histories obtained from caregivers, a thorough clinical examination, and a complete radiographic skeletal survey.

The radiologist has an important role in identifying the number, age, and severity of fractures. Skeletal surveys are indicated for all children less than 2 yr of age when child abuse is suspected *(39)*. Bone scintigraphy with technetium-99m-labeled bisphosphonate may help to disclose injuries that are not readily visible on the radiographic skeletal survey, including periosteal injuries, fresh rib fractures, and bony injuries in a complex area such as the pelvis *(40)*.

Table 2
Sources of Variability in Densitometry Evaluation of Bone and Body Mass for Children With Special Needs

Source of variability	Considerations	Recommendations
Software	*DXA*: standard software packages are not designed for use in infants or children. Adult software may underestimate BMC and BMD.	• Pediatric software and corresponding reference data must be ordered separately from the manufacturer.
Operator	*DXA*: beware of inconsistent or incorrect external calibration of the instrument.	• Perform daily calibration with the manufacturer-supplied phantom. • Maintain consistent placement of the external calibration standard.
Subject	*Altered posture*: whole-body BMC measured in the lateral position differs by ±7.5%. The frog-leg position slightly overestimates BMC, and the semi-lateral position slightly underestimates it. Fat mass may vary by 5–11%, depending on position *(11)*. *Altered posture*: knee flexion contractures do not appear to significantly affect DXA measures of BMC, fat, or lean mass *(11)*. *Covering*: clothing may increase soft tissue values, specifically lean mass *(26)*.	• Develop corrective equations from a larger study cohort. Note that the precision of the measurement is not affected when the positioning is reproducible. Therefore, the measured rates of change for longitudinal evaluations will be reliable, but pediatric reference ranges may not be appropriate. • Consider an alternative measurement site such as the distal femur *(10)*. • Assess what the child is wearing. If measuring only the proximal femur, the lower body garment can be removed. If not, have the child change into a cotton gown. • Document the type, amount, and weight of covering used for each subject.

Movement artifacts: children with spastic movements or limited cognitive ability may have trouble holding still during the scan. Movement can increase quantitative values for both fat and lean mass (26).

- Assess the child for movement prior to scan.
- Determine whether the caregiver will remain in the room and will be able to help.
- Avoid abrupt movements or load noises: reflexes are often hyperactive and will illicit greater-than-normal response.
- Stabilize legs with sand bags or tape, or have someone hold them.
- Consider sedation if the child is unable to lie still.

Feeding artifacts: (IV or enteral) recent bolus can impact lean mass values (26).

- Perform scan at least 30 minutes after bolus feeding.

Radiographic contrast artifacts: can effect bone and body mass values (26).

Tubing artifacts (i.e., intravenous lines, feeding tubes, nasal cannula, and monitor leads) these can increase bone and body mass values (26).

- Perform scan prior to any radiographic studies or 2 weeks after such a study.
- Remove tubing if possible; adjust the region of interest to exclude the tubing artifact.

Orthopedic fixation device artifacts: (i.e., implanted rods or screws; splints) these can falsely increase bone mass values (10).

- Remove splints if possible when measuring the lumbar spine or the whole body.
- Consider an alternative measurement site such as the proximal femur or the distal radius.

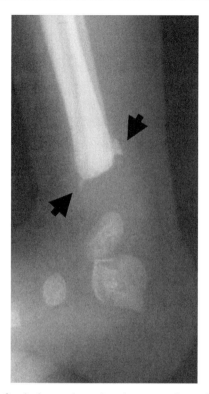

Fig. 7. Radiograph of an infant's lower leg, showing metaphyseal fractures of the distal tibia (arrows).

Although virtually any fracture can result from an NAI, certain fractures are considered to be more suggestive of abuse. These include metaphyseal fractures (Fig. 7), posterior rib fractures (Fig. 8), scapular fractures, spinous process fractures, sternal fractures, complex skull fractures, and diaphyseal spiral fractures.

Detailed discussion of skeletal injuries due to abuse is beyond the scope of this chapter, but a useful reference source is Kleinman's *Diagnostic Imaging of Child Abuse (41).*

Osteogenesis Imperfecta

Osteogenesis imperfecta (OI) is the most common bone condition that must be considered in the differential diagnosis of an infant with unexplained fractures. It is a heterogeneous group of inherited disorders characterized by bone fragility. In most patients, OI is caused by mutations in the *COL1A1* and *COL1A2* genes that encode for the pro-α-1(I) and pro-α-2(I) chains of type I collagen. Most forms of OI are inherited as an autosomal-dominant trait; however, up to 25% of children with OI have new germ-line mutations.

The clinical course of OI is extremely variable, ranging from stillbirth as a result of multiple intrauterine fractures to a lifelong absence of fractures *(42).* Other clinical features of OI may include short stature, dentinogenesis imperfecta, fragile skin with increased tendency to bruising, a blue or grey scleral color, joint laxity, and presenile deafness.

Using clinical, radiographic, and genetic criteria, Sillence and colleagues *(43)* have classified OI into four major types. OI type I is the mildest phenotype and results from

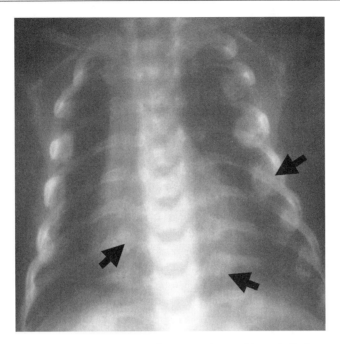

Fig. 8. Radiograph of an infant's chest, showing posterior and lateral rib fractures (arrows).

stop codon mutations in the *COL1A1* and *COL1A2* genes that lead to reduced amounts of normal type I collagen. Subjects with OI type I have blue-grey sclerae, normal teeth, and normal or near-normal stature. Fractures tend to decrease after puberty and skeletal deformities are rare.

OI types II to IV arise from point mutations in the *COL1A1* and *COL1A2* genes that lead to the production of structurally abnormal collagen. OI type II is the most severe form of the disease, and most patients die *in utero* or shortly after birth. Patients with OI type III have limb deformities from numerous fractures occurring *in utero* and characteristic facies. Individuals with OI type IV have white sclerae, but some have yellowish opalescent teeth (i.e., dentinogenesis imperfecta). The severity of bone disease in subjects with OI type IV is variable; some have fractures *in utero* leading to deformities, whereas others suffer only a few fractures throughout their lives.

More recently, Glorieux and colleagues have described OI types V, VI, and VII, which do not arise from mutations of type I collagen *(44–46)* These types of OI have distinctive clinical and radiological features and therefore are not likely to be confused with NAI.

Radiological features in milder types of OI may be nonspecific but include slender bones with thin cortices and osteopenia. Wormian bones measuring 6×4 mm or larger in size and more than 10 in number around the lambdoid suture on skull radiographs are more strongly suggestive of OI.

The milder forms of OI, especially type IV, may be difficult to diagnose clinically if classical radiological features of the disease are absent and no other family members are affected. Unexplained fractures in infants with such forms of OI may be confused with NAI. In such cases, electrophoretic studies of collagen excreted from cultured skin fibroblasts may be helpful. Approximately 85% of subjects with clinical or radiological features of OI will have either abnormal amounts or structure of type 1 collagen *(47)*.

The value of genetic testing to differentiate OI from NAI has been examined. Steiner et al. *(48)* found that 6 of 48 children with possible NAI had laboratory evidence of OI. Five of the six children with abnormal collagen also had clinical signs of OI. The authors concluded that routine genetic testing for OI in the setting of unexplained fractures was not warranted because most children with OI can be identified clinically by an experienced clinician. Normal collagen studies in up to 15% of subjects with obvious clinical features of OI also limit the usefulness of this test. Despite these factors and the expense and time required to perform genetic testing for OI, courts may require these studies in some cases of suspected NAI.

The Role of Bone Densitometry in the Assessment of an Infant With Multiple Unexplained Fractures

As mentioned previously, milder phenotypes of OI, especially type IV, may be difficult to differentiate from NAI. In cases in which parents deny harming their children, it is not uncommon for the parents and their legal representatives to inquire as to whether measurement of BMD will help in differentiating normal children who have been victims of NAI from those with milder forms of OI.

DXA measurements of BMD in older children and adults with OI have provided conflicting results. Paterson and Mole *(49)* found BMD to be within the reference range in most adults with type I or type IV OI. In contrast, others *(50–53)* reported that areal BMD (aBMD) in children with OI was significantly lower than that of age-matched controls.

Lund et al. *(54)* measured whole-body and lumbar spine BA, BMC, and aBMD in 63 subjects with both mild and severe types of OI. Their study cohort included 24 children (17 males), aged 5–18 yr, of whom 15 were classified as having OI type I or OI type IV. The authors used the approach of Mølgaard et al. *(55)* to determine whether (1) the subject's height was appropriate for age (looking for "short bones"), (2) the BA was appropriate for height (looking for "narrow bones"), and (3) the BMC was appropriate for bone area (looking for "light bones").

They compared these findings with quantitative and qualitative defects in type 1 collagen produced by subjects' cultured skin fibroblasts. Mean aBMD for age in both children and adults was low in patients with OI type III or IV and/or a qualitative collagen defect. Reduced BMC for age in OI children was due to reduced height (short bones) and reduced BMC for BA (light bones). In contrast, their BA for height was normal (normal bone width). Forty percent of all subjects studied and 75% of those with either OI type I, a quantitative collagen defect, or both had aBMD for age values within the reference range. The fact that OI subjects suffered recurrent fractures despite normal or only slightly low aBMD for age suggests that impaired skeletal mineralization was not the only cause of bone fragility.

The authors concluded that DXA has limited value in the assessment of recurrent fractures because aBMD in OI can be normal and because there are few pediatric reference data for children under the age of 2 yr, the period when fractures due to NAI are most prevalent.

Very few studies have measured BMD in infants with the milder forms of OI (i.e., type I and type IV) that would be considered in the differential diagnosis of fractures due to NAI. One small study of 14 children with OI by Miller and Hangartner recommended that the investigation of the infant with unexplained fractures should include assessment of

BMD by quantitative computed tomography (QCT) *(56)*. However, few centers have QCT scanners capable of measuring volumetric BMD in infants, and there is a paucity of age and gender reference data to allow calculation of Z-scores. Larger studies are needed to confirm the authors' preliminary findings.

Bishop and colleagues *(57)* compared aBMD of the lumbar spine by DXA in infants with fractures due to OI and those whose fractures were thought to have occurred nonaccidentally. They found that lumbar spine aBMD of infants less than 6 mo of age in both groups were within the reference range and were not significantly different. There was considerable overlap in BMD between subjects with and without OI who were up to 2 yr of age. In follow-up examinations, however, the increment in lumbar spine aBMD in OI infants was significantly lower ($27/cm^2/yr$) than that of non-OI infants ($115/cm^2/yr$). The authors concluded that a single BMD measurement was not helpful in differentiating between infants whose fractures resulted from OI vs NAI. Longitudinal aBMD measurements, however, may be helpful in discriminating between normal infants and those with milder OI phenotypes.

In summary, for the majority of infants with unexplained fractures, the diagnosis of NAI or OI can be reached with a detailed clinical history, a thorough clinical examination by a clinician experienced in bone disorders, and a skeletal survey interpreted by an experienced pediatric radiologist. DXA measurements do not help to distinguish healthy infants who have been victims of abuse from those with milder types of OI. Genetic testing for mutations in *COL1A1* and *COL1A2* should only be undertaken in rare cases in which diagnosis of NAI remains in doubt even after a painstaking clinical and radiological evaluation.

SUMMARY POINTS

- The acquisition and interpretation of DXA results in children with physical and cognitive disabilities present special challenges.
- Use of DXA measurement in infants is currently limited to research studies because of the lack of established universal reference data.
- General guidelines are provided in Table 2 for the minimization of practical and technical situations that may affect densitometry results in infants and children with physical and cognitive deficits.
- Contractures and deformities may prevent positioning the patient for a whole-body scan in a fully supine position. If a whole-body measurement is warranted, a reasonable result can be achieved (i.e., ±5% BMC) if the child is placed in a more comfortable body positions.
- Concerns regarding whether the lumbar spine accurately reflects other regions of the skeleton where children with physical disabilities tend to fracture has led to the study of alternative sites for bone assessment by DXA (e.g., the distal femur). However, the lack of reference data for newer instrument models (e.g. fan beam mode) limits the current clinical usefulness of this particular scan.
- Osteogenesis imperfecta is the most common bone condition and should be considered in the diagnosis of an infant with unexplained fractures and suspected NAI.
- The milder forms of OI, especially type IV, may be difficult to diagnose clinically, especially if classical radiological features of the disease are absent and no other family members are affected. In such cases, electrophoretic studies of collagen excreted from cultured skin fibroblasts may be helpful. Routine genetic testing is not warranted.

- Red flags for NAI include unexplained multiple fractures in nonambulatory infants, physical findings inconsistent with the history provided by the caregiver or the development of the child, delay in seeking medical attention, and other signs of physical, emotional, or sexual abuse.
- The most useful radiographic studies in cases of suspected NAI include a skeletal survey and possibly a technetium-99m-labeled bisphosphonate bone scan.
- DXA has been shown to have limited value in differentiating between NAI and mild forms of OI in young children with unexplained fractures.

REFERENCES

1. Vestergaard P, Kristensen K, Bruun JM, et al. Reduced bone mineral density and increased bone turnover in Prader-Willi syndrome compared with controls matched for sex and body mass index: a cross-sectional study. J Pediatr 2004;144:614–619.
2. Mandel K, Atkinson S, Barr RD, Pencharz P. Skeletal morbidity in childhood acute lymphoblastic leukemia. J Clin Oncol 2004;22:1215–1221.
3. Fewtrell MS. Growth and nutrition after discharge. Semin Neonat 2003;8:169–176.
4. Buntain HM, Greer RM, Schluter PJ, et al. Bone mineral density in Australian children, adolescents and adults with cystic fibrosis: a controlled cross sectional study. Thorx 2004;59:149–155.
5. Mora S, Zamproni I, Beccio S, Bianchi R, Giacomet V, Vigano A. Longitudinal changes of bone mineral density and metabolism in antiretroviral-treated human immunodeficiency virus-infected children. J Clin Endocrinol Metab 2004; 89:24–28.
6. Misra M, Miller KK, Bjornson J, et al. Alterations in growth hormone secretory dynamics in adolescent girls with anorexia nervosa and effects on bone metabolism. J Clin Endocrinol Metab 2003;88:5615–5623.
7. Daniels MW, Wilson DM, Paguntalan HG, Hoffman AR, Bachrach LK. Bone mineral density in pediatric transplant recipients. Transplantation 2003;27;76:673–678.
8. Barden EM, Kawchak DA, Ohene-Frempong K, Stallings VA, Zemel BS. Body composition in children with sickle cell disease. Am J Clin Nutr 2002;76(1):218–225.
9. Henderson RC. The correlation between dual-energy x-ray absorptiometry measures of bone density in the proximal femur and lumbar spine of children. Skeletal Radiol 1997;26:544–547.
10. Henderson RC, Lark RK, Newman JE, et al. Pediatric reference data for dual x-ray absorptiometric measures of normal bone density in the distal femur. AJR 2002;439–443.
11. Lark RK, Henderson RC, Renner JB, et al. Dual x-ray absorptiometry assessment of body composition in children with altered body posture. J Clin Densitometry 2001;4:325–335.
12. Moyer-Mileur LJ, Brunstetter V, McNaught TP, Gill G, Chan GM. Daily physical activity program improves growth and bone mineralization in preterm, VLBW infants. Pediatrics 2000;106:1088–1092.
13. Koo WWK. Body composition measurement during infancy. Am NY Acad Sci 2000;904:383–392.
14. Koo WWK, Walters J, Bush AJ, Chesney RW, Carlson SE. Dual energy x-ray absorptiometry studies of bone mineral status in newborn infants. J Bone Miner Res 1996;11:997–1002.
15. Lapillonne A, Braillon P, Claris O, Chatelain PG, Delmas PD, Salle BL. Body composition in appropriate and in small for gestational age infants. Acta Paediatr 1997;86:196–200.
16. Specker BL, Beck A, Kalkwarf H, Ho M. Randomized trial of varying mineral intake on total body bone mineral accretion during the first year of life. Pediatrics 1997;99:e12.
17. Rigo J, Nyamugabo K, Picaud JC, Gerard P, Peltain C, DeCurtis M. Reference values of body composition obtained by dual energy x-ray absorptiometry in preterm and term neonates. J Pediatr Gastroenterol Nutr 1998;27:184–190.
18. Mehta KC, Specker BL, Bartholmey S, Giddens J, Mo ML. Trial on timing of introduction to solids and food type on infant growth. Pediatrics 1998;102:569–573.
19. Rawlings DJ, Cooke RJ, McCormick K, Griffin IJ, Faulkner K, Wells JC, Smith JS, Robinson SJ. Body composition of preterm infants during infancy. Arch Dis Child Fetal Neonatal Ed 1999;80:F188–191.
20. Brunton JA, Saigal S, Atkinson SA. Growth and body composition in infants with bronchopulmonary dysplasia up to 3 months corrected age: a randomized trial of a high-energy nutrient-enriched formula fed after hospital discharge. J Pediatr 1998;133:340–345.
21. Butte N, Heinz C, Hopkinson J, Wong W, Shypailo R, Ellis K. Fat mass in infants and toddlers: comparability of total body water, total body potassium, total body electrical conductivity, and dual energy x-ray absorptiometry. J Pediatr Gastroenterol Nutr 1999;29:184–189.

22. Koo WWK, Hockman EM. Physiologic predictors of lumbar spine bone mass in neonates. Pediatr Res 2000;48:485–489.
23. Koo WWK, Walter JC, Hockman EM. Body composition in human infants at birth and postnatally. J Nutr 2000;130:2188–2194.
24. Sievanen H, Backstrom MC, Kuusela AL, Ikonen J, Maki M. Dual energy x-ray absorptiometry of the forearm in preterm and term infants: evaluation of the methodology. Pediatr Res 1999;45(1):100–105.
25. Zadik Z, Price D, Diamond G. Pediatric reference curves for multi-site quantitative ultrasound and its modulators. Osteoporosis Intl 2003;14:857–862.
26. Specker BL, Namgung R, Tsang RC. Bone mineral acquisition in utero and during infancy and childhood, in Marcus R, Feldman D, Kelsey J, eds. *Osteoporosis*, vol. 1. San Diego: Academic, 2001; 599–620.
27. Chan GM, McNaught T. Relation of forearm bone and soft tissues to infant's body composition. J Clin Densitometry 2001;41:221–224.
28. Koo WWK, Walters J, Bush AJ. Technical considerations of dual energy x-ray absorptiometry-based bone mineral measurements for pediatric studies. J Bone Min Res 1995;10:1998–2004.
29. Atkinson SA, Randall-Simpson J. Factors influencing body composition of premature infants at term-adjusted age. Ann New York Acad Sci 2000;904:393–399.
30. Koo WWK, Hockman EM, Hammami M. Dual energy x-ray absorptiometry measurements in small subjects: conditions affecting clinical measurements. J Am Coll Nutr 2004;23:212–219.
31. Picaud JC, Duboeuf F, Vey-Marty V, Delmas P, Clanis C, Salle BL, Rigo J. First all-solid pediatric phantom for dual x-ray absorptiometry in infants. J Clin Densitometry 2003;6:17–23.
32. Lee JJK, Lyne ED. Pathologic fractures in severely handicapped children and young adults. J Pediatr Orthop 1990;10:497–500.
33. McIvor WC, Samilson RL. Fractures in patients with cerebral palsy. J Bone Joint Surg Am 1966;48:858–866.
34. Lock TR, Aronson DD. Fractures in patients who have myelomeningocele. J Bone Joint Surg Am 1989;71:1153–1157.
35. Robin GC. Fracture in poliomyelitis in children. J Bone Joint Surg Am 1966;48:1048–1054.
36. Harcke HT, Taylor A, Bachrach S, Miller F, Henderson RC. Lateral femoral scan: an alternative method for assessing bone mineral density in children with cerebral palsy. Pediatr Radiol 1998;28:241–246.
37. Henderson RC, Lark RK, Newman JE, et al. Pediatric reference data for dual x-ray absorptiometric measures of normal bone density in the distal femur. AJR 2002;178:439–443.
38. Leventhal JM, Thomas SA, Rosenfield NS, Markowitz RI. Fractures in young children. Distinguishing child abuse from unintentional injuries. Am J Dis Child 1993;147(1):87–92.
39. American Academy of Pediatrics. Diagnostic imaging of child abuse. Pediatrics 2000;105:1345–1348.
40. Conway JJ, Collins M, Tanz RR, et al. The role of bone scintigraphy in detecting child abuse. Semin Nucl Med 1993;23:321–333.
41. Lachman RS, Krakow D, Kleinman PK. Differential diagnosis II: osteogenesis imperfecta, in *Diagnostic Imaging of Child Abuse*, 2nd ed. Kleinman PK Ed. Missouri: Mosby, 1998;197–213.
42. Shapiro JR, Stover ML, Burn VE, et al. An osteopenic nonfracture syndrome with features of mild osteogenesis imperfecta associated with the substitution of a cysteine for glycine at triple helix position 43 in the pro alpha 1 (I) chain of type I collagen. J Clin Invest 1992;89:567—573.
43. Sillence D, Senn A and Danks D. Genetic heterogeneity in osteogenesis imperfecta. J Med Genet 1979;16:101–106.
44. Glorieux FH, Rauch F, Plotkin H, et al. Type V osteogenesis imperfecta: a new form of brittle bone disease. J Bone Miner Res 2000;15:1650–1658.
45. Glorieux FH, Ward LM, Rauch F, Lalic L, Roughley PJ, Travers R. Osteogenesis imperfecta type VI: a form of brittle bone disease with a mineralization defect. J Bone Miner Res 2002;17:30–38.
46. Ward LM, Rauch F, Travers R, et al. Osteogenesis imperfecta type VII: an autosomal recessive form of brittle bone disease. Bone 2002;31:12–18.
47. Byers PH. Disorders of collagen biosynthesis and structure, in Scriver CR, Beaudet AL, Sly WS, Valle D, eds. *The Metabolic and Mmolecular Basis of Inherited Disease*, 7th ed. New York: McGraw-Hill, 1995; 4029—4078.
48. Steiner RD, Pepin M, Byers PH. Studies of collagen synthesis and structure in the differentiation of child abuse from osteogenesis imperfecta. J Pediatr 1996;128:542–547.
49. Paterson CR, Mole PA. Bone density in osteogenesis imperfecta may well be normal. Postgrad Med J 1994;70:104–107.

50. Davie, M, Haddaway M. Bone mineral content and density in healthy subjects and in osteogenesis imperfecta. Arch Dis Child 1994;70:331–334.
51. Glorieux, F, Lanoue, G, Chabot, G, Travers R. Bone mineral density in osteogenesis imperfecta. J Bone Min Res 1994;9:225–225.
52. Zionts LE, Nash JP, Rude R, Ross T, Stott NS. Bone mineral density in children with mild osteogenesis imperfecta. J Bone Joint Surg Br 1995;77B:143–147.
53. Cepollaro, C, Gonnelli, S, Pondrelli, C, et al. Osteogenesis imperfecta: bone turnover, bone density, and ultrasound parameters. Calcif Tissue Int 1999;65:129–132.
54. Lund AM, Mølgaard C, Muller J, Skovby F. Bone mineral content and collagen defects in osteogenesis imperfecta. Acta Pædiatr 1999;88:1083–1088.
55. Mølgaard C, Thomsen BL, Prentice A, Cole TJ, Michaelsen KF. Whole body bone mineral content in healthy children and adolescents. Arch Dis Child 1997;76:9–15.
56. Miller ME, Hangartner TN. Bone density measurements by computed tomography in osteogenesis imperfecta-type 1. Osteoporos Int 1999;9:427–432.
57. Bishop NJ, Plotkin H, Lanoue G, Chabot G, Glorieux FH. When is a fracture child abuse? Bone 23(5):F198(Abstract).

10 Research Considerations

Mary B. Leonard, MD, MSCE,
and Moira Petit, PhD

CONTENTS

INTRODUCTION
SPINE
HIP
WHOLE BODY
THE FUNCTIONAL BONE–MUSCLE UNIT
SUMMARY POINTS
REFERENCES

INTRODUCTION

The preceding chapters of this text are primarily dedicated to the optimal acquisition and interpretation of dual-energy x-ray absorptiometry (DXA) scans in children in clinical practice. In addition to these techniques, many investigators have proposed novel methods for scan acquisition and analysis in order to overcome the limitations of DXA and to improve estimates of bone strength. Although these techniques are not yet available for clinical use, consideration of research strategies highlights the potential limitations of conventional DXA techniques and may aid in the interpretation of clinical scan results. This chapter summarizes these methods, cites examples of research applications in healthy children and children with chronic disease, and considers the potential strengths and weaknesses of these techniques.

DXA techniques traditionally focus on posteroanterior (PA) or anteroposterior (AP) projections of the spine and the hip. However, alternative scanning and analytic techniques have been advocated at these sites in order to provide estimates of volumetric density and three-dimensional structure and to improve fracture discrimination. Furthermore, algorithms have been developed to assess bone mass in the context of muscle mass and the functional bone–muscle unit.

From: *Current Clinical Practice: Bone Densitometry in Growing Patients: Guidelines for Clinical Practice*
Edited by: A. J. Sawyer, L. K. Bachrach, and E. B. Fung © Humana Press Inc., Totowa, NJ

SPINE

It is well recognized that DXA estimates of vertebral bone mineral density (BMD) are confounded by bone size in children and adults (1). Lumbar spine DXA provides an estimate of areal BMD (aBMD; in g/cm^2) that does not adjust for the depth of bone. Bones of larger width and height also tend to be thicker. Because bone thickness is not factored into DXA estimates of BMD, reliance on aBMD inherently underestimates the bone density of shorter individuals. That is, a child with smaller bones may appear to have a mineralization disorder (Iowa BMD) despite having a normal volumetric BMD (vBMD). This clearly introduces an important artifact in children with chronic diseases associated with growth delay. Furthermore, the projected bone mineral content (BMC) within the AP or PA projection of vertebrae includes the superimposed vertebral spinous processes.

These limitations are highlighted in a recent report that compared DXA aBMD and quantitative computed tomography (QCT) vBMD Z-scores for the spine in 200 healthy children and 200 chronically ill children (2). The hypothesis of the study was that aBMD measurements as measured by DXA would result in the overdiagnosis of low bone mass (defined as a Z-score <–2.0) in children with poor growth. Consistent with this hypothesis, a significantly greater proportion of children were classified as having low bone mass by the criteria of DXA aBMD Z-scores (76 of 400) compared with the number identified as low using QCT vBMD Z-scores QCT (25 of 400); discrepancies in aBMD and vBMD were more common among children below the fifth percentile for height and/ or weight for age. Using QCT as the standard for this comparison, the specificity of a DXA aBMD Z-score of less than –2.0 was 94% among healthy children but only 74% among the chronically ill children. That is, among the 179 ill children with QCT Z-scores greater than –2.0, 47 (26%) had DXA Z-scores less than –2.0.

Estimates of Spine Volumetric BMD Based on the PA or AP Scan

The confounding effect of skeletal size on DXA measures is well recognized, and two analytic strategies have been proposed to estimate vertebral vBMD from projected PA (e.g., Hologic scanners) or AP (e.g., GE Lunar scanners) bone dimensions and BMC. The technique developed by Carter et al. (3) for calculating vBMD (termed bone mineral apparent density [BMAD]) is based on the observation that vertebral BMC is scaled proportionately to the projected bone area to the 1.5 power; therefore, BMAD is defined as BMC/(area)$^{1.5}$.

Kroger et al. (4,5) proposed an alternative estimate of vertebral volume: the lumbar body is assumed to have a cylindrical shape, and volume of the cylinder is calculated as

$$(\pi)(radius^2)(height)$$

which is equivalent to

$$(\pi)[(width/2)^2](area/width)$$

Therefore, vBMD is calculated as

$$(aBMD)(4)/[(\pi)(width)]$$

using vertebral width and aBMD from the AP projection.

This approach was validated by comparison with magnetic resonance imaging (MRI) measurements of vertebral dimensions in 32 adults (6); DXA-derived vBMD correlated moderately well with BMD based on MRI-derived estimates of vertebral volume (R = 0.665). Of note, the Kroger studies were conducted with a Lunar DPX scanner. This approach cannot be applied to DXA scans obtained with a Hologic scanner because measures of vertebral width are not provided by Hologic software.

These two approaches have been used in numerous pediatric studies to assess the effects of puberty *(7,8)*, ethnicity *(9–11)*, gene polymorphisms *(12)*, and weight-bearing physical activity *(13–15)* on spine vBMD in healthy children. They have also been used to assess the effects of calcium deficiency and milk avoidance *(16,17)* and hypovitaminosis D *(18)*, and to assess the effects of varied chronic disorders associated with poor growth such as Turner's syndrome *(19)*, cystic fibrosis *(20–22)*, hypogonadism *(23)*, growth hormone disorder *(24–26)*, prematurity *(27)*, Cushing's syndrome *(28)*, thalassemia *(29)*, diabetes mellitus *(30)*, solid-organ transplantation *(31)*, and childhood leukemia *(32,33)*. In addition, these approaches have been used to assess the effects of bisphosphonate *(34)* and growth hormone therapy *(24,26)*.

In the earliest study of BMAD in children, Katzman et al. *(7)* concluded that 50% of the pubertal increase in spine BMC in adolescent females was the result of bone expansion rather than an increase in BMC per unit volume. The reported pattern of changes in bone size and density during puberty was consistent with studies using spine QCT *(35)*.

The Bone Mineral Density in Childhood Study *(36)* recently reported the results of a comparison of spine QCT and varied DXA-based estimates of vBMD in 124 children and adolescents. The authors considered two approaches to decrease the influence of bone size on DXA BMD results: (1) BMAD, and (2) aBMD divided by bone height. The highest correlations were observed for QCT BMC and DXA BMC (R^2 = 0.94). DXA aBMD was only moderately correlated with QCT vBMD (R^2 = 0.39).

Illustrating the confounding effect of bone size on aBMD, the correlation between DXA aBMD and QCT estimates of bone volume (R^2 = 0.68) was greater than the correlation between DXA aBMD and QCT vBMD. The two strategies to adjust for bone size resulted in only slight improvements in the correlations with QCT vBMD (BMAD, R^2 = 0.49; aBMD/bone height: R^2 = 0.55).

Of note, the correlations were especially poor among children in the early stages of pubertal development. For example, the correlation between BMAD and QCT vBMD was only R^2 = 0.13 in Tanner stages 1–3, compared with 0.60 in Tanner stages 4 and 5. Only after multiple regression techniques were used to correct aBMD for puberty, age, weight, height, and bone age was the correlation between DXA and QCT improved (R^2 = 0.91).

It is not known if these volumetric techniques provide better estimates of fracture risk compared with aBMD in healthy children or children with chronic disease. To our knowledge, no studies have assessed BMAD in children with vertebral compression fractures. Fracture studies in children have been largely limited to forearm fractures, the most common fracture site in childhood.

Multiple studies in healthy children reported that spine BMAD and aBMD were lower in wrist and forearm fracture cases compared with controls *(37–39)*. The lower aBMD in the fracture subjects compared with controls was not attributed to smaller bone size because the BMAD values were also lower.

A recent prospective cohort study of fractures at any site provided some support for BMAD measures as predictors of new fracture *(39)*. In young girls with and without a history of prior distal forearm fractures, the risk of new fractures at any site was significantly increased for each one-standard-deviation decrease in BMAD (hazard ratio [HR]

1.34; 95% confidence interval [CI] 1.02, 1.75) for spine BMAD, but the effect did not achieve statistical significance for spine aBMD (HR 1.33; 95% CI 0.97, 1.82). However, given the substantial overlap in the confidence intervals and the comparable hazard ratios, it is unclear whether BMAD improves fracture prediction compared with aBMD. Future studies using receiver operating characteristic (ROC) curves are needed to determine the sensitivity and specificity of spine aBMD and BMAD in the assessment of spine fracture risk in children, as well as fracture risk at other sites.

Studies in adults suggested that estimates of vBMD did not improve fracture prediction compared with aBMD (40,41). In an in vitro assessment of vertebral body breaking strength in adults specimens, aBMD and BMAD provided comparable estimates of bone strength (41). Jergas et al. (42) reported the results of a comparison of aBMD, BMAD, and spine QCT for fracture discrimination in 260 postmenopausal women. Consistent with the confounding effect of subject height on aBMD, aBMD was correlated with height, whereas BMAD and QCT BMD were not correlated with height. The associations with vertebral fracture were stronger for QCT (odds ratio [OR] 3.17; 95% CI 1.90, 5.27), compared with BMAD (OR 1.68, 95% CI 1.14, 2.48) and aBMD (OR 1.47, 95% CI 1.02, 2.13).

In conclusion, BMAD has provided insight into the differential effects of age, maturation, ethnicity, nutrition, and disease processes on bone size and vBMD in children. However, significantly more research is needed to validate these findings compared with three-dimensional imaging techniques and to determine the sensitivity and specificity of these techniques for fracture prediction in healthy children and in children with varied chronic diseases.

Lateral Spine BMD

Spine aBMD is used to assess the predominantly trabecular vertebral bodies; however, the projected vertebral area includes the superimposed spinous processes. Lateral spine scans isolate the vertebral body from the cortical bone in these posterior elements (Fig. 1). Although this technique allows one to limit the region of interest to the vertebral body, this advantage must be balanced against the potential errors introduced by the greater thickness and in homogeneity of the surrounding soft tissue.

Prior studies have demonstrated that vertebral trabecular vBMD increases significantly during growth and maturation, whereas cortical vBMD remains relatively constant (43,44). Therefore, in theory, isolation of the predominantly trabecular vertebral body on the lateral spine may highlight growth-related increases in trabecular BMC. This potential benefit of lateral scans is analogous to reports in the elderly that lateral DXA was significantly more sensitive than PA DXA to age-related bone loss in males and females (45–47).

Few studies have assessed lateral spine scans in children (48–56). In 1995, normative data for PA (L2–L4) and lateral (L2–L3) lumbar spine were published from 778 healthy children in Argentina, as measured with a Norland XR-26 scanner (48). Studies of the changes in AP and lateral aBMD with growth and maturation have produced varied results.

Sabatier et al. (49) compared AP and lateral spine BMD in a cross-sectional study of 574 healthy females, ages 10–24 yr. Both AP and lateral BMD increased markedly between the ages of 10 and 14 yr; however, between 14 and 17 yr, AP BMD increased

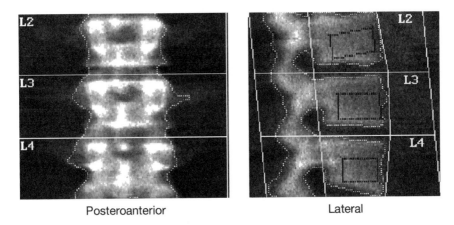

Posteroanterior   Lateral

Fig. 1. Paired posteroanterior and lateral lumbar spine dual-energy x-ray absorptiometry.

and lateral BMD was not associated with age. In contrast, Plotkin et al. *(50)* reported that PA and lateral BMD increased from Tanner stages 1 through 3, but then there were no further differences between stages 3 and 5. Wu et al. *(56)* compared PA and lateral BMD in 1286 children and young adults (ages 6–24 yr). Lateral BMD was comparable in males and females until age 14, after which lateral BMD was greater in males. This gender difference was attributed to differences in height. Henry et al. *(55)* reported that lateral spine BMC increased steeply with age in males and females, peaking at age 22 yr in men and at age 26 yr in women.

These large, descriptive studies have demonstrated the variable patterns in PA and lateral BMC and aBMD. However, the benefits of lateral scans in the assessment of childhood chronic disease remain untested.

Paired PA-Lateral Spine Estimates of Volumetric BMD

Another approach is to use paired PA-lateral vertebral scans (Fig. 1) to measure vertebral width, height, and depth in order to estimate bone volume and vBMD. Although this approach requires an additional scan, the paired PA-lateral scans offer two advantages for the assessment of vertebral vBMD. First, the addition of the lateral spine scan permits direct measurement of bone depth, as opposed to estimating depth from the PA dimensions. Second, the lateral image is edited to isolate the vertebral body, excluding the BMC within the cortical spinous processes. Studies in adults have demonstrated that paired PA-lateral scans provide better discriminatory capability for vertebral fracture than BMAD or PA aBMD *(42)*.

The estimates based on the paired PA-lateral scans are calculated automatically with manufacturer software that assumed the vertebral body was an elliptical cylinder *(57)*. The width of the vertebrae on the PA scan is used as an estimate of the major axis of the ellipse, and the depth of the vertebrae on the lateral scan is used as the estimate of the minor axis of the ellipse. Volume is calculated as

$$[(\pi/4)(\text{PA vertebral width})(\text{lateral depth})(\text{vertebral height})]$$

BMC measured on the lateral scan is then divided by this estimate of volume to generate "width-adjusted vBMD."

We have identified three studies that used this approach in children *(53,55,56)*. The first two examined and compared changes in PA aBMD, lateral aBMD, and vBMD in large cross-sectional samples of healthy children. Henry et al. *(55)* reported that vBMD increased gradually during growth in childhood and into young adulthood in both sexes. Wu et al. *(56)* also reported gradual increases in vBMD, with no gender differences across the 6- to 24-yr age range.

In the third study, PA aBMD, lateral aBMD, and vBMD were examined as clinical outcomes in a randomized clinical trial of gonadotropin-releasing hormone agonist with and without calcium supplementation *(53)*. Bone measures were assessed at baseline (mean age 7.3 ± 0.91 yr), at the end of the intervention (mean age 11.3 ± 0.97 yr), and at the time of final height (mean age 16.2 ± 1.9 yr). The vBMD was significantly higher in the calcium-supplemented group at the end of treatment period and at final evaluation compared with the group that did not receive calcium. The differences in PA aBMD and lateral aBMD between the groups at the end of treatment period and at final evaluation did not achieve statistical significance. The percentage changes between the start and end of the treatment period and between the start of treatment and final evaluations were significant for PA aBMD and vBMD; no results were provided for lateral aBMD.

Although this study suggests that paired PA-lateral estimates of vBMD may be more sensitive to disease and treatment effects, additional studies are needed to determine the best outcome for clinical trials and for the monitoring of patients.

HIP

Femoral Neck BMAD

A formula for BMAD has also been developed for the femoral neck in order to normalize BMC to a derived bone reference volume *(7)*.

femoral neck BMAD = (femoral neck BMC)/(femoral neck bone area)^2

This approach has been used in a variety of studies in children *(7,10,31,38,58)* and adults *(59,60)*. Comparable decrements in hip aBMD and hip BMAD were reported in healthy boys with a history of forearm fracture, as compared with controls *(38)*. Cauley et al. *(61)* recently reported that hip aBMD and hip BMAD were significantly lower in adults with vertebral compression fractures compared to controls. The predicted probability of having a vertebral fracture at a given hip aBMD level differed in men and women. In contrast, the probability of fracture at a given BMAD was similar in men and women, suggesting that measures of bone mass that partially correct for gender differences in bone size may yield universal estimates of fracture risk in adults.

In 1996, van der Meulen et al. *(62)* estimated cross-sectional geometric properties of the femoral midshaft from DXA scans. Two geometry-based structural indicators, the section modulus and whole bone strength index, were calculated to assess the structural characteristics of the femur. Femoral strength, as described by these structural indicators, increased dramatically from childhood through young adulthood. To our knowledge, neither of these two techniques has been validated using three-dimensional imaging modalities.

Hip Structural Analysis

In 1990, Beck et al. *(63)* introduced the hip structural analysis (HSA) technique to derive femoral neck geometry from DXA bone mineral image data. This approach is based on the principals developed by Martin and Burr *(64)*. A series of experiments with an aluminum phantom, with cadaver femora, and with sequential computed tomography (CT) cross-sectional images were used to validate HSA-computed femoral neck cross-sectional areas (CSAs), and cross-sectional moments of inertia (CSMIs), a measure of bone strength. Breaking strengths of cadaveric femora were measured with a materials testing system and showed better agreement with HSA-predicted strength ($r = 0.89$) than femoral neck aBMD ($r = 0.79$). It is important to note that this approach makes a number of assumptions. For example, estimates of cortical thickness assume that the cross-section is a circular annulus, the narrow neck region is assumed to have 60% of the measured bone area in the cortex, and the shaft region is assumed to be entirely cortical bone. The HSA approach has not been validated in children.

Since its introduction, the HSA approach has been used in more than 30 publications in adults, ranging from studies of the effects of gender *(65)*, race *(60,66)*, physical performance and muscle function *(67,68)*, gene polymorphisms *(69,70)*, aging *(71)*, and teriparatide therapy *(72)*.

The HSA technique has also been used to provide insight into geometric changes that result in apparent increases in hip aBMD in healthy children, athletes, and obese children *(73–80)* For example, Petit et al. *(76)* reported that a 7-mo randomized exercise intervention resulted in significantly greater increases in femoral neck and intertrochanteric aBMD in early pubertal females. Underpinning these changes were increased bone cross-sectional area and reduced endosteal expansion. Changes in subperiosteal dimensions did not differ. These structural changes significantly improved section modulus (i.e., bending strength) at the femoral neck. The research team subsequently reported that the intervention resulted in greater bone expansion on the periosteal and the endosteal surfaces of the narrow neck, resulting in greater section modulus *(78)*.

Other HSA studies have demonstrated sexual dimorphism of the femoral neck during the adolescent growth spurt *(80)*. The gender differences in bending strength were explained by differences in height and lean body mass. HSA has also been used to demonstrate a significant relationship between physical activity and femoral neck section modulus in healthy children *(73,79,81)*, as well as greater indices of axial strength and bending strength in gymnasts, as compared with controls *(77)*. Finally, a recent HSA study reported that the greater bone mass in obese children was due to significantly greater section modulus compared with nonobese controls, and the greater bone strength was appropriately adapted to lean mass and height *(74)*.

We are unaware of any studies that used the HSA technique to evaluate the impact of childhood disease or pharmacological interventions on bone structure.

WHOLE BODY

As detailed previously, geometric algorithms have been developed to estimate vBMD in the hip and spine—sites with relatively simple geometry. Unfortunately, these approaches cannot readily applied to the complex shape of the whole skeleton, and the biomechanical significance of BMC relative to bone area across the entire skeleton is not known.

Multiple sources of pediatric DXA reference data are now available for the calculation of whole-body bone Z-scores. These include gender-specific centile curves, age- and height-specific means and standard deviations, and Z-score prediction models *(82–89)*. Despite the recent widespread availability of whole-body reference data, there is a lack of consensus regarding the most appropriate strategy for the interpretation of two-dimensional whole-body DXA BMC and bone area results across children of differing body size and body composition. Proposed strategies include assessing bone area relative to height and BMC relative to bone area *(84)*, assessing BMC relative to height and age *(82)*, assessing BMC relative to body weight or lean mass *(90–92)*, and multistaged prediction models for BMC incorporating age, ethnicity, height, weight, bone area, and pubertal stage *(89)*.

Cortical bone comprises 80% of the skeletal bone mass; therefore, whole-body DXA BMC and area reflect predominantly cortical bone mass and dimensions. The primary function of cortical bone is mechanical strength. Leonard et al. *(93)* recently compared whole-body BMC, projected area, and aBMD with peripheral QCT (pQTC) measures of cortical geometry, vBMD, and bending strength in 150 healthy children in order to develop analytic strategies for the assessment of whole-body DXA that describe the biomechanical characteristics of cortical bone across a wide range of body sizes. DXA bone area for height and BMC for height were both strongly and positively associated with pQCT cortical cross-sectional area and bending strength relative to length (all $p <$ 0.0001). This suggested that decreases in DXA bone area for height or DXA BMC for height represented narrower bones with less resistance to bending. DXA BMC for age ($p < 0.01$) and aBMD ($p < 0.05$) for age were moderately correlated with strength. DXA BMC for bone area was weakly associated with pQCT bone strength, and in females only. Therefore, normalizing whole-body DXA bone area for height and BMC for height provided the best measures of bone dimensions and strength. DXA BMC normalized for bone area was a poor indicator of bone strength.

Studies assessing the ability of these varied strategies to discriminate between fracture and nonfracture cases have not been performed, and these are imperative in order to identify the best analytic approach to the interpretation of whole-body DXA data for research and clinical applications. This is especially important as GE Lunar recently introduced pediatric software that will generate Z-scores for whole-body bone area for height and whole-body BMC for bone area, and Hologic recently presented reference data for whole-body BMC relative to height *(94)*.

One other consideration in performing whole-body scans is whether to exclude or include the data obtained from scanning the skull region. The skull provides a larger proportion of total-body BMC in younger children, and this proportion decreases with age. Therefore, the technique of evaluating whole-body DXA results without the skull may be more sensitive in detecting changes in BMC or BMD over time *(93, 95–97)*. This technique has been used in prior studies and is available in new software from the manufacturers *(98)*.

THE FUNCTIONAL BONE–MUSCLE UNIT

According to Wolff's law, bone grows in response to the magnitude and direction of the forces to which it is subjected *(99)*. This response keeps mechanically-induced deformation of bone (i.e., strain) at a set point. This capacity of bone to respond to mechanical loading with increased bone strength is greatest during growth *(100)*; mechanical signals that are osteogenic in the young skeleton fail to stimulate bone formation in the mature skeleton *(101)*. Hormones and nutrients influence mechanical loads by influencing linear growth and muscle mass and may alter the muscle–bone set point *(102)*. These relationships dictate that studies of bone health in childhood should incorporate assessment of muscle.

The very high correlation between muscle mass and BMC is well recognized in children and adults *(103)*. Numerous investigators advocate a multistage algorithm for the assessment of DXA bone data relative to muscle mass in children *(104–106)*. In 2002, Schoenau et al. *(106)* proposed a simple diagnostic algorithm to evaluate musculoskeletal adaptation as an index of the "functional bone–muscle unit." This functional approach addresses two questions: (1) is muscle force (or mass) adequate for body size (because muscle force is largely determined by body height *[107,108]*, muscle parameters should be related to body height); and (2) is bone strength normally adapted to muscle force.

The results can then be divided into four diagnostic groups. In the first group, muscle force is adequate for height and BMC is normally adapted to the muscle forces, representing a normal system. In the second group, muscle is adequate for height but BMC is lower than expected for muscle force; this represents a "primary bone defect." In the third group, muscle force is low for height and BMC is adapted adequately to the decreased mechanical load. This means that BMC is presumably too low for height, and a "secondary bone defect" is diagnosed. In the fourth group, muscle force is low for height and BMC is even lower than expected for the reduced muscle force; this indicates a "mixed bone defect" (i.e., primary and secondary).

Multiple sources of DXA reference data are now available for the assessment of the functional bone muscle unit in healthy children. Crabtree et al. *(61)* provided gender- and maturation-specific prediction equations for lean body mass for height and BMC for lean mass for the whole body and the lumbar spine based on 646 healthy children, ages 5–18 yr. Hogler et al. *(104)* reported gender-specific reference curves for lean mass for height and the ratio of BMC to lean mass in 459 healthy children.

The assessment of the functional bone–muscle unit has been reported in varied pediatric conditions, including renal transplant recipients *(109)* and children with chronic renal failure *(106)*, juvenile idiopathic arthritis *(110)*, neuromuscular disease ,*(105)*, osteogenesis imperfecta *(105)*, anorexia nervosa *(104)*, growth hormone deficiency *(104)*, Turner's syndrome *(111)*, and Crohn's disease *(96)*. Future studies are needed to assess appropriate interventions to improve bone health in children with a dysfunctional bone muscle unit.

SUMMARY POINTS

- Multiple strategies have been proposed to estimate vBMD in the spine; however, it is not known if these techniques improve fracture prediction in children.
- Lateral spine scans isolate the predominantly trabecular vertebral body; however, the sensitivity and specificity of lateral spine scans for the diagnosis of bone disorders have not been tested in children.
- HSA provides estimates of bone structure and has proved useful in the assessment of physical activity interventions; however, this technique has not been validated in children.
- A large number of analytic strategies for the assessment of whole- body BMC have been developed. Future studies are needed to assess the value of these approaches for fracture prediction and measuring response to therapy.
- The functional bone–muscle unit algorithms provide insight into the classification of pediatric bone disorders and the investigation of pathophysiological processes. However, it remains to be determined if "secondary bone disorders" truly represent bone deficits that are caused by muscle deficits, as opposed to independent disease effects on muscle and bone.

REFERENCES

1. Prentice A, Parsons TJ, Cole TJ. Uncritical use of bone mineral density in absorptiometry may lead to size-related artifacts in the identification of bone mineral determinants. Am J Clin Nutr 1994;60(6):837–842.
2. Wren TA, Liu X, Pitukcheewanont P, Gilsanz V. Bone densitometry in pediatric populations: discrepancies in the diagnosis of osteoporosis by DXA and CT. J Pediatr 2005;146(6):776–779.
3. Carter DR, Bouxsein ML, Marcus R. New approaches for interpreting projected bone densitometry data. J Bone Miner Res 1992;7(2):137–145.
4. Kroger H, Kotaniemi A, Kroger L, Alhava E. Development of bone mass and bone density of the spine and femoral neck—a prospective study of 65 children and adolescents. Bone Miner 1993;23(3):171–182.
5. Kroger H, Kotaniemi A, Vainio P, Alhava E. Bone densitometry of the spine and femur in children by dual-energy x-ray absorptiometry. Bone Miner 1992;17:75–185.
6. Kroger H, Vainio P, Nieminen J, Kotaniemi A. Comparison of different models for interpreting bone mineral density measurements using DXA and MRI technology. Bone 1995;17(2):157–159.
7. Katzman DK, Bachrach LK, Carter DR, Marcus R. Clinical and anthropometric correlates of bone mineral acquisition in healthy adolescent girls. J Clin Endocrinol Metab 1991;73(6):1332–1339.
8. Haapasalo H, Kannus P, Sievanen H, et al. Development of mass, density, and estimated mechanical characteristics of bones in Caucasian females. J Bone Miner Res 1996;11(11):1751–1760.
9. Bhudhikanok GS, Wang MC, Eckert K, Matkin C, Marcus R, Bachrach LK. Differences in bone mineral in young Asian and Caucasian Americans may reflect differences in bone size. J Bone Miner Res 1996;11(10):1545–1556.
10. Wang MC, Aguirre M, Bhudhikanok GS, et al. Bone mass and hip axis length in healthy Asian, black, Hispanic, and white American youths. J Bone Miner Res 1997;12(11):1922–1935.
11. Bachrach LK, Hastie T, Wang MC, Narasimhan B, Marcus R. Bone mineral acquisition in healthy Asian, Hispanic, black, and Caucasian youth: a longitudinal study. J Clin Endocrinol Metab 1999;84(12):4702–4712.
12. Boot AM, van der Sluis IM, de Muinck Keizer-Schrama SM, et al. Estrogen receptor alpha gene polymorphisms and bone mineral density in healthy children and young adults. Calcif Tissue Int 2004;74(6):495–500.
13. Ward KA, Roberts SA, Adams JE, Mughal MZ. Bone geometry and density in the skeleton of pre-pubertal gymnasts and school children. Bone 2005;36(6):1012–1018.
14. Dyson K, Blimkie CJ, Davison KS, Webber CE, Adachi JD. Gymnastic training and bone density in pre-adolescent females. Med Sci Sports Exerc 1997;29(4):443–450.
15. Morris FL, Naughton GA, Gibbs JL, Carlson JS, Wark JD. Prospective ten-month exercise intervention in premenarcheal girls: positive effects on bone and lean mass. J Bone Miner Res 1997;12(9):1453–1462.
16. Pettifor JM, Moodley GP. Appendicular bone mass in children with a high prevalence of low dietary calcium intakes. J Bone Miner Res 1997;12(11):1824–1832.
17. Rockell JE, Williams SM, Taylor RW, Grant AM, Jones IE, Goulding A. Two-year changes in bone and body composition in young children with a history of prolonged milk avoidance. Osteoporos Int 2005;16:1016–1023.
18. Lehtonen-Veromaa MK, Mottonen TT, Nuotio IO, Irjala KM, Leino AE, Viikari JS. Vitamin D and attainment of peak bone mass among peripubertal Finnish girls: a 3-year prospective study. Am J Clin Nutr 2002;76(6):1446–1453.
19. Neely EK, Marcus R, Rosenfeld RG, Bachrach LK. Turner syndrome adolescents receiving growth hormone are not osteopenic. J Clin Endocrinol Metab 1993;76(4):861–866.
20. Bhudhikanok GS, Wang MC, Marcus R, Harkins A, Moss RB, Bachrach LK. Bone acquisition and loss in children and adults with cystic fibrosis: a longitudinal study. J Pediatr 1998;133(1):18–27.
21. Bhudhikanok GS, Lim J, Marcus R, Harkins A, Moss RB, Bachrach LK. Correlates of osteopenia in patients with cystic fibrosis. Pediatrics 1996;97(1):103–111.
22. Sood M, Hambleton G, Super M, Fraser WD, Adams JE, Mughal MZ. Bone status in cystic fibrosis. Arch Dis Child 2001;84(6):516–520.
23. Takahashi Y, Minamitani K, Kobayashi Y, Minagawa M, Yasuda T, Niimi H. Spinal and femoral bone mass accumulation during normal adolescence: comparison with female patients with sexual precocity and with hypogonadism. J Clin Endocrinol Metab 1996;81(3):1248–1253.
24. Boot AM, Engels MA, Boerma GJ, Krenning EP, De Muinck Keizer-Schrama SM. Changes in bone mineral density, body composition, and lipid metabolism during growth hormone (GH) treatment in children with GH deficiency. J Clin Endocrinol Metab 1997;82(8):2423–2428.

25. Bachrach LK, Marcus R, Ott SM, et al. Bone mineral, histomorphometry, and body composition in adults with growth hormone receptor deficiency. J Bone Miner Res 1998;13(3):415–421.

26. van der Sluis IM, Boot AM, Hop WC, De Rijke YB, Krenning EP, de Muinck Keizer-Schrama SM. Long-term effects of growth hormone therapy on bone mineral density, body composition, and serum lipid levels in growth hormone deficient children: a 6-year follow-up study. Horm Res 2002;58(5):207–214.

27. Backstrom MC, Kouri T, Kuusela AL, et al. M. Bone isoenzyme of serum alkaline phosphatase and serum inorganic phosphate in metabolic bone disease of prematurity. Acta Paediatr 2000;89(7):867–873.

28. Abad V, Chrousos GP, Reynolds JC, et al. Glucocorticoid excess during adolescence leads to a major persistent deficit in bone mass and an increase in central body fat. J Bone Miner Res 2001;16(10):1879–1885.

29. Bielinski BK, Darbyshire P, Mathers L, Boivin CM, Shaw NJ. Bone density in the Asian thalassaemic population: a cross-sectional review. Acta Paediatr 2001;90(11):1262–1266.

30. Salvatoni A, Mancassola G, Biasoli R, et al. Bone mineral density in diabetic children and adolescents: a follow-up study. Bone 2004;34(5):900–904.

31. Daniels MW, Wilson DM, Paguntalan HG, Hoffman AR, Bachrach LK. Bone mineral density in pediatric transplant recipients. Transplantation 2003;76(4):673–678.

32. van der Sluis IM, van den Heuvel-Eibrink MM, Hahlen K, Krenning EP, de Muinck Keizer-Schrama SM. Bone mineral density, body composition, and height in long-term survivors of acute lymphoblastic leukemia in childhood. Med Pediatr Oncol 2000;35(4):415–420.

33. Lequin MH, van der Shuis IM, Van Rijn RR, et al. Bone mineral assessment with tibial ultrasonometry and dual-energy x-ray absorptiometry in long-term survivors of acute lymphoblastic leukemia in childhood. J Clin Densitom 2002;5(2):167–173.

34. Gandrud LM, Cheung JC, Daniels MW, Bachrach LK. Low-dose intravenous pamidronate reduces fractures in childhood osteoporosis. J Pediatr Endocrinol Metab 2003;16(6):887–892.

35. Gilsanz V, Roe TF, Mora S, Costin G, Goodman WG. Changes in vertebral bone density in black girls and white girls during childhood and puberty. N Engl J Med 1991;325(23):1597–1600.

36. Wren TA, Liu X, Pitukcheewanont P, Gilsanz V. Bone acquisition in healthy children and adolescents: comparisons of dual-energy x-ray absorptiometry and computed tomography measures. J Clin Endocrinol Metab 2005;90(4):1925–1928.

37. Ma D, Jones G. The association between bone mineral density, metacarpal morphometry, and upper limb fractures in children: a population-based case-control study. J Clin Endocrinol Metab 2003;88(4):1486–1491.

38. Goulding A, Jones IE, Taylor RW, Williams SM, Manning PJ. Bone mineral density and body composition in boys with distal forearm fractures: a dual-energy x-ray absorptiometry study. J Pediatr 2001;139(4):509–515.

39. Goulding A, Jones IE, Taylor RW, Manning PJ, Williams SM. More broken bones: a 4-year double cohort study of young girls with and without distal forearm fractures. J Bone Miner Res 2000;15(10):2011–2018.

40. Hui SL, Slemenda CW, Carey MA, Johnston CC Jr. Choosing between predictors of fractures. J Bone Miner Res 1995;10(11):1816–1822.

41. Tabensky AD, Williams J, DeLuca V, Briganti E, Seeman E. Bone mass, areal, and volumetric bone density are equally accurate, sensitive, and specific surrogates of the breaking strength of the vertebral body: an in vitro study. J Bone Miner Res 1996;11(12):1981–1988.

42. Jergas M, Breitenseher M, Gluer CC, Yu W, Genant HK. Estimates of volumetric bone density from projectional measurements improve the discriminatory capability of dual x-ray absorptiometry. J Bone Miner Res 1995;10(7):1101–1110.

43. Gilsanz V, Kovanlikaya A, Costin G, Roe TF, Sayre J, Kaufman F. Differential effect of gender on the sizes of the bones in the axial and appendicular skeletons. J Clin Endocrinol Metab 1997;82(5):1603–1607.

44. Gilsanz V, Skaggs DL, Kovanlikaya A, et al. Differential effect of race on the axial and appendicular skeletons of children. J Clin Endocrinol Metab 1998;83(5):1420–1427.

45. Zmuda JM, Cauley JA, Glynn NW, Finkelstein JS. Posterior-anterior and lateral dual-energy x-ray absorptiometry for the assessment of vertebral osteoporosis and bone loss among older men. J Bone Miner Res 2000;15(7):1417–1424.

46. Finkelstein JS, Cleary RL, Butler JP, et al. A comparison of lateral versus anterior-posterior spine dual energy x-ray absorptiometry for the diagnosis of osteopenia. J Clin Endocrinol Metab 1994;78(3):724–730.

47. Grampp S, Genant HK, Mathur A, et al. Comparisons of noninvasive bone mineral measurements in assessing age-related loss, fracture discrimination, and diagnostic classification. J Bone Miner Res 1997;12(5):697–711.

48. Zanchetta JR, Plotkin H, Alvarez Filgueira ML. Bone mass in children: normative values for the 2–20-year-old population. Bone 1995;16(4 Suppl):393S–399S.

49. Sabatier JP, Guaydier-Souquieres G, Laroche D, et al. Bone mineral acquisition during adolescence and early adulthood: a study in 574 healthy females 10–24 years of age. Osteoporos Int 1996;6(2):141–148.

50. Plotkin H, Nunez M, Alvarez Filgueira ML, Zanchetta JR. Lumbar spine bone density in Argentine children. Calcif Tissue Int 1996;58(3):144–149.

51. Yu W, Qin M, Xu L, et al. Normal changes in spinal bone mineral density in a Chinese population: assessment by quantitative computed tomography and dual-energy x-ray absorptiometry. Osteoporos Int 1999;9(2):179–187.

52. Hangartner TN, Skugor M, Landoll JD, Matkovic V. Comparison of absorptiometric evaluations from total-body and local-regional skeletal scans. J Clin Densitom 2000;3(3):215–225.

53. Antoniazzi F, Zamboni G, Bertoldo F, et al. Bone mass at final height in precocious puberty after gonadotropin-releasing hormone agonist with and without calcium supplementation. J Clin Endocrinol Metab 2003;88(3):1096–1101.

54. Liao EY, Wu XP, Luo XH, et al. Establishment and evaluation of bone mineral density reference databases appropriate for diagnosis and evaluation of osteoporosis in Chinese women. J Bone Miner Metab 2003;21(3):184–192.

55. Henry YM, Fatayerji D, Eastell R. Attainment of peak bone mass at the lumbar spine, femoral neck and radius in men and women: relative contributions of bone size and volumetric bone mineral density. Osteoporos Int 2004;15:263–273.

56. Wu XP, Yang YH, Zhang H, et al. Gender differences in bone density at different skeletal sites of acquisition with age in Chinese children and adolescents. J Bone Miner Metab 2005;23(3):253–260.

57. Blake GM, Warner HW, Fogelman I. The Evaluation of Osteoporosis: Dual Energy X-ray Absorptiometry and Ultra Sound in Clinical Practice, 2nd ed. London: Blackwell Science, 1999.

58. Arabi A, Nabulsi M, Maalouf J, et al. Bone mineral density by age, gender, pubertal stages, and socio-economic status in healthy Lebanese children and adolescents. Bone 2004;35(5):1169–1179.

59. Tracy JK, Meyer WA, Flores RH, Wilson PD, Hochberg MC. Racial differences in rate of decline in bone mass in older men: The Baltimore Men's Osteoporosis Study. J Bone Miner Res 2005;20(7):1228–1234.

60. Cauley JA, Lui LY, Stone KL, et al. Longitudinal study of changes in hip bone mineral density in Caucasian and African-American women. J Am Geriatr Soc 2005;53(2):183–189.

61. Cauley JA, Zmuda JM, Wisniewski SR, et al. Bone mineral density and prevalent vertebral fractures in men and women. Osteoporos Int 2004;15(1):32–37.

62. van der Meulen MC, Ashford MW, Jr., Kiratli BJ, Bachrach LK, Carter DR. Determinants of femoral geometry and structure during adolescent growth. J Orthop Res 1996;14(1):22–29.

63. Beck TJ, Ruff CB, Warden KE, Scott WW, Jr., Rao GU. Predicting femoral neck strength from bone mineral data. A structural approach. Invest Radiol 1990;25(1):6–18.

64. Martin RB, Burr DB. Non-invasive measurement of long bone cross-sectional moment of inertia by photon absorptiometry. J Biomech 1984;17(3):195–201.

65. Duan Y, Beck TJ, Wang XF, Seeman E. Structural and biomechanical basis of sexual dimorphism in femoral neck fragility has its origins in growth and aging. J Bone Miner Res 2003;18(10):1766–1774.

66. Nelson DA, Pettifor JM, Barondess DA, Cody DD, Uusi-Rasi K, Beck TJ. Comparison of cross-sectional geometry of the proximal femur in white and black women from Detroit and Johannesburg. J Bone Miner Res 2004;19(4):560–565.

67. Uusi-Rasi K, Sievanen H, Heinonen A, Beck TJ, Vuori I. Determinants of changes in bone mass and femoral neck structure, and physical performance after menopause: a 9-year follow-up of initially peri-menopausal women. Osteoporos Int 2005;16(6):616–622.

68. Szulc P, Beck TJ, Marchand F, Delmas PD. Low skeletal muscle mass is associated with poor structural parameters of bone and impaired balance in elderly men—The MINOS study. J Bone Miner Res 2005;20(5):721–729.

69. Moffett SP, Zmuda JM, Oakley JI, et al. Tumor necrosis factor-alpha polymorphism, bone strength phenotypes, and the risk of fracture in older women. J Clin Endocrinol Metab 2005;90(6):3491–3497.

70. Rivadeneira F, Houwing-Duistermaat JJ, Beck TJ, et al. The influence of an insulin-like growth factor I gene promoter polymorphism on hip bone geometry and the risk of nonvertebral fracture in the elderly: The Rotterdam Study. J Bone Miner Res 2004;19(8):1280–1290.

71. Wang XF, Duan Y, Beck TJ, Seeman E. Varying contributions of growth and ageing to racial and sex differences in femoral neck structure and strength in old age. Bone 2005;36(6):978–986.

72. Uusi-Rasi K, Semanick LM, Zanchetta JR, et al. Effects of teriparatide [rhPTH (1–34)] treatment on structural geometry of the proximal femur in elderly osteoporotic women. Bone 2005;36(6):948–958.

73. Lloyd T, Beck TJ, Lin HM, et al. Modifiable determinants of bone status in young women. Bone 2002;30(2):416–421.

74. Petit MA, Beck TJ, Shults J, Zemel BS, Foster BJ, Leonard MB. Proximal femur bone geometry is appropriately adapted to lean mass in overweight children and adolescents. Bone 2005;36(3):568–576.

75. Petit MA, Beck TJ, Lin HM, Bentley C, Legro RS, Lloyd T. Femoral bone structural geometry adapts to mechanical loading and is influenced by sex steroids: The Penn State Young Women's Health Study. Bone 2004;35(3):750–759.

76. Petit MA, McKay HA, MacKelvie KJ, Heinonen A, Khan KM, Beck TJ. A randomized school-based jumping intervention confers site and maturity-specific benefits on bone structural properties in girls: a hip structural analysis study. J Bone Miner Res 2002;17(3):363–372.

77. Faulkner RA, Forwood MR, Beck TJ, Mafukidze JC, Russell K, Wallace W. Strength indices of the proximal femur and shaft in prepubertal female gymnasts. Med Sci Sports Exerc 2003;35(3):513–518.

78. MacKelvie KJ, Petit MA, Khan KM, Beck TJ, McKay HA. Bone mass and structure are enhanced following a 2-year randomized controlled trial of exercise in prepubertal boys. Bone 2004;34(4):755–764.

79. Janz KF, Burns TL, Levy SM, et al. Everyday activity predicts bone geometry in children: The Iowa Bone Development Study. Med Sci Sports Exerc 2004;36(7):1124–1131.

80. Forwood MR, Bailey DA, Beck TJ, Mirwald RL, Baxter-Jones AD, Uusi-Rasi K. Sexual dimorphism of the femoral neck during the adolescent growth spurt: a structural analysis. Bone 2004;35(4):973–981.

81. Lloyd T, Petit MA, Lin HM, Beck TJ. Lifestyle factors and the development of bone mass and bone strength in young women. J Pediatr 2004;144(6):776–782.

82. Ellis KJ, Shypailo RJ, Hardin DS, et al. Z score prediction model for assessment of bone mineral content in pediatric diseases. J Bone Miner Res 2001;16(9):1658–1664.

83. Faulkner RA, Bailey DA, Drinkwater DT, McKay HA, Arnold C, Wilkinson AA. Bone densitometry in Canadian children 8–17 years of age. Calcif Tissue Int 1996;59(5):344–351.

84. Molgaard C, Thomsen BL, Prentice A, Cole TJ, Michaelsen KF. Whole body bone mineral content in healthy children and adolescents. Arch Dis Child 1997;76(1):9–15.

85. Binkley TL, Specker BL, Wittig TA. Centile curves for bone densitometry measurements in healthy males and females ages 5–22 yr. J Clin Densitom 2002;5(4):343–353.

86. Hannan WJ, Tothill P, Cowen SJ, Wrate RM. Whole body bone mineral content in healthy children and adolescents. Arch Dis Child 1998;78(4):396–397.

87. Maynard LM, Guo SS, Chumlea WC, et al. Total-body and regional bone mineral content and areal bone mineral density in children aged 8–18 y: The Fels Longitudinal Study. Am J Clin Nutr 1998;68(5):1111–1117.

88. van der Sluis IM, de Ridder MA, Boot AM, Krenning EP, de Muinck Keizer-Schrama SM. Reference data for bone density and body composition measured with dual energy x ray absorptiometry in white children and young adults. Arch Dis Child 2002;87(4):341–347; discussion 341–347.

89. Horlick M, Wang J, Pierson RN, Jr., Thornton JC. Prediction models for evaluation of total-body bone mass with dual-energy x-ray absorptiometry among children and adolescents. Pediatrics 2004;114(3):e337–345.

90. Tothill P, Hannan WJ. Bone mineral and soft tissue measurements by dual-energy x-ray absorptiometry during growth. Bone 2002;31(4):492–496.

91. Goulding A, Taylor RW, Jones IE, McAuley KA, Manning PJ, Williams SM. Overweight and obese children have low bone mass and area for their weight. Int J Obes Relat Metab Disord 2000;24(5):627–632.

92. Crabtree NJ, Boivin CM, Shaw NJ. Can body size related normative data improve the diagnosis of osteoporosis in children? (Abstract). J Bone Min Res 2001;16 (Suppl 1):S560.

93. Leonard MB, Shults J, Elliott DM, Stallings VA, Zemel BS. Interpretation of whole body dual energy x-ray absorptiometry measures in children: comparison with peripheral quantitative computed tomography. Bone 2004;34(6):1044–1052.

94. Zemel BS, Leonard MB, Kalkwarf HJ, et al. Reference data for the whole body, lumbar spine and proximal femur for American children relative to age, gender and body size. J Bone Miner Res (Abstract) 2004;231.

95. Taylor A, Konrad PT, Norman ME, Harcke HT. Total body bone mineral density in young children: influence of head bone mineral density. J Bone Miner Res 1997;12:652–655.

96. Burnham JM, Shults J, Semeao E, et al. Whole body BMC in pediatric Crohn disease: independent effects of altered growth, maturation, and body composition. J Bone Miner Res 2004;19(12):1961–1968.

97. Leonard MB, Feldman HI, Shults J, Zemel BS, Foster BJ, Stallings VA. Long-term, high-dose glucocorticoids and bone mineral content in childhood glucocorticoid-sensitive nephrotic syndrome. N Engl J Med 2004;351(9):868–875.

98. Landoll JD, Barden HS, Wacher WK, et al. Pediatric skeletal assessment in Duchenne muscular dystrophy. Bone 2005;36 (Suppl 1):S76.

99. Rauch F, Schoenau E. The developing bone: slave or master of its cells and molecules? Pediatr Res 2001;50(3):309–314.   100.   Parfitt AM. The two faces of growth: benefits and risks to bone integrity. Osteoporos Int 1994;4(6):382–398.

101. Rubin CT, Bain SD, McLeod KJ. Suppression of the osteogenic response in the aging skeleton. Calcif Tissue Int 1992;50(4):306–313.

102. Schiessl H, Frost HM, Jee WS. Estrogen and bone-muscle strength and mass relationships. Bone 1998;22(1):1–6.

103. Ferretti JL, Capozza RF, Cointry GR, et al. Gender-related differences in the relationship between densitometric values of whole-body bone mineral content and lean body mass in humans between 2 and 87 years of age. Bone 1998;22(6):683–690.

104. Hogler W, Briody J, Woodhead HJ, Chan A, Cowell CT. Importance of lean mass in the interpretation of total body densitometry in children and adolescents. J Pediatr 2003;143(1):81–88.

105. Crabtree NJ, Kibirige MS, Fordham JN, et al. The relationship between lean body mass and bone mineral content in paediatric health and disease. Bone 2004;35(4):965–972.

106. Schoenau E, Neu CM, Beck B, Manz F, Rauch F. Bone mineral content per muscle cross-sectional area as an index of the functional muscle-bone unit. J Bone Miner Res 2002;17(6):1095–1101.

107. Parker DF, Round JM, Sacco P, Jones DA. A cross-sectional survey of upper and lower limb strength in boys and girls during childhood and adolescence. Ann Hum Biol 1990;17(3):199–211.

108. Round JM, Jones DA, Honour JW, Nevill AM. Hormonal factors in the development of differences in strength between boys and girls during adolescence: a longitudinal study. Ann Hum Biol 1999;26(1):49–62.

109. Ruth EM, Weber LT, Schoenau E, et al. Analysis of the functional muscle-bone unit of the forearm in pediatric renal transplant recipients. Kidney Int 2004;66(4):1694–1706.

110. Bechtold S, Ripperger P, Dalla Pozza R, Schmidt H, Hafner R, Schwarz HP. Musculoskeletal and functional muscle-bone analysis in children with rheumatic disease using peripheral quantitative computed tomography. Osteoporos Int 2005;16(7):757–763.

111. Hogler W, Briody J, Moore B, Garnett S, Lu PW, Cowell CT. Importance of estrogen on bone health in Turner syndrome: a cross-sectional and longitudinal study using dual-energy x-ray absorptiometry. J Clin Endocrinol Metab 2004;89(1):193–199.

11 Looking to the Future of Pediatric Bone Densitometry

Nicholas J. Bishop, MD, Aenor J. Sawyer, MD, and Mary B. Leonard, MD, MSCE

CONTENTS

INTRODUCTION
THE FUTURE OF DXA: WHO SHOULD BE TESTED?
ANALYSES OF DXA DATA BEYOND BONE MASS
PEDIATRIC DXA SOFTWARE
ADJUSTING FOR BODY SIZE AND SKELETAL MATURITY
VERTEBRAL MORPHOMETRY
COMPARISON OF DXA WITH OTHER TECHNIQUES
SUMMARY
SUMMARY POINTS
REFERENCES

INTRODUCTION

The earlier chapters of this book provide a clear view of the current state of the use of dual-energy x-ray absorptiometry (DXA) in children. The purpose of this chapter is to highlight those areas in which we believe that significant advances in bone densitometry are likely to be forthcoming over the next 5–10 yr. These changes will likely improve the performance of DXA and alternative noninvasive methods of assessing bone health in pediatric subjects.

This chapter focuses on several key areas of investigation that are needed to increase the utility of DXA as a clinical tool in the care of children. These include the following: (1) refining the clinical indications for DXA in the growing patient, (2) determining the relationship of DXA data to bone strength and to fracture risk, (3) optimizing pediatric-specific software, (4) evaluating appropriate adjustment techniques for body size and skeletal maturity, (5) developing vertebral morphometry for children, and (6) comparing DXA to other densitometry techniques.

From: *Current Clinical Practice: Bone Densitometry in Growing Patients: Guidelines for Clinical Practice*
Edited by: A. J. Sawyer, L. K. Bachrach, and E. B. Fung © Humana Press Inc., Totowa, NJ

THE FUTURE OF DXA: WHO SHOULD BE TESTED?

There are established guidelines for performing DXAs and criteria for the diagnosis and treatment of osteoporosis in older adults. Guidelines are also emerging for the testing and treatment of less common adult cases of "secondary osteoporosis," which are the result of myriad chronic illnesses and medications. However, deciding which children warrant bone densitometry and how the findings should guide therapy is far from established.

One potential group of pediatric patients to evaluate by DXA includes children with fractures. Fractures in children are common. According to Landin (1), 42% of boys and 27% of girls will have a fracture by age 16. Evidence from large data sets, such as the UK General Practice Research Database (2), indicates that fracture frequency rises gradually during childhood and is most common around the time of peak height velocity in either gender. The geographical distribution of fractures in childhood is similar to that seen for adult hip fracture in the elderly, suggesting that fracture in childhood might represent a risk factor for adult osteoporosis (2). Children who have had at least one fracture (at any site) are two- to threefold more likely to sustain another fracture in childhood or adolescence (3).

Does this mean that every child with a fracture should have a DXA scan? It would seem logical to develop an approach similar to that used in adults which considers other clinical factors for poor bone health in deciding who to study. Risk factors including older age, low body weight, a family history of osteoporosis, prior anticonvulsant or glucocorticoid therapy, or a history of a fragility fracture are weighed before ordering a DXA. Based on current data, performing DXA on every child with a fracture is *not* being proposed. Clinical factors that might influence the decision to perform a scan include the number of fractures, the fracture pattern or type, history of chronic illness, family history of osteoporosis, and poor diet and exercise patterns. Large studies are essential, however, to establish an association of any of these factors with poor peak bone mass or increased fracture risk. It is unknown whether the same factors, which, in combination with bone mass, might predict fracture in children who are otherwise healthy, would likewise apply to chronically ill children These questions can likely be addressed using fracture registries, with standardized data collection and tracking, performed longitudinally. Although much is yet unknown, it is clear from the work of Goulding et al. (3) that every child with a fracture should be clinically assessed for risk factors and counselled on the determinants of healthy bone development.

The decision to perform a DXA scan in an otherwise healthy child with a history of a low-impact fracture is problematic. Ma et al. (4) reported that the majority of fractures in healthy youths resulted from low-energy falls at home. Cross-sectional, prospective, and retrospective studies have identified clinical factors associated with fracture in these children. These include obesity (5,6), increased time spent watching television (7), lower levels of breast-feeding (8), and age and gender (9). Further characterization of risk factors for fracture in healthy children is needed in order to determine which subjects at risk would benefit from a DXA scan. Importantly, studies are needed to assess the predictive value of bone mass measurements by DXA for both short-term fracture risk and peak bone mass.

The completion of DXA scans in all children at risk constitutes screening; screening should only be performed in conditions in which there is an accepted treatment recognized for the disease and in which the screening procedure is reasonably safe and sufficiently sensitive and specific *(10)*. To date, the medical, psychological, and financial costs of false-positive results for osteopenia in children have not been addressed; to undertake such studies, however, will require considerable planning and networking across multiple centers. There is also a lack of studies to delineate the financial and social impact of recurrent childhood fractures. However, the costs of adult osteoporosis have been documented, and it is feasible that, by optimizing the bone health of children, the devastating effects of osteoporosis at any age will be lessened.

It has been stated that bone mass in childhood determines peak bone mass, which, in turn, is a major determinant of adult osteoporosis and fragility fractures. These concepts, although logical, are being challenged and bear further investigation. This would require longitudinal studies tracking individuals from the point of peak bone mass into late adulthood. It would also be very helpful to know more about the ability of the skeleton to "catch up" once childhood bone deficits are identified and treated.

ANALYSES OF DXA DATA BEYOND BONE MASS

Future work will help define the relationship between parameters measured by DXA and bone strength as discussed in some detail in Chapter 10. Bone strength is determined not only by mass (i.e., bone mineral content [BMC] or bone mineral density [BMD]), but also by the size, geometry, microarchitecture, and material properties of the bone. Although these parameters are not directly assessed by DXA, several models to approximate them have been developed. For example, hip structural analysis utilizes measurements of cortical thickness and bone width from the proximal hip scan to estimate biomechanical expressions of bone strength. The challenge ahead will be to test these models against the likelihood of fracture Given the low frequency of hip fracture in children, this research will need to begin with in vitro models.

Further research is also needed to determine the optimal system to correct for variations in bone size and maturity among individuals at risk. It remains unclear which of the proposed schemes for adjusting axial bone mass measurements for bone size is the most applicable across the pediatric age range. The different methods will be compared, but consensus must first be reached as to the yardstick or gold standard against which these methods are to be judged. Patient registries from large pediatric centers might yield sufficient data on fractures in at-risk children to address the predictive value of these models in clinical practice.

PEDIATRIC DXA SOFTWARE

DXA manufacturers have recognized the concerns of pediatric practitioners by enhancing pediatric reference data and developing adjustments for body size. Hologic, General Electric/Lunar, and Norland have expanded age-adjusted standard deviation scores (i.e., Z-scores) for a broader range of ages and skeletal sites. Newer software also includes features such as "auto-low density" that purportedly improve edge detection (i.e., distinguishing the margins of bone and soft tissue) with minimal discrepancies in results from standard mode analysis. This would facilitate longitudinal measurements in subjects. In addition, standardization of techniques would allow comparison of data from different centers to gain knowledge of uncommon diseases. We expect that the T-score will be removed from the report page for those who are not yet young adults. Already, reference to World Health Organization (WHO) criteria for "osteoporosis" and "osteopenia," which is based on T-scores, has been eliminated from some newer software programs for subjects under age 20. As with all upgrades or changes in hardware or software, there is an impact on serial measurements. Much work must be done to allow comparisons of repeat studies on a patient when different machines or software versions are used.

ADJUSTING FOR BODY SIZE AND SKELETAL MATURITY

Although a number of approaches have been described to address the elements of variation in bone and body size and, in some instances, the potentially confounding effect of pubertal stage or bone age, there is no universally agreed on method of presenting whole body data. As with the issue of creating volumetric measurements for axial bone mass estimates, none of these various adjustment methods has been proven superior for predicting clinical outcomes. It may well be that the adjustments made to remove the confounding effect of body size are inappropriate in situations in which the underlying disease process or the condition's treatment affects body size. An example might be steroid-induced bone disease, in which linear growth slows but weight increases. How would adjustments for body size work in such a situation? Again, models designed to correct for body size or bone geometry should be validated over time against another gold standard such as future fragility fracture or in vitro testing of bone strength.

VERTEBRAL MORPHOMETRY

Some DXA instruments allow for lateral spine morphometric analysis through the rotation of the source and the detector arm. Such analyses can be used to detect vertebral compression fractures without performing standard radiographs of the spine. Other DXA devices require careful positioning of the patient to obtain a lateral scan. Software programs for vertebral morphometric analysis have been for the incorporated into software for some of the latest generation of scanners. Use of spine morphometric analysis in pediatric patients is worthy of investigation because this approach might provide the means to monitor a child for vertebral deformities and fracture with a lower radiation exposure than conventional lateral spine x-rays.

COMPARISON OF DXA WITH OTHER TECHNIQUES

As discussed in previous chapters, single- and multislice peripheral quantitative computed tomography (pQCT) is being utilized widely in the assessment of bone geometry, both in health and in disease. Combining and comparing DXA-derived data with QCT- and pQCT-derived data is likely to be commonplace over the next few years. As discussed in detail in Chapter 10, comparison of spine bone mass measurements by DXA and QCT found the highest correlation between BMC by both techniques ($r^2 = 0.94$) and the lowest for areal BMD (aBMD) by DXA and volumetric BMD by QCT ($r^2 = 0.39$). From these observations, it appears that the methods detect different parameters of bone mass (11). The findings do not establish whether one method or the other will have greater predictive value for clinical bone fragility.

DXA and pQCT are likely to be regarded in the future as complementary in terms of their use. Although each will have its proponents, pQCT cannot measure total body bone mass, and DXA cannot measure volumetric BMD of cortical or trabecular bone separately, nor can it measure cortical area or thickness. Each method provides information that the other does not. However, there is likely to be overlap in the area of bone strength estimation through comparison of hip structure analysis derived from DXA and the cross-sectional moment of inertia and strength strain index produced by pQCT. It is imperative that formal studies be conducted in children using receiver operating characteristic (ROC) techniques to determine the sensitivity and specificity of standard DXA measures of aBMD, alternative DXA measures (e.g., bone mineral apparent density [BMAD] and hip structural analysis [HSA]), and QCT measures of volumetric BMD and bone dimensions in the discrimination of fracture from nonfracture cases.

SUMMARY

DXA likely has a future in imaging children's bones and in providing quantitative assessment of bone mass. The technique is a safe, available, rapid, and precise means to assess bone mass, and the data can be exploited to provide estimates of bone size and geometry. However, continued research is needed to optimize its utility in clinical practice. The clinical interpretation of what constitutes "normal" or "sufficient" skeletal strength is challenging because it must be interpreted relative to the age and maturity of the child and to the demands placed on the skeleton by mechanical forces (including local effects of muscle).

The demands for assessment of skeletal health in children will continue to mount, and DXA will be employed to determine both bone mass and body composition. Childhood obesity has been associated with an increased risk of forearm fracture; this finding adds to concerns about health threats from the worldwide epidemic in obesity. Similarly, models of the bone–muscle unit have increased interest in assessing lean body mass by DXA and other techniques. It is likely that DXA will be one of several techniques used to make assessments of skeletal health in children for some time to come.

If the limitations of DXA are recognized, it can be optimized as a clinical tool and will play a significant role in improving the bone health of children and adults.

SUMMARY POINTS

- Future research is needed to optimize the utility of DXA in the clinical care of children and adolescents.
- The clinical factor or factors that best predict suboptimal peak bone mass or fracture must be determined from long-term prospective longitudinal studies.
- The optimal model to estimate bone geometry (such as hip structural analysis) or to adjust for bone and body size must be tested against a clinical gold standard such as fractures. Establishment of fracture registries will be valuable in addressing these questions.
- Adaptation of vertebral morphometry for younger subjects may allow monitoring for vertebral fractures with less radiation than standard lateral spine x-rays.
- Studies comparing DXA with pQCT, QCT, and other methods are likely to yield different results. Research is needed to determine the value of each in predicting clinical outcomes.
- Ongoing modifications of DXA software programs will reduce the risk of misdiagnoses by providing age- and gender-specific normative data for wider ranges of age skeletal sites. Other safeguards, such as elimination of T-scores and the WHO terms "osteopenia" and "osteoporosis" on reports for subjects under age 20, are needed as well.

REFERENCES

1. Landin LA. Fracture patterns in children. Acta Orthop Scan 1983;54(suppl 202):1–109.
2. Cooper C, Dennison EM, Leufkens HGM, Bishop N, van Staa TP. Epidemiology of childhood fractures in Britain: a study using the general practice research database. J Bone Miner Res 2004; 19(12):1976–1981.
3. Goulding A, Jones IE, Williams SM, et al. First fracture is associated with increased risk of new fractures during growth. J Pediatr 2005;146:286–288
4. Ma DQ, Jones G. Clinical risk factors but not bone density are associated with prevalent fractures in prepubertal children. J Paed Child Health 2002:38:497–500.
5. Goulding A, Jones IE, Taylor RW, Manning PJ, Williams SM. More broken bones: a 4-year double cohort study of young girls with and without distal forearm fractures. J Bone Miner Res 2000;15(10):2011–2018.
6. Skaggs DL, Loro ML, Pitukcheewanont P, Tolo V, Gilsanz V. Increased body weight and decreased radial cross-sectional dimensions in girls with forearm fractures. J Bone Miner Res 2001; 16:7:1337–1342.
7. Ma DQ, Jones G. The association between bone mineral density, metacarpal morphometry, and upper limb fractures in children: a population-based case-control study. J Clin Endocrinol Metab 2003;88(4):1486–1491.
8. Ma DQ, Jones G. Clinical risk factors but not bone density are associated with prevalent fractures in prepubertal children. J Paed Child Health 2002;38:497–500.
9. Khosla S, Melton LJ III, Dekutoski MB, Achenbach SJ, Oberg AL, Riggs Bl. Incidence of childhood distal forearm fractures over 30 years: a population-based study. JAMA 2003;290:1479–1485.
10. Wilson JM, Jungner YG. Principles and practice of mass screening for disease. Bol Oficina Sanit Panam 1968;65(4):281–393.
11. Wren TAL, Liu X, Pitukcheewanont P, Gilsanz V. Bone acquisition in healthy children and adolescents: comparisons of dual-energy x-ray absorptiometry and computed tomography measures. J Clin Endocrinol Metab 2005;90:1925–1928.

Appendix A
Resources

Table 1
Information for National and International Societies

American Dietetic Association Nutrition Resources
120 Riverside Plaza, Suite 200
Chicago, IL 60606-6995
Tel: (800) 877-1600
Fax: (312) 899-4873
http://www.eatright.org

American Society for Bone and Mineral Research
2025 M Street NW, Suite 800
Washington, DC 20036
Tel: (202) 367-1161
Fax: (202) 367-2161
E-mail: asbmr@asbmr.org
http://www.asbmr.org

Bone Biology for Kids
Written by Susan Ott, MD
Associate Professor of Medicine
University of Washington
http://www.depts.washington.edu/bonebio/

BoneKEy-Osteovision
http://www.bonekey-ibms.org

Centers for Disease Control and Prevention
1600 Clifton Road
Atlanta, GA 30333 Tel: (404) 639-3311
Tel: (404) 639-3534 (public inquiries)
Tel: (800) 311-3435 (public inquiries, toll-free)
http://www.cdc.gov

The Dairy Council
Henrietta House
17/18 Henrietta Street
London WC2E 8QH
Tel: 020-735-4030
Fax: 020-7240-9679
E-mail: info@dairycouncil.org.uk
http://www.milk.co.uk

From: *Current Clinical Practice: Bone Densitometry in Growing Patients: Guidelines for Clinical Practice*
Edited by: A. J. Sawyer, L. K. Bachrach, and E. B. Fung © Humana Press Inc., Totowa, NJ

Table 1 (Continued)

Foundation for Osteoporosis Research and Education (FORE)
300 27th Street, Suite 103
Oakland, CA 94612
Tel: (888) 266-3015
Tel: (510) 832-2663
Fax: (510) 208-7174
E-mail: info@fore.org
http://www.fore.org

International Bone and Mineral Society (IBMS)
2025 M Street NW, Suite 800
Washington, DC 20036-3309
Tel: (202) 367-1121
Fax: (202) 367-2121
http://www.ibmsonline.org

International Osteoporosis Foundation (IOF)
Swiss Office
5 Rue Perdtemps
1260 Nyon Switzerland
Tel: 41-22-994-0100
Fax: 41-22-994-0101]
E-mail: info@osteofound.org
http://www.osteofound.org

International Society for Clinical Densitometry (ISCD)
342 North Main Street
West Hartford, CT 06117-2507
Tel: (860) 586-7563
Fax: (860) 586-7550
E-mail: iscd@iscd.org
http://www.iscd.org

Internet course on Assessment of Pediatric Bone Fragility
John Shepherd, PhD
Emily von Scheven, MD
University of California, San Francisco
Tel: (415) 353-4556
E-mail: john.shepherd@radiology.ucsf.edu

Kids and Their Bones: A Guide for Parents
http://www.niams.nih.gov/hi/topics/osptoporosis/kidbones.htm
Revised, December 2005
National Institute of Arthritis and Musculoskeletal and Skin Disease

Milk Matters Calcium Education Campaign
31 Center Drive, Room 2A32
Bethesda, MD 20892
Tel: (301) 496-5133
Fax: (301) 496-7101
E-mail: NICHDmilkmatters@mail.nih.gov

National Dairy Council
10255 W. Higgins Road, Suite 900
Rosemont, IL 60018
http://www.nationaldairycouncil.org

(continued)

National Institutes of Health, Osteoporosis, and Related Bone Diseases,
National Resource Center
2 AMS Circle Bethesda, MD 20892-3676
Tel: (800) 624-BONE (toll-free)
Tel: (202) 223-0344
Fax: (202) 293-2356
TTY: (202) 466-4315
E-mail: niamsboneinfo@mail.nih.gov
http://www.osteo.org

National Organization for Rare Disorders (NORD)
55 Kenosia Avenue
P.O. Box 1968
Danbury, CT 06813-1968
Tel: (800) 999-6673 (toll-free)
Tel: (203) 744-0100
Fax: (203) 798-2291
E-mail: orphan@raredisease.org
http://www.rarediseases.org *(last revised 10/04)*

National Osteoporosis Foundation
1232 22nd Street NW
Washington, DC 20037-1292
Tel: (202) 223-2226
Fax: (202) 223-2237
http://www.nof.org

National Osteoporosis Society (NOS)
United Kingdom
Camerton, Bath BA2 0PJ
Tel: 01-76-147-1771
Fax: 01-76-147-1104
E-mail: info@nos.org.uk
http://www.nos.org.uk

Northern California Institute for Bone Health Inc.
3100 Telegraph Ave., Suite 3000
Oakland, CA 94609
Tel: (510) 625-9100

Nutrition Explorations: Kids
http://www.nutritionexplorations.org/kids/main.asp

Osteogenesis Imperfecta Foundation
804 West Diamond Avenue, Suite 210
Gaithersburg, MD 20878
Tel: (800) 981-BONE (toll-free)
Tel: (301) 947-0083
Fax: (301) 947-0456
http://www.oif.org

Osteoporosis Society of Canada
1090 Don Mills Road, Suite 301
Toronto, Ontario M3C 3R6
Tel: (416) 696-2663
Fax: (416) 696-2673

(continued)

Table 1 (Continued)

Osteoporosis Society of Canada (continued)
Toll-free (English): 1-800-463-6842 (in Canada only)
Toll-free (French): 1-800-977-1778 (in Canada only)
E-mail: info@osteoporosis.ca
http://www.osteoporosis.ca

Paget Foundation
120 Wall Street, Suite 1602
New York, NY 10005
Tel: (800) 23-PAGET (toll-free)
Tel: (212) 509-5335
Fax: (212) 509-8492
E-mail: pagetfdn@aol.com
http://www.paget.org

Pediatric Bone Health Consortium
Director: Aenor J. Sawyer, MD
Children's Hospital & Research Center of Oakland
747 52nd Street
Oakland, CA 94609
Tel: (510) 428-3000
http://www.kidsbones.org
http://www.kidsbones.com

Powerful Bones. Powerful Girls. (The National Bone Health Campaign)
Division of Nutrition and Physical Activity
National Center for Chronic Disease Prevention and Health Promotion
Centers for Disease Control and Prevention
4770 Buford Highway, NE, MS/K-24
Atlanta, GA 30341-3717
Tel: (770) 488-5820
Fax: (770) 488-6000
E-mail: powerfulbones@cdc.gov
http://www.cdc.gov/powerfulbones

A Report of the Surgeon General: Bone Health and Osteoporosis
October, 2004
http://www.surgeongeneral.gov/library/bonehealth/

U.S. National Library of Medicine
8600 Rockville Pike
Bethesda MD 20894
Tel: (800) 272-4787 (toll-free)
Tel: (301) 496-6308
http://www.nlm.nih.gov

Table 2
Manufacturer Contact Information

General Electric Medical Systems, Lunar
726 Heartland Trial
Madison, WI 53717-1915
Tel: (888) 795-8627 (toll-free)
Tel: (608) 828-3663
Fax: (608) 826-7102
E-mail: info@gemedicalsystems.com
http://www.gemedicalsystems.com

Hologic, Inc
35 Crosby Drive
Bedford, MA 01730-1401
Tel: (800) 343-9729 (toll-free)
Tel: (781) 999-7300
Fax: (781) 280-0669
E-mail: support@hologic.com
http://www.hologic.com

Norland, CooperSurgical, Inc.
W6340 Hackbarth Road
Fort Atkinson, WI 53538
Tel: (800) 563-9504 (toll-free)
Tel: (920) 563-9504
Fax: (920) 563-8626
http://www.coopersurgical.com

Table 3
Makes and Models of Central X-Ray Densitometers Currently in Use

Manufacturer	Model	X-ray beam geometry	Detector
General Electric MedicalSystems/Lunar (Madison, WI)	DPX-IQ	Pencil beam	NaI
	DPX-MD, DPX-MD+	Pencil beam	NaI
	DPX-NT	Pencil beam	NaI
	Expert-XL	Fan beam	Dual-energy solid state
	Prodigy	Narrow-fan beam	Cadmium-zinc-telluride
Hologic, Inc. (Bedford, MA)	QDR-2000	Fan beam	Multi-element detector array
	QDR-4500 (C, W, SL, A)	Fan beam	Multi-element detector array
	QDR-Delphi (C, W, SL, A)	Fan beam	Multi-element detector array
	QDR-Discovery (C, W, SL, A)	Fan beam	Multi-element detector array
Norland/CooperSurgical (Fort Atkinson, WI)	XR-26, XR-36, XR-46	Pencil beam	Two NaI scintillation detectors
	Excell, Excell plus	Pencil beam	Two NaI scintillation detectors

For more information regarding these instruments, please contact the manufacturers directly.

Table 4
Useful Bone Densitometry Reference Texts

Adams J, Shaw N, eds. *A Practical Guide to Bone Densitometry in Children.* Camerton, Bath, UK: National Osteoporosis Society, 2004.
ISBN: N/A Handbook

Bonjour JP, Tsang RC, eds. *Nutrition and Bone Development. Nestle Nutrition Workshop Series, V. H.*
Philadelphia, PA: Lippincott Williams & Wilkins, 1998.
ISBN: 0-78171-753-1

Bonnick SL, ed. *Bone Densitometry in Clinical Practice: Application and Interpretation*, 2nd ed. Totowa, NJ: Humana, 2004.
ISBN: 1-58829-275-4

Bonnick SL, Lewis LA. *Bone Densitometry for Technologists.* Totowa, NJ: Humana, 2001.
ISBN: 1-58829-020-4

Favus MJ, ed. *Primer on the Metabolic Bone Diseases and Disorders of Mineral Metabolism, 5th ed.* Philadelphia: Lippincott Williams & Wilkins, 2003.
ISBN: 0-97447-820-2

Fordam JN, ed. *Manual of Bone Densitometry Measurements: An Aid to the Interpretation of Bone Densitometry Measurements in a Clinical Setting.* London: Springer-Verlag, 2000.
ISBN: 1-85233-278-6

Glorieux FH, Pettifor JM, Juppner H, eds. *Pediatric Bone: Biology and Diseases.* London: Academic, 2003.
ISBN: 0-12286-551-0

Holick MF, Dawson-Hughes B. *Nutrition and Bone Health.* Totowa, NJ: Humana Press, 2004
ISBN: 1-58829-248-7

Office of the Surgeon General. Bone Health and Osteoporosis: A Report of the Surgeon General. Washington DC: U.S. Department of Health and Human Services, Public Health Service, 2004.

Blake GM, Wahner HW, Fogelman I, eds. *The Evaluation of Osteoporosis: Dual Energy X-Ray Absorptiometry and Ultrasound in Clinical Practice*, 2nd Edition. London: Martin Dunitz Ltd, 1999.
ISBN: 1-85317-472-6

Table 5
Provision of Educational and Training Courses Available for Dual-Energy X-Ray Absorptiometry

There is no universal certification course of competence in bone densitromerty or pediatric bone densitometry. There is significant variability in requirements for licensing and training in bone densitometry for technologists and other clinical practitioners. These requirements will vary by state or country of origin. Regulations are subject to change. In order to find the most up-to-date requirements for your region, contact the International Society for Clinical Densitometry (ISCD).

ISCD offers educational courses in bone densitometry and certification examinations for technicians who perform the exams, as well as medical professionals who interpret scans. Details regarding this training are available on their website (http://www.iscd.org). They are also able to refer you to regional training areas. The National Osteoporosis Society of the United Kingdom also offers certification courses. See their website for more information: http://www.nos.org.uk

Table 6
Sampling of Radiation Dosages

	Effective dose (μSv)
Radioisotope bone scan	3000
Planar lumbar spine radiograph	700
Transatlantic flight, with return trip	80
Dental bitewing	60
Chest radiograph	12–50
US airline flight, New York to San Francisco, with return trip	40
Exposure by airline crew flying New York to Tokyo (polar route), per day	25
Average dose to US nuclear industry employee, per day	6.6
Naturally occurring background radiation, per day	4–8
Hand radiograph	0.17
Average dose for dual-energy x-ray absorptiometry, per scan (fan beam scanners)[a]	0.05–8.0

[a]Please refer to Chapter 3, Table 1 for more detail on manufacturers and scan-specific radiation dosages. Data taken from the following sources:

World Nuclear Association. Radiation and the Nuclear Fuel Cycle, March 2005. Available at http://world-nuclear.org/info/inf05.htm.

Hart D et al. National Radiological Protection Board, Oxon, 2002.

Huda W, Gkanatsios NA. Radiation dosimetry for extremity radiographs. Health Phys 1998;75: 492–499.

Faulkner KG, Gluer CC, Genant HK. Radiation dosages from bone densitometry: Comparisons using the effective dose equivalent. International Conference on Osteoporosis. November 1991, Japan. Poster #152.

Operations Manuals from the DXA manufacturers, Hologic, Lunar/GE, Norland.

Table 7
Anthropometric Techniques: Assessment of Weight and Height

Weight
Equipment:
- An electronic or beam balance scale or wheelchair electronic scale: should be calibrated regularly and set to zero between readings
Technique:
- Children should wear an examination gown or lightweight clothing without shoes or orthopedic apparatuses
- Infants should be weighed without clothing or diapers
- Children should be weighed to the nearest 0.1 kg; infants, to the nearest 0.01 kg

Stature
(for children without contractures or scoliosis who can stand independently)
Equipment:
- Digital or electronic stadiometer (calibrated daily) is ideal; otherwise, use a sturdy board with secured tape measure and two stable paddle boards for the head and feet set at 90°. Measurements should be to the nearest 0.1 cm.
- Head paddle, firmly perpendicular to the backboard (should glide smoothly)
- Heel plate, in alignment with the backboard
- Solid flooring (not carpeting)
Technique:
- Stature measurements begin with children ≥2 yr of age
- Child must be able to stand unsupported and should be without significant scoliosis or contractures
- Child should be relaxed, with arms at sides
- Weight should be evenly placed on both feet
- Feet should be against the heel plate and as close together as is comfortable
- Heels, buttocks, shoulders, and head should be touching the back of the stadiometer
- The head should be held with the Frankfurt plane (an imaginary line from the upper margin of the ear to the lower margin of the eye socket) parallel to the floor
- With obesity or kyphosis, standard position may not be possible; positioning of feet and head should align the spine as erect as possible
- Hair clips must be removed from top of head
- Lower paddle gently to top of head; any pressure lowering the paddle will alter child's posture
- Use a foot stool to view reading at eye level, when necessary
- Repeat

Length
(for children aged < 2 yr or any child unable to stand independently)
Equipment:
- Digital infantometer (calibrated daily) is ideal; otherwise, use a sturdy board with secured tape measure and two stable paddle boards for the head and foot set at 90°. Measurements should be to the nearest 0.1 cm.
Technique:
- Requires two people to hold and position the child correctly: one person (the parent can assist) holds the head gently but firmly against the headboard, cupping the cheeks and the back of the head
- Position the head with the Frankfurt plane perpendicular to the board
- The torso should rest flat on the length board, with the midline centered on the board
- Legs should be extended gently but firmly, with the knees flat and the hips even
- With the feet together and flexed at a 90° angle, glide the foot board to the heel
- Best measurements are obtained when the child is relaxed—keep toys on hand for distraction
- Repeat

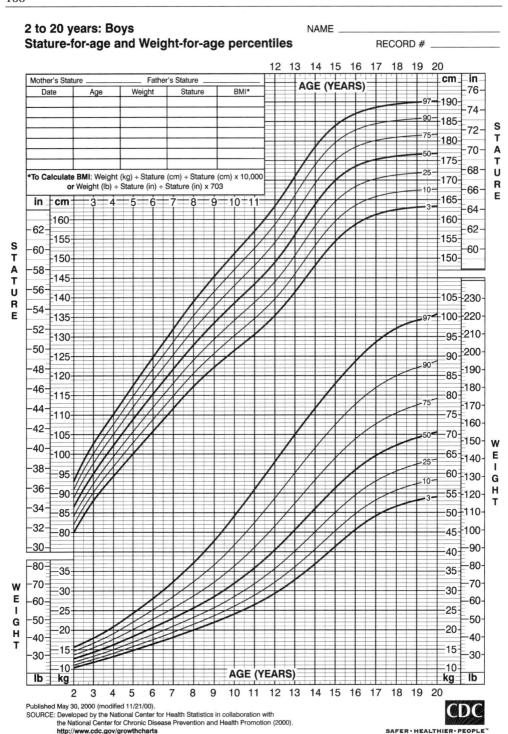

Fig. 1. Centers for Disease Control pediatric growth chart for boys aged 2 to 20 yr: stature-for-age and weight-for-age percentiles.

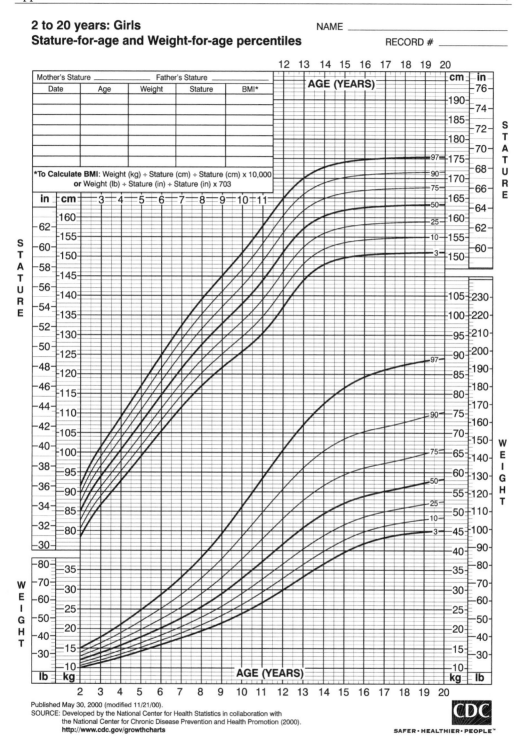

Fig. 2. Centers for Disease Control pediatric growth chart for girls aged 2 to 20 yr: stature-for-age and weight-for-age percentiles.

CDC Growth Charts: United States

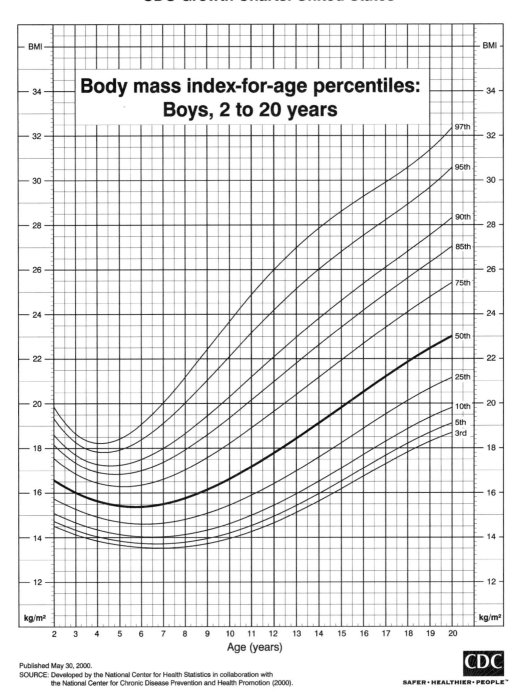

Fig. 3. Centers for Disease Control pediatric growth chart for boys aged 2 to 20 yr: body mass index-for-age percentiles.

CDC Growth Charts: United States

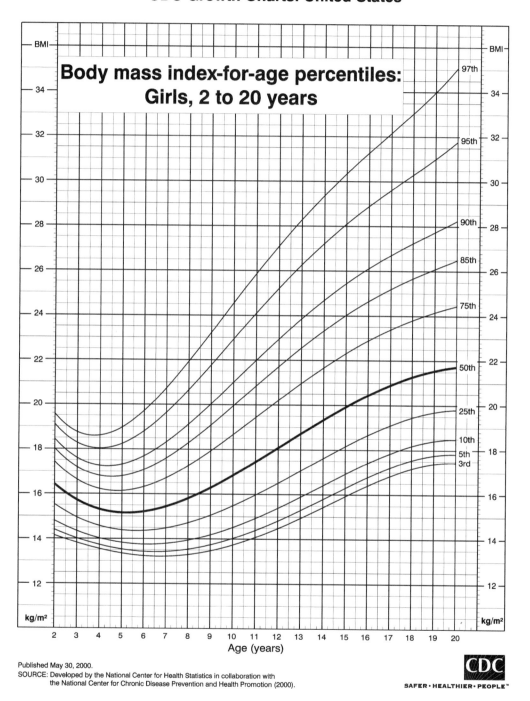

Published May 30, 2000.
SOURCE: Developed by the National Center for Health Statistics in collaboration with
the National Center for Chronic Disease Prevention and Health Promotion (2000).

Fig. 4. Centers for Disease Control pediatric growth chart for girls aged 2 to 20 yr: body mass index-for-age percentiles.

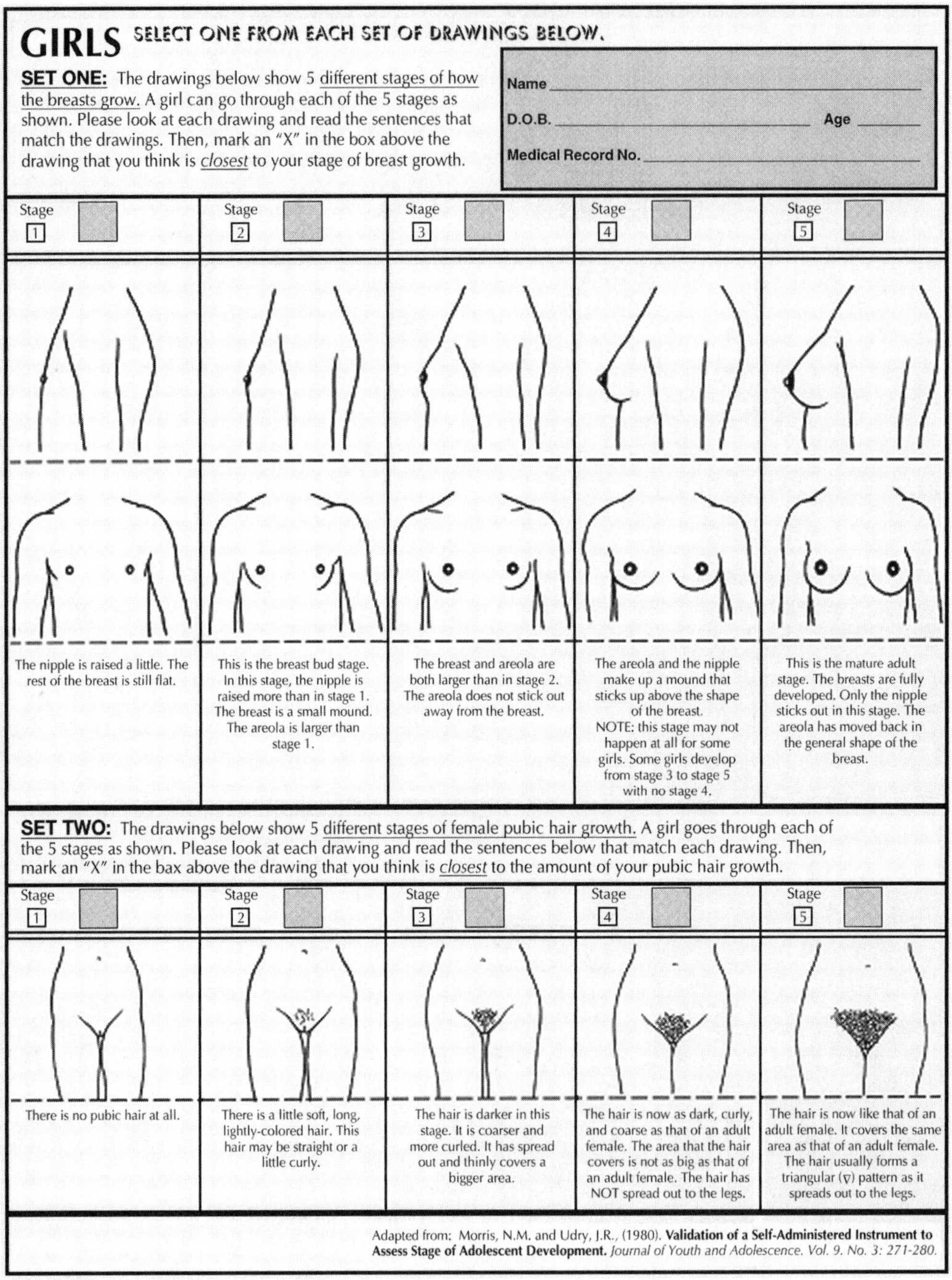

GIRLS SELECT ONE FROM EACH SET OF DRAWINGS BELOW.

SET ONE: The drawings below show 5 different stages of how the breasts grow. A girl can go through each of the 5 stages as shown. Please look at each drawing and read the sentences that match the drawings. Then, mark an "X" in the box above the drawing that you think is *closest* to your stage of breast growth.

Name _____

D.O.B. _____ Age _____

Medical Record No. _____

Stage 1 — The nipple is raised a little. The rest of the breast is still flat.

Stage 2 — This is the breast bud stage. In this stage, the nipple is raised more than in stage 1. The breast is a small mound. The areola is larger than stage 1.

Stage 3 — The breast and areola are both larger than in stage 2. The areola does not stick out away from the breast.

Stage 4 — The areola and the nipple make up a mound that sticks up above the shape of the breast. NOTE: this stage may not happen at all for some girls. Some girls develop from stage 3 to stage 5 with no stage 4.

Stage 5 — This is the mature adult stage. The breasts are fully developed. Only the nipple sticks out in this stage. The areola has moved back in the general shape of the breast.

SET TWO: The drawings below show 5 different stages of female pubic hair growth. A girl goes through each of the 5 stages as shown. Please look at each drawing and read the sentences below that match each drawing. Then, mark an "X" in the box above the drawing that you think is *closest* to the amount of your pubic hair growth.

Stage 1 — There is no pubic hair at all.

Stage 2 — There is a little soft, long, lightly-colored hair. This hair may be straight or a little curly.

Stage 3 — The hair is darker in this stage. It is coarser and more curled. It has spread out and thinly covers a bigger area.

Stage 4 — The hair is now as dark, curly, and coarse as that of an adult female. The area that the hair covers is not as big as that of an adult female. The hair has NOT spread out to the legs.

Stage 5 — The hair is now like that of an adult female. It covers the same area as that of an adult female. The hair usually forms a triangular (∇) pattern as it spreads out to the legs.

Adapted from: Morris, N.M. and Udry, J.R., (1980). **Validation of a Self-Administered Instrument to Assess Stage of Adolescent Development.** *Journal of Youth and Adolescence. Vol. 9. No. 3: 271-280.*

Fig. 5. Self-administered pubertal assessment form: girls. Adapted from Morris NM and Udry JR. J Youth Adol 1980;9(3);271–280.

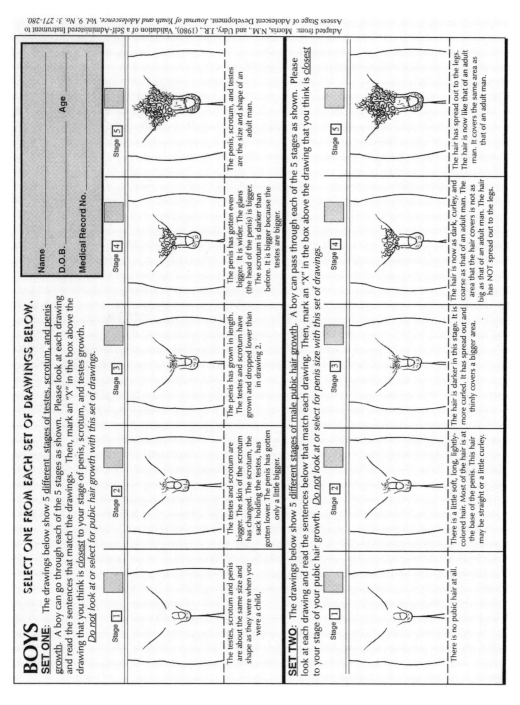

Fig. 6. Self-administerd pubertal assessment form: boys. Adapted from Morris NM and Udry JR. J Youth Adol 1980;9(3); 271–280.

193

school entry screen and body mass index [BMI]

The National Screening Committee recommends that the height and weight of every boy in the United Kingdom be measured at, or around, school entry and the data stored for the calculation of BMI for public health and the National Minimum Dataset purposes. A boys BMI centile chart [birth – 18yrs] is available. It also features waist circumference centiles as a second measurement to confirm fatness more conclusively. The International Obesity Task Force definitions of paediatric overweight/obesity [from 2-18yrs] are superimposed over the UK centiles to facilitate international comparison. A BMI chart can of course be used to monitor under-nutrition as well as over-nutrition. The charts may be purchased in packs of 20, 50 and 100 upwards.

growth assessment at school

If two growth assessments have not been recorded pre-school, two further assessments should be made after the school entry check and preferably within the next 12 months to establish normal/abnormal growth. Approximately 20% of growth-related disorders may not be identifiable until the school years because of their late onset or their association with puberty.

ADULT HEIGHT POTENTIAL

(a) ....cm

(b) ....cm

(c) ....cm

(d) ....cm

(e) ....cm   (f) ....centile

(g) ....centile — ....centile

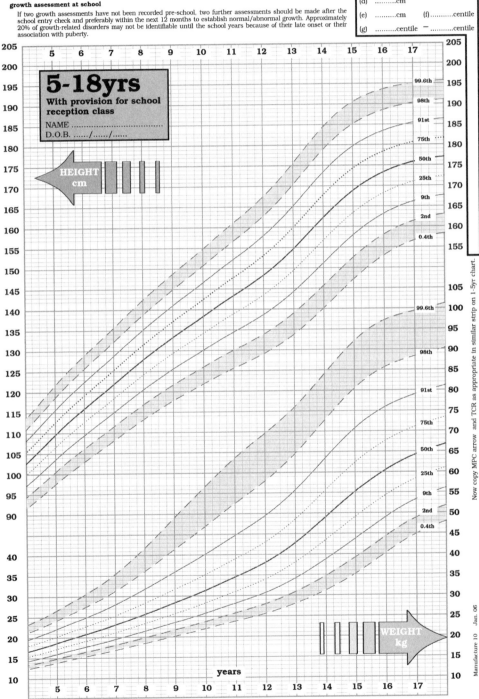

Fig. 7. Boys.

school entry screen and body mass index [BMI]

The National Screening Committee recommends that the height and weight of every girl in the United Kingdom be measured at, or around, school entry and the data stored for the calculation of BMI for public health and the National Minimum Dataset purposes. A girls BMI centile chart [birth – 18yrs] is available. It also features waist circumference centiles as a second measurement to confirm fatness more conclusively. The International Obesity Task Force definitions of paediatric overweight/obesity [from 2-18yrs] are superimposed over the UK centiles to facilitate international comparison. A BMI chart can of course be used to monitor under-nutrition as well as over-nutrition. The charts may be purchased in packs of 20, 50 and 100 upwards.

growth assessment at school

If two growth assessments have not been recorded pre-school, two further assessments should be made after the school entry check and preferably within the next 12 months to establish normal/abnormal growth. Approximately 20% of growth-related disorders may not be identifiable until the school years because of their late onset or their association with puberty.

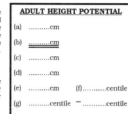

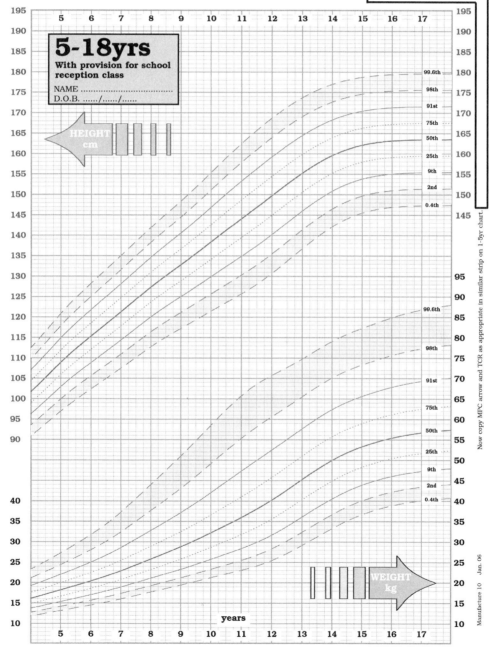

Fig. 8. Girls.

Appendix B
Equations and Calculations

Table 1
Universal Standardized Equations

Posteroanterior Spine BMD Conversions Among Central DXA Devices

Hologic QDR-2000 = (0.906 × Lunar DPX-L) − 0.025

Hologic QDR-2000 = (0.912 × Norland XR-26) + 0.088

Lunar DPX-L = (1.074 × Hologic QDR-2000) + 0.054

Lunar DPX-L = (0.995 × Norland XR-26) + 0.135

Norland XR-26 = (0.983 × Lunar DPX-L) − 0.112

Norland XR-26 = (1.068 × Hologic QDR-2000) − 0.07

Equations to Convert Manufacturer-Specific BMD (in g/cm^2) for Spine to Standardized BMD (sBMD) in mg/cm^2

sBMD = 1000 (1.0761 × Norland XR-26 BMD$_{spine}$)

sBMD = 1000 (0.9522 × Lunar DPX-L BMD$_{spine}$)

sBMD = 1000 (1.0755 × Hologic QDR-2000 BMD$_{spine}$)

Equations to Convert Manufacturer-Specific BMD (in g/cm^2) for Total Hip to Standardized BMD (sBMD) in mg/cm^2

sBMD = 1000 [(1.012 × Norland XR-26 BMD$_{hip}$) + 0.026]

sBMD = 1000 [(0.979 × Lunar DPX-L BMD$_{hip}$) − 0.031]

sBMD = 1000 [(1.008 × Hologic QDR-2000 BMD$_{hip}$) + 0.006]

Note: although specific models of the central dual-energy x-ray absoptiometry (DXA) devices are noted in the equations, the formulas may be used to convert bone mineral density (BMD) measured on any model for a given manufacturer to the BMD for a model of the other manufacturer. However, it must be recognized that these formulas were generated from data obtained on adult patients only. Also, the errors inherent in these conversions are too great to allow for serial monitoring of BMD to be useful among different manufacturers.

All equations are multiplied by 1000 to express the standardized BMD (sBMD) as described by Genant HK, Grampp S, Gluer CC, Faulkner KG, Jergas M, Engelke K, Hagiwara S, Van Kuijk C. Universal standardization for dual x-ray absorptiometry: Patient and phantom cross-calibration results. J Bone Miner Res 1994;9:1503–1514; Genant HK. Universal standardization for dual x-ray absorptiometry: patient and phantom cross-calibration results. J Bone Miner Res 1995;10:997–998; and Hanson J. Standardization of femur BMD. J Bone Miner Res 1997;12:1316–1317.

From: *Current Clinical Practice: Bone Densitometry in Growing Patients: Guidelines for Clinical Practice*
Edited by: A. J. Sawyer, L. K. Bachrach, and E. B. Fung © Humana Press Inc., Totowa, NJ

Table 2
Important Calculations and Conversions

English to Metric:
Length: 1 in. = 2.54 cm
Weight   1 lb = 0.45 kg

Metric to English:
Length: 1 cm = 0.39 in.
Weight: 1 kg = 2.2 lb

Temperature:
$°F = (1.8 \times °C) + 32$

Radiation Dosages:
Gray = Gy
Sieverts = Sv
1 mrad = 10 µGy
1 mREM = 10 µSv

Z-score: (observed – mean)
        Standard deviation

The number of standard deviations by which the measured value departs from the mean value of individuals matched for age and gender.

T-score: (observed – mean)
        Standard deviation

The number of standard deviations by which the measured value departs from the mean value of a group of healthy 25- to 35-yr-old individuals.

Appendix C
Pediatric Normative Data

From: *Current Clinical Practice: Bone Densitometry in Growing Patients: Guidelines for Clinical Practice*
Edited by: A. J. Sawyer, L. K. Bachrach, and E. B. Fung © Humana Press Inc., Totowa, NJ

Table 1
Summary of Published Pediatric Reference Data Available for DXA Scanners

Reference	DXA type	N =	Age	Sex	Exclusions	Ethnicity	Sites
Glastre C, et al. (1) Metab 1990;70:5:1330–1333	Hologic QDR 1000	135	1–15	M/F	No treatment for bone metabolism; chronic disease; growth problems	White	Spine (L1-L4),
Southard RN, et al. (2) 1991;179:735–738.	Hologic 1000	218	1–19	M/F	Endocrine, growth, renal, or nutritional problems; premises; patients using medications; patients with more than two fractures	Black, white (U.S.)	Spine (L1-L4)
Bonjour JP, et al. (3) J Clin Endo Metab 1991;73:555–563.	Hologic 1000	207	9–18	M/F	Weight or height < 3% or > 97% for age; chronic disease; GI or malabsorption; bone disease; drugs; intense exercise	White (Switzerland)	Femoral neck, spine (L2–L4)
Molgaard C, et al. (4) Arch Dis Child 1997;76:9–15.	Hologic 1000 (pencil beam)	343	5–19	M/F	Chronic disease; medications that affect BMD	White (Denmark)	Whole body (adjustments for heights, area)
Bachrach LK, et al. (5) J Clin Endo Metab 1999;84:4701–4712	Hologic 1000W (pencil beam)	423 (longitudinal)	9–25	M/F	Medical conditions; medications that affect BMD	Asian, black, Hispanic, white	Femoral neck, total hip, whole body, spine (L2–L4)
Henderson RC, et al. (6) Am J Roent 2002;178:439–443.	Hologic 1000, 2000 (pencil beam)	256	3–18	M/F	Medical conditions; medicals or injuries that could affect BMB	n = 212 white, n = 25 black, n = 19 other (U.S.)	Distal femur (forearm software used for analysis)
Faulkner RA, et al. (7) Calcif Tissue Int 1993;53:7–12.	Hologic 2000 Array mode	234 (cross-sectional)	8–16	M/F		White (Canada)	Femoral neck, whole body, spine (L1–L4)
Faulkner RA, et al. (8) Calcif Tissue Int 1996;59:344–351.	Hologic 2000	234 (longitudinal)	8–17	M/F			(L1–L4)
Taylor A, et al. (9) J Bone Min Res 1997;12:652–655.	Hologic 2000 Array mode	94	2–9	M/F	Unusual diet; weight or height < 5% or > 95% for age	Mostly white, n = 10 black	Whole body

(continued)

Reference	Instrument/scan mode	N	Age	M/F	Inclusion: "Healthy"	Race	Site
Ellis KJ, et al. (10) J Bone Miner Res 2001;16:1658–1664.	Hologic 2000 Array mode	982 healthy + 106 with chronic disease	5–18	M/F		White, black, Hispanic; plus chronic diseases; CF; JDM; LD, RS,HIV	Whole body (Z-scores corrected for size)
Van Coeverden. (11) J Bone Miner Res 2001;16:774–778.	Hologic 2000 Array mode	151	9–12	F		White	Forearm
Binkley TL, et al. (12) J Clin Dens 2002;5:343–353.	Hologic 4500	231	5–22	M/F		Mostly white	Total body BMC
Lu PW, et al. (13) J Bone Miner Res 1994;9:1451–1458	Lunar DPX cross-sectional and longitudinal	266	4–27	M/F		White (Australia)	Spine (L1–L4), femoral neck, whole body
Lu PW, et al. (14) J Clin Endo Metab 1996;81:1586–1590	Lunar DPX	209	5–27	M/F		White (Australia)	Spine (L1–L4), femoral neck, and volumetric BMD calculated
Maynard LM, et al. (15) Am J Clin Nutr 1998;68:1111–1117.	Lunar DPX	148 longitudinal	8–18	M/F		White (U.S.)	Whole body
Hogler W, et al. (16) J Pediatr 2003;143:81–88.	Lunar DPX	646	5–18	M/F		White	Total body (corrected for lean body mass)
Fonseca AS, et al. (17) Braz J Med Biol Res 2001;34:347–352.	Lunar DPX Medium mode scan	255	6–14	M/F	Endocrine problems, asthma, short stature, obesity, premies treatment with steroids, fractures >2	White (Brazil)	Spine (L2–L4), BMC, BMD
del Rio L, et al. (18) Pediatr Res 1994;35:362–366.	Lunar DPX-L	471	3 mo to 21 years	M/F		White (Spain)	Spine (L2–L4)

Table 1 (*continued*)

Summary of Published Pediatric Reference Data Available for DXA Scanners

Reference	DXA type	N =	Age	Sex	Exclusions	Ethnicity	Sites
Crabtree NJ, et al. (*19*) Bone 2004;35:965–972.	Lunar DPX-L pencil beam)	646	5–18	M/F		Unkown (U.K.)	Spine, whole body (corrected for lean body mass)
Boot AM, et al. (*20*) J Clin Endo Metab 1997;82:57–62/	Lunar DPX-L/PED	500	4–20	M/F	Diabetes; thyroid or liver problems; taking heparin, steroids, or anticonvulsants; CF; bone disease	Mostly white, n = 21 black, n = 35 Asian (Netherlands)	Whole body, spine (L2–L4)
van der Sluis IM, et al. (*21*) Arch Dis Child 2002;87:341–347	Lunar DPXL/PED	444	4–20	M/F		White (Netherlands)	Whole body, spine (L1-4), BMD and BMAD, body composition
Zanchetta JR, et al. (*22*) Bone 1995;16:393S–399S.	Norland XR-26	778	2–20	M/F	Inclusion: "Healthy"	White (Argentina)	Whole body, spine, femoral neck, radius, trochanter
Plotkin H, et al. (*23*) Calcif Tissue Int 1996;58:144–149.	Norland XR-26	433	2–20	F	Inclusion: "Healthy"	White (Argentina)	L2-L4, adjusted for height

Note: Only published manuscripts are included in this summary table; abstract citations from scientific meetings are not included. If information regarding the subjects, the scans performed, or instrument details used within a study was too limited, the citation was not included.

Table 2
Pediatric Normative Data Available for Hologic Systems

Hologic, Inc. Pediatric BMD Database
May 2005
Caucasian Female

Age years	AP Spine L1–L4		Proximal femur Femoral Neck		Proximal femur Gr. Trochanter		Proximal Femur Intertrochanter		Proximal Femur Total hip		Whole body	
	BMD	SD	BMD	SD	BMD	SD	BMD	SD	BMD	SD	BMD	SD
3	0.441	0.048	–	–	–	–	–	–	–	–	0.540	0.034
4	0.463	0.051	–	–	–	–	–	–	–	–	0.584	0.038
5	0.485	0.055	0.525	0.055	0.458	0.059	0.592	0.082	0.551	0.062	0.625	0.042
6	0.508	0.059	0.549	0.059	0.469	0.061	0.620	0.085	0.573	0.065	0.661	0.046
7	0.532	0.064	0.574	0.063	0.482	0.062	0.652	0.089	0.598	0.069	0.694	0.050
8	0.558	0.069	0.603	0.068	0.499	0.065	0.690	0.093	0.628	0.074	0.729	0.054
9	0.589	0.076	0.636	0.074	0.522	0.068	0.736	0.098	0.663	0.080	0.765	0.058
10	0.629	0.085	0.673	0.081	0.556	0.072	0.790	0.103	0.707	0.087	0.805	0.061
11	0.685	0.096	0.714	0.089	0.601	0.078	0.852	0.110	0.757	0.095	0.850	0.065
12	0.758	0.108	0.757	0.096	0.651	0.084	0.916	0.116	0.811	0.102	0.899	0.068
13	0.837	0.113	0.799	0.102	0.695	0.089	0.978	0.122	0.863	0.107	0.952	0.070
14	0.902	0.110	0.832	0.105	0.726	0.093	1.030	0.126	0.904	0.110	0.999	0.072
15	0.945	0.107	0.856	0.106	0.744	0.095	1.069	0.130	0.934	0.110	1.036	0.073
16	0.973	0.105	0.872	0.106	0.755	0.097	1.097	0.132	0.954	0.109	1.063	0.073
17	0.990	0.104	0.882	0.106	0.761	0.097	1.117	0.133	0.968	0.108	1.083	0.073
18	1.000	0.103	0.888	0.106	0.764	0.098	1.132	0.134	0.978	0.107	1.097	0.073
19	1.007	0.103	0.892	0.105	0.765	0.098	1.144	0.135	0.985	0.107	1.107	0.074
20	1.012	0.102	0.895	0.105	0.765	0.098	1.153	0.135	0.990	0.106	1.115	0.074

(continued)

Table 2 (*continued*)
Pediatric Normative Data Available for Hologic Systems

Hologic, Inc. Pediatric BMD Database
May 2005
Caucasian male

Age years	AP Spine L1–L4		Proximal femur Femoral Neck		Proximal femur Gr. Trochanter		Proximal Femur Intertrochanter		Proximal Femur Total hip		Whole body	
	BMD	SD	BMD	SD	BMD	SD	BMD	SD	BMD	SD	BMD	SD
3	0.454	0.046	–	–	–	–	–	–	–	–	0.560	0.037
4	0.473	0.049	–	–	–	–	–	–	–	–	0.602	0.040
5	0.491	0.051	0.540	0.054	0.484	0.065	0.601	0.062	0.572	0.060	0.642	0.044
6	0.510	0.054	0.582	0.060	0.509	0.064	0.653	0.069	0.612	0.064	0.679	0.047
7	0.529	0.056	0.620	0.066	0.552	0.064	0.700	0.076	0.649	0.069	0.713	0.051
8	0.549	0.060	0.654	0.072	0.552	0.065	0.743	0.082	0.682	0.073	0.750	0.054
9	0.574	0.064	0.685	0.078	0.570	0.066	0.783	0.088	0.714	0.078	0.787	0.058
10	0.606	0.071	0.714	0.083	0.586	0.068	0.823	0.095	0.745	0.083	0.823	0.062
11	0.642	0.082	0.744	0.089	0.604	0.073	0.864	0.103	0.777	0.090	0.859	0.066
12	0.686	0.095	0.777	0.095	0.638	0.084	0.910	0.112	0.816	0.098	0.895	0.070
13	0.742	0.109	0.814	0.103	0.688	0.101	0.964	0.123	0.863	0.107	0.936	0.074
14	0.808	0.119	0.855	0.111	0.741	0.114	1.024	0.134	0.914	0.117	0.983	0.080
15	0.878	0.124	0.895	0.120	0.787	0.122	1.085	0.144	0.966	0.127	1.034	0.086
16	0.942	0.124	0.934	0.128	0.825	0.127	1.145	0.153	1.015	0.135	1.085	0.092
17	0.992	0.122	0.969	0.137	0.854	0.130	1.199	0.160	1.060	0.141	1.130	0.097
18	1.033	0.121	1.001	0.144	0.878	0.132	1.248	0.166	1.100	0.147	1.170	0.103
19	1.067	0.120	1.031	0.152	0.900	0.135	1.294	0.171	1.138	0.151	1.206	0.107
20	1.098	0.119	1.060	0.160	0.922	0.136	1.339	0.175	1.175	0.155	1.241	0.112

Note. Reference values developed from 1444 spine, 1047 hip, and 1948 whole body exams of healthy US white children using Hologic 4500 or Delphi systems. (From Kelly TL, Specker BL, Binkley T, et al. Pediatric BMD reference database for US white children. Bone 2005;36(suppl 1):S30. AP, anteroposterior; BMD, bone mineral density (g/cm²); SD, standard deviation.

Table 3
Pediatric Normative Data Available for Lunar Systems

Lunar Pediatric BMD Reference Values
Caucasian Female

Age (years)	Whole body Including head		Whole body Excluding Head		Spine L1-L4	
	g/cm²	SD	g/cm²	SD	g/cm²	SD
5	0.793	0.02	0.622	0.04	0.624	0.06
6	0.806	0.04	0.648	0.05	0.644	0.07
7	0.819	0.05	0.674	0.06	0.664	0.08
8	0.832	0.06	0.700	0.07	0.684	0.09
9	0.845	0.07	0.726	0.07	0.704	0.09
10	0.885	0.08	0.767	0.08	0.772	0.10
11	0.925	0.08	0.808	0.08	0.840	0.11
12	0.965	0.08	0.849	0.08	0.908	0.11
13	1.005	0.09	0.890	0.09	0.976	0.12
14	1.045	0.09	0.931	0.09	1.044	0.12
15	1.085	0.08	0.972	0.09	1.112	0.13
16	1.125	0.08	1.013	0.09	1.180	0.13
17	1.125	0.08	1.013	0.08	1.180	0.13
18	1.125	0.07	1.013	0.08	1.180	0.13
19	1.125	0.06	1.013	0.07	1.180	0.12

Lunar Pediatric BMD Reference Values
Caucasian Male

Age (years)	Whole body Including head		Whole Body Excluding Head		Spine L1-L4	
	g/cm²	SD	g/cm²	SD	g/cm²	SD
5	0.780	0.04	0.600	0.04	0.606	0.07
6	0.800	0.04	0.631	0.04	0.633	0.08
7	0.820	0.05	0.662	0.05	0.660	0.08
8	0.840	0.05	0.693	0.05	0.687	0.09
9	0.860	0.06	0.724	0.06	0.714	0.09
10	0.880	0.06	0.755	0.07	0.741	0.10
11	0.900	0.07	0.786	0.07	0.768	0.11
12	0.920	0.07	0.817	0.08	0.795	0.12
13	0.970	0.08	0.868	0.08	0.880	0.13
14	1.020	0.08	0.919	0.09	0.965	0.13
15	1.070	0.09	0.970	0.09	1.050	0.14
16	1.120	0.09	1.021	0.10	1.135	0.14
17	1.170	0.10	1.072	0.10	1.220	0.14
18	1.220	0.10	1.072	0.10	1.220	0.14
19	1.220	0.10	1.072	0.09	1.220	0.13

From Wacker W, Barden HS. Pediatric Reference Data for male and female total body and spine BMD and BMC. Presented at ISCD, March 2001, Dallas, TX; Barden HS, Wacker WK, Faulkner KG. Pediatric enhancements to Prodigy software: variable standard deviations and subcranial total body results. Presented at ISCD, February 2005, New Orleans, LA.

BMD, bone mineral density; SD, standard deviation.

Table 4
Pediatric Normative Data Available for Norland XR Systems

A. XR-System Reference Values

Caucasian Female

Age (Years)	AP spine L2-L4 Value	SD	Femur Femoral Neck Value	SD	Femur Trochanter Value	SD	Whole-body BMC Value (g)	SD	Whole-body BMD Value	SD	Forearm Proximal Radius Value	SD
2	0.38	0.06	0.46	0.02	0.38	0.05	344.5	79.9	0.733	0.039	0.18	0.05
3	0.42	0.04	0.50	0.06	0.42	0.11	446.4	78.6	0.747	0.076	0.22	0.10
4	0.45	0.09	0.53	0.13	0.46	0.12	503.1	92.5	0.743	0.049	0.20	0.04
5	0.52	0.24	0.58	0.20	0.49	0.18	671.3	30.1	0.782	0.077	0.22	0.08
6	0.54	0.09	0.62	0.17	0.51	0.13	716.9	24.9	0.775	0.039	0.23	0.06
7	0.52	0.10	0.63	0.14	0.53	0.12	813.1	108.4	0.797	0.048	0.21	0.05
8	0.55	0.14	0.64	0.16	0.54	0.17	878.1	171.2	0.789	0.056	0.23	0.10
9	0.59	0.13	0.65	0.14	0.55	0.16	1049.1	209.7	0.806	0.054	0.24	0.04
10	0.62	0.22	0.69	0.08	0.57	0.09	1196.9	284.2	0.832	0.090	0.25	0.05
11	0.65	0.24	0.72	0.17	0.61	0.08	1257.3	274.5	0.849	0.056	0.24	0.07
12	0.72	0.23	0.77	0.21	0.67	0.08	1532.6	393.2	0.867	0.083	0.28	0.11
13	0.87	0.28	0.87	0.22	0.73	0.09	1963.7	430.3	0.964	0.101	0.31	0.14
14	0.98	0.26	0.96	0.25	0.76	0.10	2238.6	313.8	1.004	0.091	0.36	0.13
15	0.95	0.21	0.93	0.26	0.76	0.12	2228.1	384.8	1.047	0.097	0.37	0.13
16	1.00	0.24	0.94	0.27	0.76	0.10	2397.2	288.4	1.093	0.093	0.39	0.12
17	1.01	0.23	0.92	0.23	0.76	0.19	2396.9	282.9	1.092	0.078	0.39	0.13
18–20	0.97	0.23	0.95	0.33	0.76	0.25	2368.1	349.2	1.075	0.079	0.39	0.12

Caucasian Male

Age (Years)	AP spine L2-L4		Femur Femoral Neck		Femur Trochanter		Whole-body BMC		Whole-body BMD		Forearm Proximal Radius	
	Value	SD	Value	SD	Value	SD	Value (g)	SD	Value	SD	Value	SD
2	0.42	0.13	0.52	0.15	0.45	0.08	431.3	41.8	0.688	0.047	0.19	0.04
3	0.48	0.07	0.54	0.10	0.48	0.16	494.2	49.2	0.748	0.063	0.21	0.05
4	0.47	0.07	0.57	0.08	0.50	0.12	526.6	82.3	0.786	0.075	0.22	0.05
5	0.50	0.10	0.65	0.12	0.56	0.14	665.0	77.0	0.806	0.046	0.22	0.03
6	0.54	0.09	0.70	0.15	0.57	0.14	723.8	34.7	0.801	0.091	0.23	0.07
7	0.56	0.12	0.71	0.15	0.61	0.14	855.9	96.3	0.816	0.048	0.24	0.06
8	0.59	0.10	0.73	0.15	0.64	0.17	1024.3	166.9	0.823	0.042	0.25	0.10
9	0.59	0.12	0.75	0.17	0.62	0.15	1023.0	161.7	0.828	0.055	0.26	0.07
10	0.61	0.16	0.77	0.16	0.64	0.19	1186.0	225.0	0.851	0.074	0.28	0.13
11	0.63	0.16	0.78	0.17	0.64	0.16	1334.7	219.1	0.856	0.015	0.28	0.07
12	0.62	0.23	0.80	0.16	0.67	0.16	1438.8	251.5	0.878	0.067	0.26	0.07
13	0.71	0.21	0.86	0.22	0.78	0.12	1779.7	311.9	0.933	0.013	0.33	0.20
14	0.79	0.33	0.90	0.24	0.81	0.24	2094.6	339.6	0.966	0.020	0.32	0.15
15	0.96	0.24	1.01	0.22	0.90	0.21	2364.9	323.4	0.994	0.081	0.36	0.14
16	1.01	0.18	1.09	0.27	0.96	0.27	2663.5	235.5	1.096	0.080	0.39	0.11
17	1.06	0.25	1.15	0.34	0.96	0.25	2825.2	309.2	1.135	0.104	0.45	0.15
18–20	1.09	0.35	1.16	0.35	0.94	0.31	2964.9	344.8	1.165	0.106	0.47	0.11

Data collected from 433 girls and 345 boys between the ages of 2 and 20 yr.
AP, anteroposterior; BMC, bone mineral content; BMD, bone mineral density; SD, standard deviation.
(From ref. 22.)

Table 5
Web-Based Pediatric Normative Data for the Hologic 1000

Please refer to the following website:

http://www-stat-class.stanford.edu/pediatric-bones
The Stanford "Applet" displays gender- and ethnicity-specific curves for bone mineral density for whole body, femoral neck, total hip, and lumbar spine (L2–L4). Both areal bone mineral density (aBMD) and estimates of volumetric bone mineral apparent density (BMAD) are displayed. BMAD was calculated using bone area and bone mineral content (BMC) as described These normative data were collected from a convenience sample of 423 healthy American youth (ages 9–25 years) enrolled in a longitudinal study of bone mineral acquisition. Details regarding the study cohort and protocol have been published (ref. 5)

Table 6
Pediatric Normative Data Avalable for Lateral Distal Femur

Females

	ROI 1			ROI 2			ROI 3		
Age	Mean ROI 1 BMD	SD	Normal range	Mean ROI 2 BMD	SD	Normal range	Mean ROI 3 BMD	SD	Normal range
3	0.597	0.058	0.481–0.713	0.558	0.055	0.448–0.668	0.592	0.054	0.485–0.700
4	0.625	0.067	0491–0.759	0.596	0.063	0.469–0.723	0.628	0.062	0.504–0.751
5	0.652	0.075	0.502–0.727	0.635	0.071	0.493–0.777	0.688	0.069	0.530–0.806
6	0.680	0.082	0.515–0.845	0.675	0.078	0.520–0.830	0.713	0.076	0.561–08.64
7	0.710	0.089	0.532–0.888	0.716	0.084	0.548–0.884	0.761	0.082	0598–0.925
8	0.741	0.095	0.551–0.931	0.760	0.090	0.581–0.939	0.813	0.087	0.639–0.988
9	0.774	0.101	0.572–0.976	0.806	0.095	0.616–0.996	0.868	0.093	0.683–1.053
10	0.811	0.106	0598–1.024	0.854	0.100	0.654–1.054	0.925	0.098	0.729–1.120
11	0.850	0.111	0.627–1.073	0.906	0.105	0.696–1.116	0.983	0.102	0.778–1.188
12	0.893	0.116	0.660–1.126	0.961	0.110	0.741–1.181	1.042	0.107	0.828–1.256
13	0.940	0.121	0.698–1.182	1.019	0.114	0.790–1.248	1.101	0.111	0.878–1.324
14	0.992	0.126	0.741–1.243	1.082	0.119	0845–1.319	1.160	0.116	0.929–1.392
15	1.049	0.130	0.789–1.309	1.149	0.123	0.903–1.395	1.218	0.120	0.979–1.458
16	1.111	0.134	0.842–1.380	1.221	0.127	0.967–1.475	1.275	0.124	1.028–1.522
17	1.180	0.139	0.903–1.457	1.298	0.131	1.037–1.559	1.329	0.127	1.075–1.584
18	1.255	0.143	0.970–1.540	1.380	0.134	1.111–1.649	1.381	0.131	1.119–1.643

(continued)

Males

	ROI 1				ROI 2				ROI 3		
Age	Mean ROI 1 BMD	SD	Normal range		Mean ROI 2 BMD	SD	Normal range		Mean ROI 3 BMD	SD	Normal range
3	0.650	0.073	0.504–0.796		0.624	0.064	0.495–0.753		0.632	0.057	0.519–0.745
4	0.660	0.084	0.492–0.828		0.651	0.074	0.503–0.799		0.668	0.065	0.537–0.799
5	0.674	0.094	0.486–0.862		0.679	0.083	0.513–0.845		0.705	0.073	0.558–0.851
6	0.693	0.103	0.487–0.899		0.708	0.091	0.526–0.890		0.743	0.080	0.583–0.903
7	0.716	0.111	0.493–0.939		0.739	0.098	0.543–0.935		0.784	0.087	0.611–0.957
8	0.744	0.119	0.506–0.982		0.773	0.105	0.563–0.983		0.828	0.092	0.643–1.013
9	0.776	0.126	0.523–1.029		0.811	0.111	0.588–1.034		0.875	0.098	0.679–1.071
10	0.813	0.133	0.547–1.079		0.853	0.117	0.618–1.088		0.926	0.103	0.719–1.133
11	0.854	0.140	0.714–1.133		0.900	0.123	0.654–1.146		0.981	0.108	0.765–1.198
12	0.900	0.146	0.608–1.192		0.952	0.129	0.695–1.210		1.041	0.113	0.815–1.268
13	0.950	0.152	0.646–1.254		1.012	0.134	0.744–1.279		1.107	0.118	0.871–1.343
14	1.005	0.158	0.690–1.320		1.078	0.139	0.800–1.355		1.179	0.122	0.934–1.424
15	1.065	0.163	0.739–1.391		1.152	0.144	0.864–1.439		1.257	0.127	1.004–1.511
16	1.128	0.168	0.943–1.465		1.234	0.148	0.938–1.531		1.343	0.131	1.081–1.605
17	1.197	0.174	0.850–1.544		1.326	0.153	1.020–1.632		1.436	0.135	1.167–1.706
18	1.270	0.179	0.913–1.627		1.428	0.157	1.113–1.743		1.538	0.139	1.280–1.815

From ref. 6.

REFERENCES

1. Glastre C, Braillon P, David L, Cochat P, Meunier PJ, Delmas PD. Measurement of bone mineral content of the lumbar spine by dual energy x-ray absorptiometry in normal children: correlations with growth parameters. J Clin Endocrinol Metab 1990;0:1330–1333.

2. Southard RN, Morris JD, Mahan JD, et al. Bone mass in healthy children: Measurement with quantitative DXA. Radiology 1991;179:735–738.

3. Bonjour JP, Theintz G, Buchs B, Slosman D, Rizzoli R. Critical years and stages of puberty for spinal and femoral bone mass accumulation during adolescence. J Clin Endocrinol Metab 1991;73:555–563.

4. Molgaard C, Thomsen BL, Prentice A, Cole TJ, Michaelsen KF. Whole body bone mineral content in healthy children and adolescents. Arch Dis Child 1997;76(1):9–15.

5. Bachrach LK, Hastie T, Wang M-C, Narasimhan B, Marcus R. Bone mineral acquisition in healthy Asian, Hispanic, black and Caucasian youth. A longitudinal study. J Clin Endocrinol Metab. 1999,84:4702–4712.

6. Henderson RC, Lark RK, Newman JE, et al. Pediatric reference data for dual x-ray absorptiometric measures of normal bone density in the distal femur. AJR 2002,178:439–443.

7. Faulkner RA, Bailey DA, Drinkwater DT, Wilkinson AA, Houston CS, McKay HA. Regional and total body bone mineral content, bone mineral density and total body tissue composition in children 8–16 years of age. Calcif Tissue Int 1993;53:7–12. A.

8. Faulkner RA, Bailey DA, Drinkwater DT, McKay HA, Arnold C, Wilkinson AA. Bone densitometry in Canadian children 8–17 years of age. Calcif Tissue Int 1996;59(5):344–351.

9. Taylor A, Konrad PT, Norman ME, Harcke HT. Total body bone mineral density in young children: influence of head bone mineral density. J Bone Miner Res 1997;12:652–655.

10. Ellis KJ, Shypailo RJ, Hardin DS, et al. Z score prediction model for assessment of bone mineral content in pediatric diseases. J Bone Miner Res 2001;16(9):1658–1664.

11. Van Coeverden SC, De Ridder CM, Roos JC, Van't Hof MA, Netelenbos JC, Delemarre-Van de Waal HA. Pubertal maturation characteristics and the rate of bone mass development longitudinally toward menarche. J Bone Miner Res 2001;16(4):774–781.

12. Binkley TL, Specker BL, Wittig TA. Centile curves for bone densitometry measurements in healthy males and females ages 5–22 yr. J Clin Densitom 2002;5(4):343–353.

13. Lu WP, Briody JN, Ogle GD, et al. Bone mineral density of total body: spine femoral neck in children and young adults: a cross-sectional and longitudinal study. J Bone Miner Res 1994;9:1451–1458.

14. Lu PW, Cowell CT, Lloyd-Jones S, Briody JN, Howman-Giles R. Volumetric bone mineral density in normal subjects, aged 5–27 years. J Clin Endocrinol Metab 1996;81:1586–1590.

15. Maynard LM, Guo SS, Chumlea WC, et al. Total-body and regional bone mineral content and areal bone mineral density in children aged 8–18 y: The Fels Longitudinal Study. Am J Clin Nutr 1998;68(5):1111–1117.

16. Hogler W, Briody J, Woodhead HJ, Chan A, Cowell CT. Importance of lean mass in the interpretation of total body densitometry in children and adolescents. J Pediatr 2003;143(1):81–88.

17. Fonseca AS, Szejnfeld VL, Terreri MT, Goldenberg J, Ferraz MB, Hilario MO.Bone mineral density of the lumbar spine of Brazilian children and adolescents aged 6 to 14 years. Braz J Med Biol Res 2001;34(3):347–352.

18. del Rio L, Carrascosa A, Pons F, Gusinye M, Yeste D, Domenech FM. Bone mineral density of the lumbar spine in white Mediterranean Spanish children and adolescents: Changes related to age, sex, and puberty. Pediatr Res 1994;35:362–366.

19. Crabtree NJ, Kibirige MS, Fordham JN, et al. The relationship between lean body mass and bone mineral content in paediatric health and disease. Bone 2004;35(4):965–972.

20. Boot AM, De Ridder MAJ, Pols HAP, Krenning EP, De Muinck Keizer-Schrama SMPF. Bone mineral density in children and adolescents: relation to puberty, calcium intake, and physical activity. J Clin Endocrinol Metab 1997;82:57–62.

21. van der Sluis IM, de Ridder MA, Boot AM, Krenning EP, de Muinck Keizer-Schrama SM. Reference data for bone density and body composition measured with dual energy x ray absorptiometry in white children and young adults. Arch Dis Child 2002;87(4):341–347; discussion 341–347.

22. Zanchetta JR, Plotkin H, Alvarez Filgueira ML. Bone mass in children: normative values for the 2-20 year old population. Bone 1995;16:393S–399S.

23. Plotkin H, Nunez M, Alvarez Filgueira ML, Zanchetta JR. Lumbar spine bone density in Argentine children. Calcif Tissue Int 1996;58(3):144–149.

Appendix D
Forms and Handouts

From: *Current Clinical Practice: Bone Densitometry in Growing Patients: Guidelines for Clinical Practice*
Edited by: A. J. Sawyer, L. K. Bachrach, and Ellen B. Fung © Humana Press Inc., Totowa, NJ

BONE DENSITOMETRY CLINIC

DEPARTMENTAL REFERRAL FOR DXA SCAN FORM

Referring Physician: _____

Office Phone: _____

Fax Number: _____

Name of Patient: _____

Date of Birth: ____/____/_____

Medical Record #: _____

Insurance Type: _____ Authorization #: _____

Primary Diagnosis: _____ ICD-9: _____

Reason for Referral:

_____

_____

List Current Medications: _____

Fracture History?   ❏ Yes   ❏ No

    If Yes, please explain:_____

Recent bone age?   ❏ Yes   ❏ No

    If Yes, date and results: _____

When complete, please fax this form back to the Bone Density Clinic at:

_____

BONE DENSITOMETRY CLINIC: PEDIATRIC REGISTRATION QUESTIONNAIRE
CHILDREN'S HOSPITAL & RESEARCH CENTER, OAKLAND

Patient's Name (Last, First): _____   Today's Date: ____/____/_____

Patient's Gender: ❏ Male ❏ Female   Patient's Date of Birth: ____/____/_____

Ethnicity (*circle which best describes your child*):   Asian / Black / Hispanic / White

Referring Doctor: _____   Department: _____

Has your child had this type of examination before?   ❏ Yes   ❏ No

    If yes, where did you have this done?_____

    What was the approximate date of the last exam (MM/YYYY)? ___/_____

Is your child right- or left-handed?   ❏ Right   ❏ Left

Has your child ever had hip surgery?   ❏ Yes   ❏ No

    If yes, which hip was it performed on?   ❏ Right ❏ Left   ❏ Both

Does your child have curvature (scoliosis) of the spine?   ❏ Yes   ❏ No

Has your child ever broken (fractured) a bone?   ❏ Yes   ❏ No

Has your child had any exams within the last 7 days where a contrast material (x-ray dye) was used? If so, which exam? _____When was this done?_____

Does your family have a history of osteoporosis?   ❏ Yes   ❏ No
    If yes, please describe relation to patient (e.g., mother, grandmother)_____

Has your child ever taken corticosteroids (e.g., prednisone)?   ❏ Yes   ❏ No

Does your child currently take any medications?   ❏ Yes   ❏ No

    If so, please list them here:_____

For FEMALE patients only:

    Has your child begun to menstruate?   ❏ Yes   ❏ No

    If so, when was your child's last menstrual period?_____

    Is there any chance that your child may be pregnant?   ❏ Yes   ❏ No

Calcium Intake:
For each food listed below, please indicate the number of servings your child (the patient) consumes of these calcium-rich foods in a typical week.

For example:
   If you consume 0.5 cups of milk on your cereal each morning you can respond:
      Milk = 3.5 servings per week

	Serving Size	# servings per week
Milk, any type	1 cup	
Yogurt	1 cup	
Cheese	1 slice	
Pudding	½ cup	
Ice cream, frozen yogurt	1 cup	
Macaroni and cheese	1 cup	
Pizza	1 slice	
Cooked green vegetables	½ cup	
Other calcium-rich foods:		

Does your child take calcium supplements on a regular basis?   ❏ Yes   ❏ No

   If yes, how much?_____ and how frequently? _____

For Official Use Only:

Initials of Technician:_____

   Measured Height: _____ cm   Measured Weight _____ kg
   Height for age %:_____   Weight for age %: _____

   Calculated BMI (kg/m2) _____
   BMI %: _____   Forearm Length: _____ (cm)

Fracture History Explanation:_____

Other Comments:_____

CHILDREN'S BONE DENSITY QUESTIONNAIRE
(UNIVERSITY OF MANCHESTER)

Patient Information

Name: _____ DOB: _____ I.D.: _____

Primary disease: _____

Time since diagnosis: _____

Any other health problems: _____

Height: _____   Weight: _____ BMI: _____

Original Referral   **DXA Referral**

Consultant: _____   Consultant: _____

Speciality: _____   Speciality: _____

Hospital: _____   Hospital: _____

Fractures

Have you ever fractured any bones?   ❏ Yes   ❏ No

    If Yes, when, which bone, and how?_____

Have you had any persistent back pain in the last 12 months?   ❏ Yes   ❏ No

Has a family member suffered from osteoporosis?   ❏ Yes   ❏ No

    If Yes, who? _____

Mobility and Physical Activity: Mobile Patients

How much physical activity do you do per week?

    ❏ Less than 3 hours (School activity only)

    ❏ 3 to 5 hours (School and organized activities)

    ❏ More than 5 hours (sports clubs)

Have you had any periods of prolonged immobility?   ❏ Yes   ❏ No

    If Yes, when and for how long?_____

Mobility and Physical Activity: Immobile Patients

How do you usually get around?

	Never	Occasionally	Frequently	Always
Walk	❏	❏	❏	❏
Walk with crutches	❏	❏	❏	❏
Chair	❏	❏	❏	❏
Bed	❏	❏	❏	❏

Do you use a standing frame?   ❏ Yes   ❏ No

    If yes, how often? _____

Do you have regular hydrotherapy   ❏ Yes   ❏ No

    If yes, how often? _____

Do you have any other physical activity?   ❏ Yes   ❏ No

    If yes, how often? _____

Diet

Do you have any feeding or nutritional problems?   ❏ Yes   ❏ No

     If Yes, please give details: _____

If No, how much milk do you drink daily?

None	❏
0 to 1/4 pint (150 mL)	❏
1/4 to 1/2 pint (300 mL)	❏
1/2 to 3/4 pint (450 mL)	❏
3/4 to 1 pint (600 mL)	❏
More than 1 pint (600 mL)	❏

How often do you eat the following foods?

	Occasionally	1–3 times/week	Most days
Cheese	❏	❏	❏
Yogurt	❏	❏	❏
Ice cream	❏	❏	❏
Fromage frais	❏	❏	❏
Milk chocolate	❏	❏	❏
Milk pudding	❏	❏	❏

Do you take a calcium supplement?   ❏ Yes   ❏ No

Do you take a vitamin supplement?   ❏ Yes   ❏ No

Medication

Do you or have you ever taken oral corticosteroids (e.g., Prednisolone?)   ❏ Yes   ❏No

     If Yes, how much and for how long?_____

Do you take any medication for your bones (e.g., Pamidronate)   ❏ Yes   ❏ No

     If Yes, for how long? _____

Have you ever taken hormone replacement therapy (HRT) or   ❏ Yes   ❏ No

the oral contraceptive pill?

     If Yes, for how long? _____

Do you take any other medication?   ❏ Yes   ❏ No

     If Yes, for how long?_____

Puberty

Do you have any signs of puberty   ❏ Yes   ❏ No

If Yes, please fill in the appropriate information below using the pubertal self-assessment tool provided:

Girls: Boys:

Age at menarche: _____   Age at voice breaking: _____

Regular?   ❏ Yes   ❏ No   Testicular volume: _____

Pubic hair?   1 2 3 4 5   Pubic hair?   1 2 3 4 5

Breast development? 1 2 3 4 5

**(Taken from "A practical guide to bone densitometry in children"
National Osteoporosis Society, November 2004)**

CHILDREN'S HOSPITAL & RESEARCH CENTER, OAKLAND   NAME:
BONE DENSITY CLINIC   MEDICAL RECORD#:
OAKLAND, CA 94609   DOB: AGE:
                                                       ETHNICITY:

Bone Densitometry Report

REPORT DATE: TECHNOLOGIST:
SCAN DATE:
PREVIOUS SCAN DATE(S):

PATIENT HISTORY: (free text here)

ANTHROPOMETRIC DATA:
   Height (cm):   Weight (kg):   Body mass index (kg/m^2):
   Height-for-age %:   Weight-for-age %:   Body mass index %:

RESULTS:

	Spine, L1-L4	Total Hip	Whole Body	Whole Body
Type of Analysis	Array; LDS; Auto-Low	Array, R Array, L	Pediatric, Fan Beam, Auto Analysis	Body Composition
Area, cm	00.00	00.00	000.00	
BMC, g	00.00	00.00	000.00	Lean, g:
BMD, g/cm^2	0.000	0.000	0.000	Fat, g:
BMAD, g/cm^3	0.000	0.000	0.000	Fat, %:
^Z-score	0.0	0.0	0.0	

These scans were conducted on a Hologic Delphi A Bone Densitometer (Hologic, Waltham, MA)
Notable interfering factors:

_____

^ Z-scores calculated from the following reference data: (include reference here)

INTERPRETATION AND RECOMMENDATIONS:

(Free text here)

Thank you for referring this patient for a bone densitometry examination.

_____

Name and Credentials of Reporting Physician or Specialist:

Key Terms: BMC: bone mineral content; BMD: bone mineral density; BMAD: bone mineral
apparent density. Z-score: the number of standard deviations by which the measured value departs
from the mean value of individuals matched for age and gender.

THE CHILDREN'S HOSPITAL AT WESTMEAD
WESTMEAD, NEW SOUTH WALES
AUSTRALIA

MRN: *XXXXX*

Name:
Referring Dr:
Comments:
  Scan Date: **DOB:**   **Gender:**
  Age: **Height (cm):**   **Weight (kg):**   **BMI (kg/m_):**

Total Body

Standard Regions

Variable	BMD	BMC	Age Z	Height Z	Weight Z
Arms	0.000		−0.0	−0.0	−0.0
Legs	0.000		−0.0	−0.0	−0.0
Trunk	0.000		−0.0	−0.0	−0.0
Ribs	0.000				
Pelvis	0.000				
Total BMC		000.00	−0.0	−0.0	−0.0
Total BMD	0.000		−0.0	−0.0	−0.0

Other Regions

Variable	BMD	BMC	Age Z	Height Z	Weight Z
MFS - R	0.000		−0.0	−0.0	−0.0
MFS - L	0.000		−0.0	−0.0	−0.0

Femur

Standard Regions

Variable	BMD	BMC	Age Z	Height Z	Weight Z
FNeck BMC - R		0.00			
FNeck BMD - R	0.000		−0.0	−0.0	−0.0

AP Spine

Standard Regions

Variable	BMD	BMC	Age Z	Height Z	Weight Z
L2–L4 BMC		00.00	−0.0	−0.0	−0.0
L2–L4 BMD	0.000		−0.0	−0.0	−0.0

Total Body Composition/Ancillary Results:

Region	Soft Tissue (g)	LTM (g)	Fat (g)	Fat (%)	Fat% Age Z
Arms	0000.00	0000.00	0000.00	00.00	
Legs	0000.00	0000.00	0000.00	00.00	
Trunk	0000.00	0000.00	0000.00	00.00	
Total Body	0000.00	0000.00	0000.00	00.00	0.0

	Value	LTM Z	BA Z	Height Z
Bone Mineral Content (g)	0000.00	–0.0	–0.0	
Lean Tissue Mass (LTM) (g)	0000.00			0.0
Bone Area (BA) (cm_)	0000.00			–0.0

Interpretation for age:

Region	Normal	Low (–1.5 to –2.5)	Very Low	Delta Age Z	Delta Height Z	Delta Weight Z	Change in Z since:
Arms	☑						Date
Legs	☑						
Trunk		☑					
Total BMC	☑						
Total BMD	☑						
FNeck BMD - R	☑						
L2-L4 BMC	☑						
L2-L4 BMD	☑						

Technical Comments: Femoral Neck ROI = 1.0 cm

Additional Comments:

Some:
  Right Femoral neck
  L2–L4
  Total Body

Example of free text: Variables are "Normal" for age but low for body size (i.e., height, weight, bone area, or lean tissue).

Index

A

Acute lymphoblastic leukemia (ALL), fracture
risk in treatment, 2, 3
ALL, *see* Acute lymphoblastic leukemia

B

BMC, *see* Bone mineral content
BMD, *see* Bone mineral density
Bone age, estimation, 121, 122
Bone mineral content (BMC),
    dual-energy X-ray absorptiometry calculation,
        43, 116
    peak, 4
Bone mineral density (BMD),
    compartment mineral density, 17
    dual-energy X-ray absorptiometry spinal
        estimates,
        combined posteroanterior-lateral spine
            bone mineral density estimation,
            163, 164
        lateral spine bone mineral density estima-
            tion, 162, 163
        volumetric bone mineral density estima-
            tion from posteroanterior scans,
            160–162
    material mineral density, 17
    peak, 4
    reporting, *see* Dual-energy X-ray
        absorptiometry report
    total mineral density, 17, 18
Bone–muscle unit, dual-energy X-ray
    absorptiometry assessment, 166, 167

C

Calcaneum,
    dual-energy X-ray absorptiometry scans, 84
    quantitative ultrasound, 26, 28
Calcium, peak bone mass and nutrition, 6
Cerebral palsy, dual-energy X-ray
    absorptiometry scan collection, 140, 147

CF, *see* Cystic fibrosis
Computed tomography, *see* Quantitative com-
    puted tomography
Cystic fibrosis (CF), pediatric dual-energy X-ray
    absorptiometry, 63, 66

D

Diabetes, pediatric dual-energy X-ray
    absorptiometry, 63
Dual-energy X-ray absorptiometry (DXA),
    advantages and limitations, 18, 19
    attenuation formulas, 42, 43
    availability, 49
    bone age estimation, 121, 122
    bone mineral content calculation, 43, 116
    bone–muscle unit assessment, 166, 167
    central vs peripheral bone densitometry in
        osteoporosis prediction, 31, 32
    comparison with other bone densitometry
        techniques, 176, 177
    historical perspective, 41, 42
    limitations,
        bone detection algorithms, 53
        bone size confounding, 51
        projection artifacts, 51–53
        reference data standardization, 53, 54
    osteoporosis risk screening in adults, 8, 50, 51
    pediatric use,
        artifacts, 84, 86, 148, 149
        challenges, 1, 9, 10, 93, 115, 116
        edge detection, 86, 87
        follow-up scan analysis, 111, 112, 122, 123
        indications,
            chronic disease, 61, 63
            endocrine disorders, 63
            fracture, 64, 65, 149, 152
            genetic disorders, 61, 63, 152–154
            idiopathic juvenile osteoporosis, 64
            immobilization, 63, 64
            osteomalacia, 64
            osteopenia, 65

overview, 61, 62
refinement, 68, 69, 174, 175
rickets, 64
scoliosis, 64
instrument and software differences in
    analysis, 97, 98
movement effects, 87
prospects,
    body size and skeletal maturity adjust-
        ment, 176
    non-bone mass data studies, 175
    software for analysis, 175, 176
    vertebral morphometry, 176
proximal hip scan analysis,
    femoral neck bone mineral apparent
        density estimation, 164
    fundamentals, 96, 97
    hip structural analysis, 164, 165
    recommendations, 108, 110, 111
    software, 102, 104
rationale, 60, 61
scanning,
    calcaneum scans, 84
    children, 75
    distal femur scans, 83, 84
    distal radius scans, 83, 84
    history taking, 73, 74
    infants, 74, 75, 138, 139, 142, 143, 154,
        155
    patient preparation and positioning, 74,
        76–78, 80, 82, 88
    post-scan, 75, 76
    postural deformities, 140, 141, 147
    proximal hip scans, 81, 82
    room preparation, 74
    scan area, 76
    scan mode, 76, 77
    spine scans, 77, 78
    teenagers, 75
    toddlers and older infants, 75
    whole-body scans, 79–81
software upgrades for analysis, 104–107
spine scan analysis,
    combined posteroanterior-lateral spine
        bone mineral density estimation,
        163, 164
    fundamentals, 94, 95
    lateral spine bone mineral density esti-
        mation, 162, 163

recommendations, 107, 108
software, 98–101
volumetric bone mineral density esti-
    mation from posteroanterior
    scans, 160–162
timing,
    initial studies, 65–67
    follow-up studies, 68
whole-body scan analysis,
    bone mineral content, 165, 166
    fundamentals, 95, 96
    recommendations, 108
    software, 101, 102
precision,
    advantages, 50
    least significant change, 49, 134
    long-term,
        in vivo, 49
        machine precision, 49
    percent coefficient of variation, 48
    short-term,
        in vivo, 49
        machine precision, 49
principles, 18, 42, 43, 45
radiation exposure risks, 46–49
reference data, *see* Reference data, dual-
    energy X-ray absorptiometry
reporting, *see* Dual-energy X-ray
    absorptiometry report
scan time, 50
scanners, pencil beam vs fan beam, 45, 46
Z-score calculation, 117, 118, 120
Dual-energy X-ray absorptiometry report,
    elements,
        interpretation, 133, 134
        medical history, 130, 131
        patient demographics, 129, 130
        recommendations, 133, 134
        software proprietary report, 134
        technical comments, 132
        test results, 131, 132
    guidelines, 128
    overview, 127, 128
    purpose and audience, 128
DXA, *see* Dual-energy X-ray absorptiometry

E,F

Exercise, peak bone mass effects, 7, 8
Femur, 83,84

Fracture,
    chemotherapy effects, 2, 3
    pediatric dual-energy X-ray absorptiometry,
        indications, 64, 65
        infants, 154, 155
        nonaccidental injury, 149, 152
        risk prediction, 123
    pediatric epidemiology, 2

G

Glucocorticoid therapy, pediatric dual-energy
    X-ray absorptiometry, 63
Greulich and Pyle Atlas, bone age estimation,
    121

H

Hip, dual-energy X-ray absorptiometry
    distal femur scanning, 83, 84
    proximal hip scan analysis,
        femoral neck bone mineral apparent
            density estimation, 164
        fundamentals, 96, 97
        hip structural analysis, 164, 165
        recommendations, 108, 110, 111
        software, 102, 104
    proximal hip scanning, 81, 82

I

Idiopathic juvenile osteoporosis (IJO), pediatric
    dual-energy X-ray absorptiometry, 64
IJO, *see* Idiopathic juvenile osteoporosis
Immobilization, pediatric dual-energy X-ray
    absorptiometry, 63, 64
Infants, dual-energy X-ray absorptiometry
    fracture assessment, 154, 155
    guidelines for scanning, 138, 139
    older infants, 75
    variability sources, 142, 143
    young infants, 74, 75

L

LDS, *see* Legacy low-density software
Least significant change (LSC), dual-energy
    X-ray absorptiometry, 49, 134
Legacy low-density software (LDS), dual-
    energy X-ray absorptiometry spine scan
    analysis, 94, 99, 100, 104
LSC, *see* Least significant change

M,N

Magnetic resonance imaging (MRI),
    advantages of bone densitometry,
        30
    principles, 29
MRI, *see* Magnetic resonance imaging
Muscular dystrophy, dual-energy X-ray
    absorptiometry scan collection,
        140
Nutrition, *see* specific nutrients

O

OI, *see* Osteogenesis imperfecta
Osteogenesis imperfecta (OI),
    gene mutations, 152, 153
    infant assessment, 154, 155
    pediatric dual-energy X-ray absorptiometry,
        61, 63, 152–154
    types, 152, 153
Osteomalacia, pediatric dual-energy X-ray
    absorptiometry, 64
Osteopenia, pediatric dual-energy X-ray
    absorptiometry, 65
Osteoporosis,
    definition, 2, 31
    dual-energy X-ray absorptiometry for risk
        screening, 8, 50, 51
    epidemiology, 2
    peak bone mass significance, 4, 5

P

PBM, *see* Peak bone mass
Peak bone mass (PBM),
    attainment, 3, 4
    definition, 4
    determinants
        exercise, 7, 8
        heritability, 5
        nutrition,
            calcium, 6
            phosphorous, 6
            protein, 7
            vitamin D, 6, 7
        osteoporosis significance, 4, 5
Phosphorous, peak bone mass and nutrition,
    6
Protein, peak bone mass and nutrition, 7

Q

QCT, *see* Quantitative computed tomography
Quantitative computed tomography (QCT),
    axial quantitative computed tomography,
        advantages and limitations, 22
        data reporting, 20, 22
        historical perspective, 19
        scan collection, 19, 20
    peripheral quantitative computed tomography,
        advantages, 25
        bone strength studies, 26
        clinical research applications, 26
        historical perspective, 22
        scan collection, 22, 25
Quantitative ultrasound (QUS),
    advantages and limitations, 28
    historical perspective, 26
    pediatric assessment, 28
    sites of measurement, 26, 28
QUS, *see* Quantitative ultrasound

R

Radiogrammetry,
    digital X-ray radiogrammetry, 30, 31
    precision, 30
Radius, dual-energy X-ray absorptiometry
    of distal radius, 83, 84
Reference data, dual-energy X-ray
    absorptiometry,
    ethnic differences, 119, 120
    ideal characteristics, 117
    precautions, 50
    sources and selection, 118, 119
    standardization limitations, 53, 54
Rickets, pediatric dual-energy X-ray
    absorptiometry, 64

S

Scoliosis,
    dual-energy X-ray absorptiometry scan
        collection, 140

    pediatric dual-energy X-ray absorptiometry,
        64
Spine,
    axial quantitative computed tomography,
        advantages and limitations, 22
        data reporting, 20, 22
        historical perspective, 19
        scan collection, 19, 20
    dual-energy X-ray absorptiometry,
    scan analysis,
            combined posteroanterior-lateral spine
                bone mineral density estimation,
                163, 164
            fundamentals, 94, 95
            lateral spine bone mineral density
                estimation, 162, 163
            recommendations, 107, 108
            software, 98–101
            volumetric bone mineral density
                estimation from posteroanterior scans,
                160–162
        scanning, 77, 78
        vertebral morphometry, 176

T–V

Tanner Whitehouse III method, bone age
    estimation, 121
Ultrasound, *see* Quantitative ultrasound
Vitamin D, peak bone mass and nutrition, 6, 7

W

Whole-body dual-energy X-ray absorptiometry,
    scan analysis,
        bone mineral content, 165, 166
        fundamentals, 95, 96
        recommendations, 108
        software, 101, 102
    scanning, 79–81

Z

Z-score, calculation for dual-energy X-ray
    absorptiometry, 117, 118, 120